DEPRESSION SOURCEBOOK

SIXTH EDITION

Health Reference Series

DEPRESSION SOURCEBOOK

SIXTH EDITION

Provides Basic Consumer Health Information about the Prevalence, Symptoms, Diagnosis, Causes, Treatment, and Types of Depression, Including Major Depression, Atypical Depression, Bipolar Disorder, Depression during Reproductive Transitions in Women, Premenstrual Dysphoric Disorder, and Seasonal Affective Disorder, as well as the Strategies for Managing Depression

Along with Facts about Depression and Chronic Illness, Treatment-Resistant Depression and Suicide, Mental Health Medications, Therapies, and Treatments; Tips for Improving Self-Esteem, Resilience, and Quality of Life While Living with Depression; a Glossary of Terms Related to Depression; and Resources for Additional Help and Information

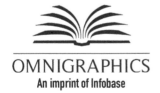

OMNIGRAPHICS
An imprint of Infobase

Bibliographic Note

Because this page cannot legibly accommodate all the copyright notices, the Bibliographic Note portion of the Preface constitutes an extension of the copyright notice.

* * *

OMNIGRAPHICS
An imprint of Infobase
132 W. 31st St.
New York, NY 10001
www.infobase.com
James Chambers, *Editorial Director*

* * *

Copyright © 2023 Infobase
ISBN 978-0-7808-2054-8
E-ISBN 978-0-7808-2055-5

Library of Congress Cataloging-in-Publication Data

Names: Chambers, James (Editor), editor.

Title: Depression sourcebook / edited by James Chambers.

Description: Sixth edition. | New York, NY: Omnigraphics, An imprint of Infobase, [2023] | Series: Health reference series | Includes index. | Summary: "Provides basic consumer health information about the causes, symptoms, diagnosis, and treatment of various forms of depression, along with coping tips and strategies for building resilience and self-esteem. Includes index, glossary of related terms, and other resources"-- Provided by publisher.

Identifiers: LCCN 2023012242 (print) | LCCN 2023012243 (ebook) | ISBN 9780780820548 (library binding) | ISBN 9780780820555 (ebook)

Subjects: LCSH: Depression, Mental--Popular works.

Classification: LCC RC537.D4455 2023 (print) | LCC RC537 (ebook) | DDC 616.85/27--dc23/eng/20230524

LC record available at https://lccn.loc.gov/2023012242
LC ebook record available at https://lccn.loc.gov/2023012243

Electronic or mechanical reproduction, including photography, recording, or any other information storage and retrieval system for the purpose of resale is strictly prohibited without permission in writing from the publisher.

The information in this publication was compiled from the sources cited and from other sources considered reliable. While every possible effort has been made to ensure reliability, the publisher will not assume liability for damages caused by inaccuracies in the data, and makes no warranty, express or implied, on the accuracy of the information contained herein.

This book is printed on acid-free paper meeting the ANSI Z39.48 Standard. The infinity symbol that appears above indicates that the paper in this book meets that standard.

Printed in the United States

Table of Contents

Preface... xiii

Part 1. Introduction to Mental Health Disorders and Depression
Chapter 1—Mental Health Basics...3
Chapter 2—Myths and Facts about Mental Health
 Disorders..7
Chapter 3—Depression: What You Need to Know 11
Chapter 4—Trends in Depression Prevalence
 and Impairment..17

Part 2. Types of Depression
Chapter 5—Major Depression..23
Chapter 6—Atypical Depression..31
Chapter 7—Bipolar Disorder (Manic-Depressive Illness)............35
Chapter 8—Disruptive Mood Dysregulation Disorder 43
Chapter 9—Persistent Depressive Disorder
 (Dysthymic Disorder) 47
Chapter 10—Psychotic Depression..53
Chapter 11—Seasonal Affective Disorder...57

Part 3. Who Develops Depression?
Chapter 12—Women and Depression 65
Chapter 13—Depression and Mental Health during
 Reproductive Transitions in Women.........................73
 Section 13.1—Depression and Anxiety
 Associated with the
 Menstrual Cycle:
 Premenstrual Syndrome....75

Section 13.2—Premenstrual Dysphoric Disorder 81
Section 13.3—Depression during Pregnancy: Risk Factors, Signs, and Symptoms 84
Section 13.4—Postpartum Depression 86
Section 13.5—What Is the Link between Menopause and Depression? 96
Chapter 14—Depression in Children and Adolescents 99
Section 14.1—Understanding Depression in Children 101
Section 14.2—Teen Depression: More than Just Moodiness 103
Chapter 15—Men and Depression 109
Chapter 16—Depression in Older Adults 117
Chapter 17—Depression in Racial and Ethnic Minorities 123
Chapter 18—Depression and Mental Health Challenges in Sexually Diverse and Gender-Diverse Populations 133
Chapter 19—Workplace Stress and Depression 143
Chapter 20—Depression and Mental Health in Correctional Facilities 149

Part 4. Risk Factors for Depression: Genetics, Trauma, and More

Chapter 21—Factors That Affect Depression Risk 155
Section 21.1—Genetic and Environmental Risk Factors 157
Section 21.2—Probing the Depression-Rumination Cycle 161
Chapter 22—Stress as a Risk Factor for Depression 167
Section 22.1—Stress and Your Health 169

   Section 22.2—Caregiver Stress:
      A Risk Factor for
      Depression 172
   Section 22.3—Parenting Stress and
      Mental Health: A
      Strong Connection 177
Chapter 23—Trauma as a Risk Factor for Depression 181
   Section 23.1—Depression, Trauma,
      and Posttraumatic
      Stress Disorder 183
   Section 23.2—Adverse Childhood
      Experiences..................... 185
Chapter 24—The Link between Depression and
   Other Mental Disorders 191
   Section 24.1—Anxiety Disorders among
      Women and Children.... 193
   Section 24.2—Eating Disorders,
      Anxiety, and
      Depression 198
Chapter 25—Depression, Substance Use, and Addiction 201
   Section 25.1—Substance Use and
      Co-occurring Mental
      Disorders......................... 203
   Section 25.2—Can Smoking Cause
      Depression? 208
   Section 25.3—Could Drinking Be
      Fueling Your
      Depression? 210
Chapter 26—Climate Change and Depression................................ 219
Chapter 27—Other Depression Triggers.. 225

Part 5. Depression and Chronic Illnesses
Chapter 28—Chronic Illness and Mental Health............................. 233
   Section 28.1—The Intersection
      of Depression and
      Chronic Illness 235

    Section 28.2—Chronic Pain and
        Depression 239
    Section 28.3—Depression and
        Fibromyalgia 242
Chapter 29—Arthritis–Mental Health Connection 247
Chapter 30—Depression and Attention Deficit
    Hyperactivity Disorder 251
Chapter 31—Depression and Brain Injury 255
Chapter 32—Depression and Cancer 261
Chapter 33—Depression and Diabetes 273
Chapter 34—Depression and Heart Disease 277
Chapter 35—Depression and Human Immunodeficiency
    Virus 283
Chapter 36—Depression and Multiple Sclerosis 287
Chapter 37—Depression and Neurological Disorders 293
    Section 37.1—Genetic Overlap between
        Alzheimer Disease and
        Depression 295
    Section 37.2—Depression, a Nonmotor
        Manifestation of
        Parkinson Disease 298
    Section 37.3—Depression in
        Epilepsy 302
Chapter 38—Depression and Stroke 307

Part 6. Diagnosis and Treatment of Depression
Chapter 39—Recognizing Signs of Depression in You
    and Your Loved Ones 315
Chapter 40—Finding and Choosing a Therapist 319
Chapter 41—Diagnosing Depression 323
Chapter 42—Psychotherapy for Depression 327
    Section 42.1—Elements of
        Psychotherapy 329
    Section 42.2—Cognitive-Behavioral
        Therapy 333

                Section 42.3—Interpersonal Therapy... 335
                Section 42.4—Acceptance and
                            Commitment Therapy... 337
Chapter 43—Mental Health Medications 341
Chapter 44—Combination Treatment...351
Chapter 45—Brain Stimulation Therapies for
            Severe Depression 355
Chapter 46—Light Therapy for Seasonal Affective Disorder 365
Chapter 47—Depression and the Placebo Effect............................367
Chapter 48—Genetic Studies May Lead to Accurate
            Medication Dose 371
Chapter 49—Brain Biofeedback for Depressive Symptoms...........377
Chapter 50—Alternative and Complementary Therapies
            for Depression 379
                Section 50.1—Use, Effectiveness, and
                            Safety of Complementary
                            and Alternative
                            Therapies......................... 381
                Section 50.2—Meditation, Mindfulness,
                            and Mental Health 389
                Section 50.3—What the Science Says
                            about Complementary
                            Health Approaches for
                            Depression 395
Chapter 51—Treating Depression in Children
            and Adolescents..403
Chapter 52—Treatment-Resistant and Relapsed Depression........409
Chapter 53—Paying for Mental Health Care..................................413

Part 7. Strategies for Managing Depression
Chapter 54—Understanding Mental Illness Stigma 419
Chapter 55—Well-Being Concepts 423
                Section 55.1—Well-Being and
                            Satisfaction with Life..... 425
                Section 55.2—Self-Management
                            Support: Beyond
                            the Medical Model......... 427

Chapter 56—Relationship between Psychological Resilience
 and Mental Health 433
    Section 56.1—Understanding
                  Individual Resilience..... 435
    Section 56.2—Building Resilience in
                  Children and Youth
                  Dealing with Trauma 440
Chapter 57—Building a Healthy Body Image and
 Self-Esteem 445
    Section 57.1—Healthy Body Image 447
    Section 57.2—How to Improve Your
                  Self-Esteem 450
Chapter 58—Dealing with the Effects of Trauma 455
Chapter 59—Stress in Disaster Responders and Recovery
 Workers 459
    Section 59.1—Depression and First
                  Responders 461
    Section 59.2—Compassion Fatigue 464
    Section 59.3—Tips for Families of
                  Returning Disaster
                  Responders 468
Chapter 60—Grief, Bereavement, and Coping with Loss 473
Chapter 61—Coping with the Holiday Blues 479
Chapter 62—Peer Support and Social Inclusion 483
Chapter 63—Helping a Family Member or Friend
 with Depression..487

Part 8. Depression and Suicide
Chapter 64—Understanding Suicide 495
Chapter 65—Suicide in the United States 499
Chapter 66—Suicidal Behavior, Risk, and Protective Factors 507
Chapter 67—Suicide among Youth and Older Adults....................511
    Section 67.1—Teen Suicide..................... 513
    Section 67.2—Suicide among Young
                  Adults 516

Section 67.3—Older Adults: Depression
and Suicide Facts 518
Chapter 68—Warning Signs of Suicide and How
to Deal with It 525
Section 68.1—Suicide Risk
Screening 527
Section 68.2—Treating People with
Suicidal Thoughts 532
Section 68.3—Preventing Suicide 535
Section 68.4—Taking Care of a
Family Member after
a Suicide Attempt........... 537
Chapter 69—Recovering from a Suicide Attempt............................545

Part 9. Additional Help and Information
Chapter 70—Glossary of Terms Related to Depression 555
Chapter 71—Directory of Organizations That Help
People with Depression and Suicidal
Thoughts...561

Index 573

Preface

ABOUT THIS BOOK

Depression is one of the most common disabling mental health problems in the world and is characterized by persistent sadness, hopelessness, trouble concentrating, excessive fatigue, and drastic changes in appetite and sleep habits. According to the recent National Institute of Mental Health (NIMH) statistics, an estimated 21 million adults in the United States have experienced at least one major depressive episode, accounting for 8.4 percent of all American adults. It is found that the prevalence of a major depressive episode is higher in adult females (10.5%) than in adult males (6.2%). Research indicates that a variety of genetic, biologic, and environmental factors contribute to the development of this chronic illness. Research also indicates that timely diagnosis and treatment help the affected manage their symptoms effectively and develop strategies for better living.

Depression Sourcebook, Sixth Edition offers basic information about the prevalence, symptoms, diagnosis, and treatment of depression. It talks about atypical depression, bipolar disorder, depression during the reproductive transitions in women, psychotic depression, and seasonal affective disorder (SAD). It examines the impact of depression on children, adolescents, men, women, older adults, minority populations, and sexually diverse and gender-diverse populations. It describes strategies for managing depression, along with information about the warning signs and prevalence of suicide. It also provides insight into complementary and alternative therapies used to improve depression symptoms. The book concludes with a glossary of terms related to depression and a directory of resources for additional help and information.

HOW TO USE THIS BOOK

This book is divided into parts and chapters. Parts focus on broad areas of interest. Chapters are devoted to single topics within a part.

Part 1: Introduction to Mental Health Disorders and Depression discusses the fundamentals of mental health and how it plays a vital role in the development and severity of mental health disorders like depression. It discusses various myths and facts about mental health disorders and provides basic information on depression. The part concludes with the statistical trends in the prevalence of depression.

Part 2: Types of Depression gives an overview of the most common types of depression and related mental health disorders, including major depression, atypical depression, bipolar disorder, disruptive mood dysregulation disorder, psychotic depression, and seasonal affective disorder (SAD).

Part 3: Who Develops Depression? provides information about gender, age, and racial disparities in the diagnosis of depression. Facts about depression in men, women, children, adolescents, pregnant women, and older adults are discussed, including depression faced by women during the reproductive transition phase. Information about the prevalence of depression in minority and sexual- and gender-diverse populations is also provided.

Part 4: Risk Factors for Depression: Genetics, Trauma, and More highlights genetic and environmental factors that can predispose a person to developing depression. It discusses the impact of trauma, substance use, and addiction on depression, including caregiver stress and climate change.

Part 5: Depression and Chronic Illnesses discusses chronic diseases that are often linked to depression, such as fibromyalgia, brain injury, cancer, diabetes, heart disease, human immunodeficiency virus (HIV), multiple sclerosis, attention deficit hyperactivity disorder (ADHD), and stroke.

Part 6: Diagnosis and Treatment of Depression describes the process of receiving a depression diagnosis, paying for mental health care, and finding and choosing a therapist. It also identifies mental health medications used to treat depression, including psychotherapy (talk therapy) and cognitive-behavioral therapy (CBT). Other forms of treatment, such as usings placebos, light therapy for seasonal affective disorder, brain stimulation therapies, and strategies for treating severe or relapsed forms of depression, are discussed.

Part 7: Strategies for Managing Depression discusses how to maintain emotional wellness in people who have depression, including stress in disaster responders and recovery workers. Information on developing resilience, improving self-esteem, as well as dealing with trauma and coping with grief, bereavement, and loss, is included.

Part 8: Depression and Suicide offers information about the prevalence of suicide among those who are affected with depression. It describes the warning signs of suicide and provides information on how to recover from a suicide attempt. It also suggests steps to overcome trauma when a family member attempts suicide.

Part 9: Additional Help and Information provides a glossary of important terms related to depression and a directory of organizations that help people with depression and suicidal thoughts.

BIBLIOGRAPHIC NOTE

This volume contains documents and excerpts from publications issued by the following U.S. government agencies: Administration for Children and Families (ACF); Centers for Disease Control and Prevention (CDC); Centers for Medicare & Medicaid Services (CMS); Child Welfare Information Gateway; Effective Health Care Program; *Eunice Kennedy Shriver* National Institute of Child Health and Human Development (NICHD); girlshealth.gov; GlobalChange.gov; MedlinePlus; Mental Illness Research, Education and Clinical Centers (MIRECC); MentalHealth.gov; National Cancer Institute (NCI); National Center for Complementary and Integrative Health (NCCIH); National Center for Posttraumatic Stress Disorder (NCPTSD); National Human Genome Research Institute (NHGRI); National Institute of Mental Health (NIMH); National Institute on Aging (NIA); National Institute on Alcohol Abuse and Alcoholism (NIAAA); National Institutes of Health (NIH); News and Events; *NIH News in Health*; Office of Minority Health (OMH); Office of the Assistant Secretary for Preparedness and Response (ASPR); Office on Women's Health (OWH); Smokefree.gov; Substance Abuse and Mental Health Services Administration (SAMHSA); U.S. Department of Health and Human Services (HHS); U.S. Department of Veterans Affairs (VA); United States Census Bureau; and Youth.gov.

It also contains original material produced by Infobase and reviewed by medical consultants.

ABOUT THE *HEALTH REFERENCE SERIES*

The *Health Reference Series* is designed to provide basic medical information for patients, families, caregivers, and the general public. Each volume provides comprehensive coverage on a particular topic. This is especially important for people who may be dealing with a newly diagnosed disease or a chronic disorder in themselves or in a family member. People looking for preventive guidance, information about disease warning signs, medical statistics, and risk factors for health problems will also find answers to their questions in the *Health Reference Series*. The *Series*, however, is not intended to serve as a tool for diagnosing illness, in prescribing treatments, or as a substitute for the physician–patient relationship. All people concerned about medical symptoms or the possibility of disease are encouraged to seek professional care from an appropriate health-care provider.

A NOTE ABOUT SPELLING AND STYLE

Health Reference Series editors use *Stedman's Medical Dictionary* as an authority for questions related to the spelling of medical terms and *The Chicago Manual of Style* for questions related to grammatical structures, punctuation, and other editorial concerns. Consistent adherence is not always possible, however, because the individual volumes within the *Series* include many documents from a wide variety of different producers, and the editor's primary goal is to present material from each source as accurately as is possible. This sometimes means that information in different chapters or sections may follow other guidelines and alternate spelling authorities. For example, occasionally a copyright holder may require that eponymous terms be shown in possessive forms (Crohn's disease vs. Crohn disease) or that British spelling norms be retained (leukaemia vs. leukemia).

MEDICAL REVIEW

Infobase contracts with a team of qualified, senior medical professionals who serve as medical consultants for the *Health Reference Series*. As necessary, medical consultants review reprinted and originally written material for currency and accuracy. Medical consultation services are provided to the *Health Reference Series* editors by:
    Dr. Vijayalakshmi, MBBS, DGO, MD
    Dr. Senthil Selvan, MBBS, DCH, MD
    Dr. K. Sivanandham, MBBS, DCH, MS (Research), PhD

HEALTH REFERENCE SERIES UPDATE POLICY

The inaugural book in the *Health Reference Series* was the first edition of *Cancer Sourcebook* published in 1989. Since then, the *Series* has been enthusiastically received by librarians and in the medical community. In order to maintain the standard of providing high-quality health information for the layperson, the editorial staff felt it was necessary to implement a policy of updating volumes when warranted.

Medical researchers have been making tremendous strides, and it is the purpose of the *Health Reference Series* to stay current with the most recent advances. Each decision to update a volume is made on an individual basis. Some of the considerations include how much new information is available and the feedback we receive from people who use the books. If there is a topic you would like to see added to the update list, or an area of medical concern you feel has not been adequately addressed, please write to: custserv@infobaselearning.com.

Part 1 | Introduction to Mental Health Disorders and Depression

Chapter 1 | Mental Health Basics

WHAT IS MENTAL HEALTH?
Mental health includes our emotional, psychological, and social well-being. It affects how we think, feel, and act. It also helps determine how we handle stress, relate to others, and make healthy choices. Mental health is important at every stage of life, from childhood and adolescence through adulthood.

Although the terms are often used interchangeably, poor mental health and mental illness are not the same. A person can experience poor mental health and not be diagnosed with a mental illness. Likewise, a person diagnosed with a mental illness can experience periods of physical, mental, and social well-being.

WHY IS MENTAL HEALTH IMPORTANT FOR OVERALL HEALTH?
Mental health and physical health are equally important components of overall health. For example, depression increases the risk of many types of physical health problems, particularly long-lasting conditions such as diabetes, heart disease, and stroke. Similarly, the presence of chronic conditions can increase the risk of mental illness.

CAN YOUR MENTAL HEALTH CHANGE OVER TIME?
Yes, it is important to remember that a person's mental health can change over time, depending on many factors. When the demands placed on a person exceed their resources and coping abilities, their mental health could be impacted. For example, if someone is

working long hours, caring for a relative, or experiencing economic hardship, they may experience poor mental health.

HOW COMMON ARE MENTAL ILLNESSES?
Mental illnesses are among the most common health conditions in the United States.
- More than 50 percent will be diagnosed with a mental illness or disorder at some point in their lifetime.
- One in five Americans will experience a mental illness in a given year.
- One in five children, either currently or at some point during their life, has had a seriously debilitating mental illness.
- One in twenty-five Americans lives with a serious mental illness, such as schizophrenia, bipolar disorder, or major depression.

WHAT CAUSES MENTAL ILLNESS?
There is no single cause for mental illness. A number of factors can contribute to the risk of mental illness, such as:
- early adverse life experiences, such as trauma or a history of abuse (e.g., child abuse, sexual assault, witnessing violence, etc.)
- experiences related to other ongoing (chronic) medical conditions, such as cancer or diabetes
- biological factors or chemical imbalances in the brain
- use of alcohol or drugs
- having feelings of loneliness or isolation[1]

MENTAL HEALTH AND WELLNESS
Positive mental health allows people to:
- realize their full potential
- cope with the stresses of life

---

[1] "About Mental Health," Centers for Disease Control and Prevention (CDC), June 28, 2021. Available online. URL: www.cdc.gov/mentalhealth/learn/index.htm. Accessed February 15, 2023.

Mental Health Basics

- work productively
- make meaningful contributions to their communities

Ways to maintain positive mental health include:
- getting professional help if you need it
- connecting with others
- staying positive
- getting physically active
- helping others
- getting enough sleep
- developing coping skills[2]

---

[2] "What Is Mental Health?" MentalHealth.gov, February 28, 2022. Available online. URL: www.mentalhealth.gov/basics/what-is-mental-health. Accessed February 15, 2023.

Chapter 2 | Myths and Facts about Mental Health Disorders

MENTAL HEALTH PROBLEMS AFFECT EVERYONE
- **Myth:** Mental health problems do not affect you.
  Fact: Mental health problems are actually very common. In 2020, about:
  - one in five American adults experienced a mental health issue
  - one in six young people experienced a major depressive episode
  - one in twenty Americans lived with a serious mental illness, such as schizophrenia, bipolar disorder, or major depression

  Suicide is a leading cause of death in the United States. In fact, it was the second leading cause of death for people aged 10–24. It accounted for the loss of more than 45,979 American lives in 2020, nearly double the number of lives lost to homicide.
- **Myth:** Children do not experience mental health problems.
  Fact: Even very young children may show early warning signs of mental health concerns. These mental health problems are often clinically diagnosable and can be a product of the interaction of biological, psychological, and social factors.

Half of all mental health disorders show the first signs before a person turns 14 years old, and three-quarters of mental health disorders begin before the age of 24.

Unfortunately, only half of children and adolescents with diagnosable mental health problems receive the treatment they need. Early mental health support can help a child before problems interfere with other developmental needs.

- **Myth:** People with mental health problems are violent and unpredictable.

  Fact: The vast majority of people with mental health problems are no more likely to be violent than anyone else. Most people with mental illness are not violent, and only 3–5 percent of violent acts can be attributed to individuals living with a serious mental illness. In fact, people with severe mental illnesses are over 10 times more likely to be victims of violent crime than the general population. You probably know someone with a mental health problem and do not even realize it because many people with mental health problems are highly active and productive members of our communities.

- **Myth:** People with mental health needs, even those who are managing their mental illness, cannot tolerate the stress of holding down a job.

  Fact: People with mental health problems are just as productive as other employees. Employers who hire people with mental health problems report good attendance and punctuality as well as motivation, good work, and job tenure on par with or greater than other employees.

  When employees with mental health problems receive effective treatment, it can result in:
  - lower total medical costs
  - increased productivity
  - lower absenteeism
  - decreased disability costs

- **Myth:** Personality weakness or character flaws cause mental health problems. People with mental health problems can snap out of it if they try hard enough.

Myths and Facts about Mental Health Disorders

Fact: Mental health problems have nothing to do with being lazy or weak, and many people need help to get better. Many factors contribute to mental health problems, including:
- biological factors, such as genes, physical illness, injury, or brain chemistry
- life experiences, such as trauma or a history of abuse
- family history of mental health problems

People with mental health problems can get better, and many recover completely.

HELPING INDIVIDUALS WITH MENTAL HEALTH PROBLEMS
- **Myth:** There is no hope for people with mental health problems. Once a friend or family member develops mental health problems, he or she will never recover.
  Fact: Studies show that people with mental health problems get better and many recover completely. Recovery refers to the process in which people are able to live, work, learn, and participate fully in their communities. There are more treatments, services, and community support systems than ever before, and they work.
- **Myth:** Therapy and self-help are a waste of time. Why bother when you can just take a pill?
  Fact: Treatment for mental health problems varies depending on the individual and could include medication, therapy, or both. Many individuals work with a support system during the healing and recovery process.
- **Myth:** You cannot do anything for a person with a mental health problem.
  Fact: Friends and loved ones can make a big difference. In 2020, only 20 percent of adults received any mental health treatment in the past year, which included 10 percent who received counseling or therapy from a professional. Friends and family can be important influences to help someone get the treatment and services they need by:
  - reaching out and letting them know you are available to help

- helping them access mental health services
- learning and sharing the facts about mental health, especially if you hear something that is not true
- treating them with respect, just as you would anyone else
- refusing to define them by their diagnosis or using labels such as "crazy" instead of using person-first language
- **Myth:** Prevention does not work. It is impossible to prevent mental illnesses.
  Fact: Prevention of mental, emotional, and behavioral disorders focuses on addressing known risk factors such as exposure to trauma that can affect the chances that children, youth, and young adults will develop mental health problems. Promoting the social-emotional well-being of children and youth leads to:
  - higher overall productivity
  - better educational outcomes
  - lower crime rates
  - stronger economies
  - lower health-care costs
  - improved quality of life (QOL)
  - increased life span
  - improved family life[1]

---

[1] "Mental Health Myths and Facts," MentalHealth.gov, February 28, 2022. Available online. URL: www.mental-health.gov/basics/health-myths-facts. Accessed March 10, 2023.

Chapter 3 | **Depression: What You Need to Know**

WHAT IS DEPRESSION?
Everyone feels sad or low sometimes, but these feelings usually pass with a little time. Depression (also called "major depressive disorder" or "clinical depression") is different. It can cause severe symptoms that affect how you feel, think, and handle daily activities, such as sleeping, eating, or working. It is an illness that can affect anyone regardless of age, race, income, culture, or education. Research suggests that genetic, biological, environmental, and psychological factors play a role in depression.

Depression may occur with other mental disorders and other illnesses, such as diabetes, cancer, heart disease, and chronic pain. Depression can make these conditions worse, and vice versa. Sometimes, medications taken for these illnesses cause side effects that contribute to depression symptoms.

WHAT ARE THE DIFFERENT TYPES OF DEPRESSION?
Two common forms of depression are:
- major depression, which includes symptoms of depression most of the time for at least two weeks that typically interfere with one's ability to work, sleep, study, and eat
- persistent depressive disorder (dysthymia), which often includes less severe symptoms of depression that last much longer, typically for at least two years

Other forms of depression include:
- perinatal depression, which occurs when a woman experiences major depression during pregnancy or after delivery (postpartum depression)
- seasonal affective disorder, which comes and goes with the seasons, typically starting in late fall and early winter and going away during spring and summer
- depression with symptoms of psychosis, which is a severe form of depression where a person experiences psychosis symptoms, such as delusions (disturbing, false fixed beliefs) or hallucinations (hearing or seeing things that others do not see or hear)

Individuals diagnosed with bipolar disorder (formerly called "manic depression" or "manic-depressive illness") also experience depression.

WHAT ARE THE SIGNS AND SYMPTOMS OF DEPRESSION?
Common symptoms of depression include:
- persistent sad, anxious, or "empty" mood
- feelings of hopelessness or pessimism
- feelings of irritability, frustration, or restlessness
- feelings of guilt, worthlessness, or helplessness
- loss of interest or pleasure in hobbies or activities
- decreased energy, fatigue, or being "slowed down"
- difficulty concentrating, remembering, or making decisions
- difficulty sleeping, early morning awakening, or oversleeping
- changes in appetite or unplanned weight changes
- aches or pains, headaches, cramps, or digestive problems without a clear physical cause and that do not ease even with treatment
- suicide attempts or thoughts of death or suicide

DOES DEPRESSION LOOK THE SAME IN EVERYONE?
Depression can affect people differently, depending on their age.
- Children with depression may be anxious, cranky, pretend to be sick, refuse to go to school, cling to a parent, or worry that a parent may die.
- Older children and teens with depression may get into trouble at school, sulk, be easily frustrated, feel restless, or have low self-esteem. They may also have other disorders, such as anxiety and eating disorders, attention deficit hyperactivity disorder (ADHD), or substance use disorder (SUD). Older children and teens are more likely to experience excessive sleepiness (called "hypersomnia") and increased appetite (called "hyperphagia"). In adolescence, females begin to experience depression more often than males, likely due to biological, life cycle, and hormonal factors unique to women.
- Younger adults with depression are more likely to be irritable, complain of weight gain and hypersomnia, and have a negative view of life and the future. They often have other disorders, such as generalized anxiety disorder (GAD), social phobia, panic disorder, and SUD.
- Middle-aged adults with depression may have more depressive episodes, decreased libido, middle-of-the-night insomnia, or early morning awakening. They may also more frequently report having gastrointestinal symptoms such as diarrhea or constipation.
- Older adults with depression commonly experience sadness or grief or may have other less obvious symptoms. They may report a lack of emotions rather than a depressed mood. Older adults are also more likely to have other medical conditions or pain that may cause or contribute to depression. In severe cases, memory and thinking problems (called "pseudodementia") may be prominent.

HOW IS DEPRESSION DIAGNOSED?

To be diagnosed with depression, an individual must have five depression symptoms every day, nearly all day, for at least two weeks. One of the symptoms must be a depressed mood or a loss of interest or pleasure in almost all activities. Children and adolescents may be irritable rather than sad.

If you think you may have depression, talk to your health-care provider. Primary care providers routinely diagnose and treat depression and refer individuals to mental health professionals, such as psychologists or psychiatrists.

During the visit, your provider may ask when your symptoms began, how long they last, how often they occur, and if they keep you from going out or doing your usual activities. It may help if you make some notes about your symptoms before your visit. Certain medications and some medical conditions, such as viruses or a thyroid disorder, can cause the same depression symptoms. Your provider can rule out these possibilities by doing a physical exam, interview, and lab tests.

HOW IS DEPRESSION TREATED?

Depression treatment typically involves medication, psychotherapy, or both. If these treatments do not reduce symptoms, brain stimulation therapy may be another treatment option. In milder cases of depression, treatment might begin with psychotherapy alone, and medication is added if the individual continues to experience symptoms. For moderate or severe depression, many mental health professionals recommend a combination of medication and therapy at the start of treatment.

Choosing the right treatment plan should be based on a person's individual needs and medical situation under a provider's care. It may take some trial and error to find the treatment that works best for you.

HOW CAN YOU FIND HELP?

The Substance Abuse and Mental Health Services Administration (SAMHSA) provides the Behavioral Health Treatment Services

Depression: What You Need to Know

Locator (https://findtreatment.gov/), an online tool for finding mental health treatment and support groups in your area. For additional resources, visit the Help for Mental Illnesses webpage of the National Institute of Mental Health (NIMH; https://www.nimh.nih.gov/health/find-help).[1]

---

[1] "Depression," National Institute of Mental Health (NIMH), 2021. Available online. URL: www.nimh.nih.gov/health/publications/depression. Accessed February 16, 2023.

Chapter 4 | Trends in Depression Prevalence and Impairment

Major depression is one of the most common mental disorders in the United States. For some individuals, major depression can result in severe impairments that interfere with or limit one's ability to carry out major life activities.

The National Survey of Drug Use and Health (NSDUH) study definition of the major depressive episode is based mainly on the fifth edition of the *Diagnostic and Statistical Manual of Mental Disorders* (*DSM-5*):

- Major depressive episode is a period of at least two weeks when a person experiences a depressed mood or loss of interest or pleasure in daily activities and has a majority of specified symptoms, such as problems with sleep, eating, energy, concentration, or self-worth.
- No exclusions were made for major depressive episode symptoms caused by medical illness, substance use disorders, or medication.

PREVALENCE OF A MAJOR DEPRESSIVE EPISODE AMONG ADULTS
- Figure 4.1 shows the prevalence of a major depressive episode among U.S. adults aged 18 or older in 2020.
  - An estimated number of 21.0 million adults in the United States had at least one major depressive episode. This number represented 8.4 percent of all U.S. adults.

Depression Sourcebook, Sixth Edition

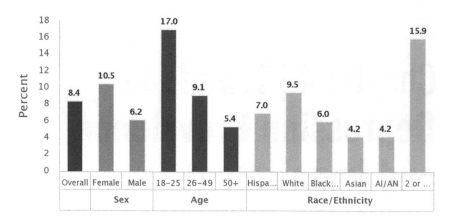

Figure 4.1. Major Depressive Episode among Adults
National Institute of Mental Health (NIMH)

- The prevalence of a major depressive episode was higher among adult females (10.5%) than that among males (6.2%).
- The prevalence of adults with a major depressive episode was the highest among individuals aged 18–25 (17.0%).
- The prevalence of a major depressive episode was highest among those who report having multiple (two or more) races (15.9%).

MAJOR DEPRESSIVE EPISODES WITH IMPAIRMENT AMONG ADULTS
- In 2020, an estimated number of 14.8 million U.S. adults aged 18 or older had at least one major depressive episode with severe impairment. This number represented 6 percent of all U.S. adults.

TREATMENT FOR A MAJOR DEPRESSIVE EPISODE AMONG ADULTS
- In 2020, an estimated 66 percent of U.S. adults aged 18 or older with a major depressive episode received treatment in the past year.

Trends in Depression Prevalence and Impairment

- Among those individuals with a major depressive episode with severe impairment, an estimated 71 percent received treatment in the past year.

PREVALENCE OF A MAJOR DEPRESSIVE EPISODE AMONG ADOLESCENTS

- Figure 4.2 shows the past year's prevalence of a major depressive episode among U.S. adolescents in 2020.
  - An estimated number of 4.1 million adolescents aged 12–17 in the United States had at least one major depressive episode. This number represented 17 percent of the U.S. population aged 12–17.
  - The prevalence of a major depressive episode was higher among adolescent females (25.2%) than that among males (9.2%).
  - The prevalence of a major depressive episode was highest among adolescents reporting two or more races (29.9%).

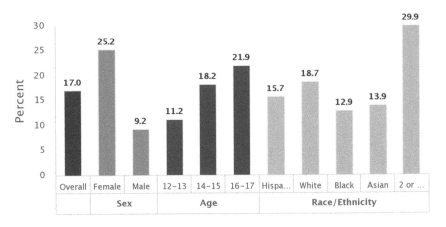

Figure 4.2. Major Depressive Episode among Adolescents

National Institute of Mental Health (NIMH)

MAJOR DEPRESSIVE EPISODE WITH IMPAIRMENT AMONG ADOLESCENTS
- In 2020, an estimated number of 2.9 million adolescents aged 12–17 in the United States had at least one major depressive episode with severe impairment in the past year. This number represented 12 percent of the U.S. population aged 12–17.

TREATMENT FOR A MAJOR DEPRESSIVE EPISODE AMONG ADOLESCENTS
- In 2020, an estimated 41.6 percent of U.S. adolescents with a major depressive episode received treatment in the past year.
- Among adolescents with a major depressive episode with severe impairment, an estimated 46.9 percent received treatment in the past year.[1]

---

[1] "Major Depression," National Institute of Mental Health (NIMH), January 2022. Available online. URL: www.nimh.nih.gov/health/statistics/major-depression#part_2565. Accessed February 17, 2023.

Part 2 | Types of Depression

Chapter 5 | Major Depression

WHAT IS MAJOR DEPRESSION?
Major depression is a medical condition distinguished by one or more major depressive episodes. A major depressive episode is characterized by at least two weeks of depressed mood or loss of interest (pleasure) and is accompanied by at least four more symptoms of depression. Such symptoms can include changes in appetite, changes in weight, difficulty in thinking and concentrating, and recurrent thoughts of death or suicide. Depression differs from feeling "blue" in that it causes severe enough problems to interfere with a person's day-to-day functioning.

People's experience with major depression varies. Some people describe it as a total loss of energy or enthusiasm to do anything. Others may describe it as constantly living with a feeling of impending doom. There are treatments that help improve functioning and relieve many symptoms of depression. Recovery is possible!

HOW COMMON IS MAJOR DEPRESSION?
Major depression is a common psychiatric disorder. It is more common in adolescent and adult women than in adolescent and adult men. Between 15 and 20 out of every 100 people (15–20%) experience an episode of major depression during their lifetime. Prevalence has not been found to be related to ethnicity, income, education, or marital status.

COURSE OF ILLNESS

The average age of onset is in the mid-20s; however, major depression can begin at any age in life. The frequency of episodes varies from person to person. Some people have isolated episodes over many years, while others suffer from frequent episodes clustered together. The number of episodes generally increases as the person grows older. The severity of the initial episode of major depression seems to indicate persistence. Episodes also seem to follow major stressors, such as the death of a loved one or a divorce. Chronic medical conditions and substance abuse may further exacerbate depressive episodes.

CAUSES OF MAJOR DEPRESSION

There is no simple answer to what causes depression because several factors play a part in the onset of the disorder. These include a genetic or family history of depression, environmental stressors, life events, biological factors, and psychological vulnerability to depression.

Research shows that the risk for depression results from the influence of multiple genes acting together with environmental factors. This is called the "stress-vulnerability model." A family history of depression does not necessarily mean children or other relatives will develop major depression. However, those with a family history of depression have a slightly higher chance of becoming depressed at some stage in their lives. Although genetic research suggests that depression can run in families, genetics alone are unlikely to cause depression. Environmental factors, such as traumatic childhood or adult life events, may act as triggers. Studies show that early childhood trauma and losses (such as the death or separation of parents) or adult life events (such as the death of a loved one, divorce, loss of a job, retirement, serious financial problems, and family conflict) can lead to the onset of depression. Subsequent episodes are usually caused by mild stressors or even none at all.

Many scientists believe the cause is biological, such as an imbalance in brain chemicals, specifically serotonin and norepinephrine. There are also theories that physical changes in the body may play a role in depression. Such physical changes can include viral

Major Depression

and other infections, heart attacks, cancer, or hormonal disorders. Personality style may also contribute to the onset of depression. People are at a greater risk of becoming depressed if they have low self-esteem, tend to worry a lot, are overly dependent on others, are perfectionists, or expect too much from themselves and others.

SYMPTOMS OF MAJOR DEPRESSION

To meet the criteria for major depressive disorder (MDD), a person must meet at least five symptoms of depression for at least a two-week period. Social, occupational, and other areas of functioning must be significantly impaired or at least require increased effort. A depressed mood caused by substances (such as drugs, alcohol, or medications) or related to another medical condition is not considered to be an MDD. MDD also cannot be diagnosed if a person has a history of manic, hypomanic, or mixed episodes (e.g., bipolar disorder) or if the depressed mood is better accounted for by schizoaffective disorder.

Not all symptoms must be present for a person to be diagnosed with depression. Five (or more) of the following symptoms have to be present during the same two-week period and represent a change from previous functioning. At least one of the symptoms must be either a depressed mood or loss of interest or pleasure.

- Depressed mood most of the day, nearly every day, as indicated by either subjective report (e.g., feels sad or empty) or observation made by others (e.g., appears tearful). In children and adolescents, this may be characterized as an irritable mood rather than a sad mood.
- Markedly diminished interest or pleasure in all, or almost all, activities most of the day, nearly every day. This includes activities that were previously found enjoyable.
- Significant weight loss when not dieting or weight gain (e.g., a change of more than 5% of body weight in a month) or a decrease or increase in appetite nearly every day.

- Insomnia or hypersomnia nearly every day. The person may have difficulty falling asleep, staying asleep, or waking early in the morning and not being able to get back to sleep. Alternatively, the person may sleep excessively (such as over 12 hours per night) and spend much of the day in bed.
- Psychomotor agitation (e.g., inability to sit still or pacing) or psychomotor retardation (e.g., slowed speech, thinking, and body movements) nearly every day. Changes in activity levels are common in depression. The person may feel agitated, "on edge," and restless. Alternatively, they may experience decreased activity levels reflected by slowness and lethargy, both in terms of the person's behavior and thought processes.
- Fatigue or loss of energy nearly every day.
- Feelings of worthlessness or excessive or inappropriate guilt nearly every day. Depressed people may feel they are worthless or that there is no hope for improving their lives. Feelings of guilt may be present about events with which the person had no involvement, such as a catastrophe, a crime, or an illness.
- Diminished ability to think or concentrate, or indecisiveness, nearly every day. A significant decrease in the ability to concentrate makes it difficult to pay attention to others or contemplate simple tasks. The person may be quite indecisive about even minor things.
- Recurrent thoughts of death (not just fear of dying), recurrent suicidal ideation without a specific plan, a specific plan for committing suicide, or a suicide attempt.

There are other psychiatric symptoms that depressed people often experience. They might complain of bodily aches and pains rather than feelings of sadness. They might report or exhibit persistent anger, angry outbursts, and an exaggerated sense of frustration over seemingly minor events. Symptoms of anxiety are also very common among people with depression. Other symptoms include hallucinations (false perceptions, such as hearing voices) and delusions (false beliefs, such as paranoid delusions). These symptoms usually disappear when the symptoms of depression have been controlled.

HOW IS MAJOR DEPRESSION DIAGNOSED?
Major depression cannot be diagnosed with a blood test, computerized axial tomography (CAT) scan, or any other laboratory test. The only way to diagnose major depression is with a clinical interview. The interviewer checks to see if the person has experienced severe symptoms for at least two weeks. If the symptoms are less severe but last over long periods of time, the person may be diagnosed with persistent depressive disorder. The clinician must also check to be sure there are no physical problems that could cause symptoms like those of major depression, such as a brain tumor or a thyroid problem.

TREATMENTS FOR MAJOR DEPRESSION
There are a variety of antidepressant medications and therapies available to those suffering from depression. Antidepressant medications help stabilize mood. People can also learn to manage their symptoms with psychotherapy. People with a milder form of depression may benefit from psychotherapy alone, while those with more severe symptoms and episodes may benefit from antidepressants. A combination of both types of treatment is often most helpful to people. The treatments listed here are ones that research has shown to be effective for people with depression. They are considered to be evidence-based practices.

Medication
The following are the five different classes of antidepressant medications:
- antidepressant class number 1: serotonin reuptake inhibitors (SSRIs)
- antidepressant class number 2: serotonin norepinephrine reuptake inhibitors (SNRIs)

- antidepressant class number 3: atypical antidepressants
- antidepressant class number 4: tricyclics and tetracyclics (TCA and TECA)
- antidepressant class number 5: monoamine oxidase inhibitors (MAOI)

Cognitive-Behavioral Therapy

Cognitive-behavioral therapy (CBT) is a well-established treatment for people with depression. CBT is a blend of two therapies: cognitive therapy and behavioral therapy. Cognitive therapy focuses on a person's thoughts and beliefs and how they influence a person's mood and actions and aims to change a person's thinking to be more adaptive and healthy. Behavioral therapy focuses on a person's actions and aims to change unhealthy behavior patterns.

CBT helps a person focus on his or her current problems and how to solve them. Both patient and therapist need to be actively involved in this process. The therapist helps the patient learn how to identify and correct distorted thoughts or negative self-talk often associated with depressed feelings, recognize and change inaccurate beliefs, engage in more enjoyable activities, relate to self and others in more positive ways, learn problem-solving skills, and change behaviors. Another focus of CBT is behavioral activation (i.e., increasing activity levels and helping the patient take part in rewarding activities that can improve mood). CBT is a structured, weekly intervention. Weekly homework assignments help the individual apply the learned techniques.

Family Psychoeducation

Mental illness affects the whole family. Family treatment can play an important role in helping both the person with depression and his or her relatives. Family psychoeducation is one way families can work together toward recovery. The family and clinician will meet together to discuss the problems they are experiencing. Families will then attend educational sessions where they will learn basic facts about mental illness, coping skills, communication skills, problem-solving skills, and ways to work together toward recovery.

Major Depression

Assertive Community Treatment
Assertive community treatment (ACT) is an approach that is most effective with individuals with the greatest service needs, such as those with a history of multiple hospitalizations. In ACT, the person receives treatment from an interdisciplinary team of usually 10–12 professionals, including case managers, a psychiatrist, several nurses and social workers, vocational specialists, substance abuse treatment specialists, and peer specialists. The team provides coverage 24 hours a day, seven days a week, and utilizes small caseloads, usually one staff for every 10 clients. Services provided include case management, comprehensive treatment planning, crisis intervention, medication management, individual supportive therapy, substance abuse treatment, rehabilitation services (i.e., supported employment), and peer support.

Electroconvulsive Therapy
Electroconvulsive therapy (ECT) is a procedure used to treat severe or life-threatening depression. It is used when other treatments, such as psychotherapy and antidepressant medications, have not worked. Electrical currents are briefly sent to the brain through electrodes placed on the head. The electrical current can last up to eight seconds, producing a short seizure. It is believed this brain stimulation helps relieve symptoms of depression by altering brain chemicals, including neurotransmitters such as serotonin and natural pain relievers called "endorphins." ECT treatments are usually done two to three times a week for two to three weeks. Maintenance treatments may be done one time each week, tapering down to one time each month. They may continue for several months to a year to reduce the risk of relapse. ECT is usually given in combination with medication, psychotherapy, family therapy, and behavioral therapy.

SIMILAR PSYCHIATRIC DISORDERS
Major depression shares symptoms with some of the other psychiatric disorders. If the person experiences very high or euphoric moods called "mania," they would be given a diagnosis of bipolar

disorder. If the person exhibits psychotic symptoms while not depressed, they might be diagnosed with schizoaffective disorder. Major depression must also be distinguished from a depressive disorder due to another medical condition. In this case, the mood disturbances are caused by physiological changes due to a medical condition.[1]

---

[1] Mental Illness Research, Education and Clinical Centers (MIRECC), "What Is Major Depression?" U.S. Department of Veterans Affairs (VA), 2015. Available online. URL: www.mirecc.va.gov/visn22/depression_education.pdf. Accessed March 1, 2023.

Chapter 6 | Atypical Depression

Atypical depression is a subtype of major depressive disorder (MDD). Although the name suggests otherwise, it is actually quite common. According to the *Diagnostic and Statistical Manual of Mental Disorders*, the main symptoms of atypical depression include moods that react strongly to environmental circumstances, overeating, oversleeping, and a sensation of heavy limbs or being weighed down. These symptoms contrast with—or are atypical of—the symptoms of another subtype, melancholic depression. Melancholic depression is usually characterized by a lack of mood reactivity, loss of appetite, insomnia, and a diminished ability to experience pleasure.

CAUSES AND SYMPTOMS OF ATYPICAL DEPRESSION

Depression happens when the brain's mood-regulating circuits (neurotransmitters) fail to work properly. Although ascertaining the precise causes of atypical depression is still a challenge, several factors can contribute to its development, including the following:
- family history of depression
- feeling a significant loss by death or divorce
- social isolation
- job loss
- long-term stress
- bipolar disorder
- anxiety
- traumatic childhood experiences
- substance abuse

- serious illness
- impaired neurotransmitter or neuroreceptor function

A symptom that is specific to atypical depression is that people tend to experience a quick mood upliftment in response to positive changes in life. To further investigate, the health-care provider will perform physical exams and tests to rule out any physical causes of these symptoms.

Here are some symptoms of atypical depression that the healthcare provider may look for:
- eating more and gaining weight
- excessive sleepiness (hypersomnia)
- feeling a heavy sensation (leaden paralysis) in the arms or legs
- being overly upset by rejection, leading to difficulties in personal and professional relationships

Other common symptoms that may manifest in atypical depression include feeling sad, hopeless, or not enjoying things that they once used to enjoy. People with atypical depression may also have difficulty concentrating or remembering things and may feel easily irritated or frustrated.

DIAGNOSIS AND TREATMENT OF ATYPICAL DEPRESSION

The first step in diagnosing atypical depression involves a complete medical examination to determine whether the patient's symptoms may have a physical cause. Hypothyroidism, for instance, may cause symptoms such as mood changes, fatigue, and weight gain due to low levels of thyroid hormones. If a physical examination and blood tests fail to reveal an underlying health condition, the doctor may recommend a psychological evaluation. A mental health professional will typically ask questions about the patient's symptoms, recent experiences, feelings, and behavior patterns and compare that information to the diagnostic criteria for atypical depression.

The treatment for atypical depression usually involves a combination of psychotherapy (talk therapy) and medications. Both treatment methods have proved effective, but treatment outcome depends on the range and severity of symptoms. Psychotherapy involves meeting with a mental health professional to identify unhealthy thoughts or behaviors, explore problematic relationships and experiences, and develop new coping and problem-solving methods.

A number of prescription medications have also proven effective in treating atypical depression. These antidepressant medications work by improving the function of brain circuits and neurotransmitters that help regulate mood. Research suggests that many patients with atypical depression respond well to monoamine oxidase inhibitors (MAOIs), whereas fewer patients experience good results with tricyclic antidepressants. All patients are different, however, so it may be necessary to try several different types or combinations of medications to find the option that works best.

References

"Atypical Depression," Cleveland Clinic, February 15, 2023. Available online. URL: https://my.clevelandclinic.org/health/diseases/21131-atypical-depression. Accessed April 26, 2023.

"Atypical Depression," Psycom, October 19, 2022. Available online. URL: www.psycom.net/depression.central.atypical.html. Accessed April 26, 2023.

"Atypical Depression," *WebMD*, November 28, 2022. Available online. URL: www.webmd.com/depression/guide/atypical-depression. Accessed April 26, 2023.

Kerr, Michael. "Atypical Depression," Healthline, March 31, 2017. Available online. URL: www.healthline.com/health/depression/atypical-depression. Accessed April 26, 2023.

Moran, Mark. "Atypical Depression: What's in a Name?" American Psychiatric Association Publishing, October 17, 2003. Available online. URL: https://psychnews.psychiatryonline.org/doi/pdf/10.1176/pn.38.2.0017. Accessed April 26, 2023.

Chapter 7 | Bipolar Disorder (Manic-Depressive Illness)

Bipolar disorder (formerly called "manic-depressive illness" or "manic depression") is a mental illness that causes unusual shifts in a person's mood, energy, activity levels, and concentration. These shifts can make it difficult to carry out day-to-day tasks.

There are three types of bipolar disorder. All three types involve clear changes in mood, energy, and activity levels. These moods range from periods of extremely "up," elated, irritable, or energized behavior (known as "manic episodes") to very "down," sad, indifferent, or hopeless periods (known as "depressive episodes"). Less severe manic periods are known as "hypomanic episodes."

- Bipolar I disorder is defined by manic episodes that last for at least seven days (nearly every day for most of the day) or by manic symptoms that are so severe that the person needs immediate medical care. Usually, depressive episodes occur as well, typically lasting at least two weeks. Episodes of depression with mixed features (having depressive symptoms and manic symptoms at the same time) are also possible. Experiencing four or more episodes of mania or depression within one year is called "rapid cycling."
- Bipolar II disorder is defined by a pattern of depressive episodes and hypomanic episodes. The hypomanic episodes are less severe than the manic episodes in bipolar I disorder.

- Cyclothymic disorder (also called "cyclothymia") is defined by recurring hypomanic and depressive symptoms that are not intense enough or do not last long enough to qualify as hypomanic or depressive episodes.

Sometimes, a person might experience symptoms of bipolar disorder that do not match the three categories listed above, and this is referred to as "other specified and unspecified bipolar and related disorders."

Bipolar disorder is often diagnosed during late adolescence (teen years) or early adulthood. Sometimes, bipolar symptoms can appear in children. Although the symptoms may vary over time, bipolar disorder usually requires lifelong treatment. Following a prescribed treatment plan can help people manage their symptoms and improve their quality of life (QOL).

SIGNS AND SYMPTOMS OF BIPOLAR DISORDER

People with bipolar disorder experience periods of unusually intense emotion and changes in sleep patterns and activity levels and engage in behaviors that are out of character for them—often without recognizing their likely harmful or undesirable effects. These distinct periods are called "mood episodes." Mood episodes are very different from the person's usual moods and behaviors. During an episode, the symptoms last every day for most of the day. Episodes may also last for longer periods, such as several days or weeks.

RISK FACTORS FOR BIPOLAR DISORDER

Researchers are studying possible causes of bipolar disorder. Most agree that there are many factors that are likely to contribute to a person's chance of having the disorder.

- **Brain structure and functioning.** Some studies show that the brains of people with bipolar disorder differ in certain ways from the brains of people who do not have bipolar disorder or any other mental disorder.

Bipolar Disorder (Manic-Depressive Illness)

Learning more about these brain differences may help scientists understand bipolar disorder and determine which treatments will work best. At this time, health-care providers base the diagnosis and treatment plan on a person's symptoms and history rather than brain imaging or other diagnostic tests.
- **Genetics.** Some research suggests that people with certain genes are more likely to develop bipolar disorder. Research also shows that people who have a parent or sibling with bipolar disorder have an increased chance of having the disorder themselves. Many genes are involved, and no one gene causes the disorder.

DIAGNOSIS OF BIPOLAR DISORDER

Receiving the right diagnosis and treatment can help people with bipolar disorder lead healthy and active lives. Talking with a health-care provider is the first step. The health-care provider can complete a physical exam and other necessary medical tests to rule out other possible causes. The health-care provider may then conduct a mental health evaluation or provide a referral to a trained mental health-care provider, such as a psychiatrist, psychologist, or clinical social worker who has experience in diagnosing and treating bipolar disorder.

Mental health-care providers usually diagnose bipolar disorder based on a person's symptoms, lifetime history, experiences, and, in some cases, family history. Accurate diagnosis in youth is particularly important.

Bipolar Disorder and Other Conditions

Many people with bipolar disorder also have other mental disorders or conditions such as anxiety disorders, attention deficit hyperactivity disorder (ADHD), misuse of drugs or alcohol, or eating disorders. Sometimes, people who have severe manic or depressive episodes also have symptoms of psychosis, which may include hallucinations or delusions. The psychotic symptoms tend to match the person's extreme mood. For example, someone having psychotic symptoms during a depressive episode may falsely believe they are financially ruined, while someone having psychotic symptoms during a manic episode may falsely believe they are famous or have special powers.

Looking at a person's symptoms over the course of the illness and examining their family history can help a health-care provider determine whether the person has bipolar disorder along with another disorder.

TREATMENTS AND THERAPIES FOR BIPOLAR DISORDER

Treatment can help many people, including those with the most severe forms of bipolar disorder. An effective treatment plan usually includes a combination of medication and psychotherapy, also called "talk therapy."

Bipolar disorder is a lifelong illness. Episodes of mania and depression typically come back over time. Between episodes, many people with bipolar disorder are free of mood changes, but some people may have lingering symptoms. Long-term, continuous treatment can help people manage these symptoms.

Medications

Certain medications can help manage symptoms of bipolar disorder. Some people may need to try different medications and work with their health-care provider to find the medications that work best.

The most common types of medications that health-care providers prescribe include mood stabilizers and atypical antipsychotics. Mood stabilizers such as lithium or valproate can help prevent mood episodes or reduce their severity. Lithium can also decrease the risk of suicide. Health-care providers may include medications that target sleep or anxiety as part of the treatment plan.

Although bipolar depression is often treated with antidepressant medication, a mood stabilizer must be taken as well—taking an antidepressant without a mood stabilizer can trigger a manic episode or rapid cycling in a person with bipolar disorder.

Bipolar Disorder (Manic-Depressive Illness)

Because people with bipolar disorder are more likely to seek help when they are depressed than when they are experiencing mania or hypomania, it is important for health-care providers to take a careful medical history to ensure that bipolar disorder is not mistaken for depression.

People taking medication should do the following:
- Talk with their health-care provider to understand the risks and benefits of the medication.
- Tell their health-care provider about any prescription drugs, over-the-counter (OTC) medications, or supplements they are already taking.
- Report any concerns about side effects to a health-care provider right away. The health-care provider may need to change the dose or try a different medication.
- Remember that medication for bipolar disorder must be taken consistently, as prescribed, even when one is feeling well.

It is important to talk to a health-care provider before stopping a prescribed medication. Stopping a medication suddenly may lead symptoms to worsen or come back.

Psychotherapy

Psychotherapy, also called "talk therapy," can be an effective part of treatment for people with bipolar disorder. Psychotherapy is a term for treatment techniques that aim to help people identify and change troubling emotions, thoughts, and behaviors. This type of therapy can provide support, education, and guidance to people with bipolar disorder and their families.

Cognitive-behavioral therapy (CBT) is an important treatment for depression, and CBT adapted for the treatment of insomnia can be especially helpful as part of treatment for bipolar depression.

Treatment may also include newer therapies designed specifically for the treatment of bipolar disorder, including interpersonal and social rhythm therapy (IPSRT) and family-focused therapy.

Other Treatment Options
Some people may find other treatments helpful in managing their bipolar symptoms:
- Electroconvulsive therapy (ECT) is a brain stimulation procedure that can help relieve severe symptoms of bipolar disorder. Health-care providers may consider ECT when a person's illness has not improved after other treatments or in cases that require rapid response, such as with people who have a high suicide risk or catatonia (a state of unresponsiveness).
- Repetitive transcranial magnetic stimulation (rTMS) is a type of brain stimulation that uses magnetic waves to relieve depression over a series of treatment sessions. Although not as powerful as ECT, rTMS does not require general anesthesia and has a low risk of negative effects on memory and thinking.
- Light therapy is the best evidence-based treatment for seasonal affective disorder (SAD), and many people with bipolar disorder experience seasonal worsening of depression or SAD in the winter. Light therapy may also be used to treat lesser forms of seasonal worsening of bipolar depression.

Unlike specific psychotherapy and medication treatments that are scientifically proven to improve bipolar disorder symptoms, complementary health approaches for bipolar disorder, such as natural products, are not based on current knowledge or evidence.

COPING WITH BIPOLAR DISORDER
Living with bipolar disorder can be challenging, but there are ways to help make it easier.
- Work with a health-care provider to develop a treatment plan and stick with it. Treatment is the best way to start feeling better.
- Follow the treatment plan as directed. Work with a health-care provider to adjust the plan as needed.

Bipolar Disorder (Manic-Depressive Illness)

- Structure your activities. Try to have a routine for eating, sleeping, and exercising.
- Try regular, vigorous exercises such as jogging, swimming, or bicycling, which can help with depression and anxiety, promote better sleep, and support your heart and brain health.
- Track your moods, activities, and overall health and well-being to help recognize your mood swings.
- Ask trusted friends and family members for help in keeping up with your treatment plan.
- Be patient. Improvement takes time. Staying connected with sources of social support can help.

Long-term, ongoing treatment can help control symptoms and enable you to live a healthy life.[1]

---

[1] "Bipolar Disorder," National Institute of Mental Health (NIMH), February 2023. Available online. URL: www.nimh.nih.gov/health/topics/bipolar-disorder. Accessed March 9, 2023.

Chapter 8 | Disruptive Mood Dysregulation Disorder

Disruptive mood dysregulation disorder (DMDD) is a condition in which children or adolescents experience persistent irritability, anger, and frequent, intense temper outbursts. Many children go through periods of moodiness, but children with DMDD experience severe symptoms and often have significant problems at home and school. They may also struggle to interact with peers. While there is no treatment specifically for DMDD, researchers are working to improve existing treatment options and identify possible new treatments.

SIGNS AND SYMPTOMS OF DISRUPTIVE MOOD DYSREGULATION DISORDER

Children and adolescents with DMDD experience:
- severe temper outbursts (verbal or behavioral), on average, three or more times per week
- outbursts and tantrums that have been ongoing for at least 12 months
- chronically irritable or angry mood most of the day, nearly every day
- trouble functioning due to irritability in more than one setting, such as at home, at school, or with peers

Youth with DMDD are typically diagnosed between the ages of 6 and 10. To be diagnosed with DMDD, a child must have experienced symptoms steadily for 12 or more months.

Depression Sourcebook, Sixth Edition

RISK FACTORS FOR DISRUPTIVE MOOD DYSREGULATION DISORDER

It is not clear how widespread DMDD is in the general population, and the exact causes of DMDD are not clear. Researchers are exploring risk factors and brain mechanisms of this disorder.

TREATMENT AND THERAPIES FOR DISRUPTIVE MOOD DYSREGULATION DISORDER

Relatively few DMDD-specific treatment studies have been conducted to date. Treatment is often based on what has been helpful for other disorders associated with irritability, such as attention deficit hyperactivity disorder (ADHD), oppositional defiant disorder (ODD), and anxiety disorders.

Treatment for DMDD generally includes certain types of psychotherapy (also called "talk therapy") and sometimes medications. In many cases, psychotherapy is considered first, with medication added later if needed. However, in some cases, providers recommend that children receive both psychotherapy and medication at the start of their treatment. Parents or caregivers should work closely with their child's health-care provider to make treatment decisions that are best for their child.

Psychotherapies

Cognitive-behavioral therapy (CBT) targets the relationship between thoughts, behaviors, and feelings and is often effective in treating anger and disruptive behavior. CBT for anger and disruptive behavior focuses on changing maladaptive thoughts. Researchers are also using CBT to help children increase their ability to tolerate frustration without having an outburst. This therapy teaches coping skills for controlling anger and ways to identify and relabel the distorted perceptions that contribute to outbursts.

Dialectical behavior therapy for children (DBT-C) teaches children skills that may help them regulate their emotions and avoid extreme or prolonged outbursts. In DBT-C, the clinician helps children learn skills that can help with regulating their moods and emotions.

Parent training teaches parents or caregivers more effective ways to respond to irritable behavior, such as anticipating events that might

Disruptive Mood Dysregulation Disorder

lead a child to have a temper outburst and working ahead to avert it. Training also focuses on the importance of predictable and consistent responses to a child's outbursts and rewards for positive behavior.

Medications

Currently, no medications are approved by the U.S. Food and Drug Administration (FDA) specifically for treating children or adolescents with DMDD. However, health-care providers may prescribe certain medications—such as stimulants, antidepressants, and atypical antipsychotics—to help relieve a child's DMDD symptoms.

- Stimulants are often used to treat ADHD, and research suggests that stimulant medications may also decrease irritability in youth.
- Antidepressants are sometimes used to treat irritability and mood problems children with DMDD may experience. One study suggests that the antidepressant citalopram, combined with the stimulant methylphenidate, can decrease irritability in youth with DMDD. It is to be noted that antidepressants may increase suicidal thoughts and behaviors in youth, who should be monitored closely by their health-care provider.
- Certain atypical antipsychotic medications are used to treat children with irritability, severe outbursts, or aggression. The FDA has approved these medications for the treatment of irritability associated with autism, and they are sometimes used to treat DMDD, too. However, due to the side effects associated with these medications, they are often used only when other approaches have not been successful.

All medications have side effects. Monitor and report your child's side effects and review the medications frequently with your child's health-care provider.[1]

---

[1] "Disruptive Mood Dysregulation Disorder," National Institute of Mental Health (NIMH), January 2023. Available online. URL: www.nimh.nih.gov/health/topics/disruptive-mood-dysregulation-disorder-dmdd/disruptive-mood-dysregulation-disorder. Accessed March 2, 2023.

Chapter 9 | Persistent Depressive Disorder (Dysthymic Disorder)

WHAT IS PERSISTENT DEPRESSIVE DISORDER?
Persistent depressive disorder (PDD) is a less severe form of major depressive disorder (MDD) and usually lasts longer than MDD. It is also called "dysthymic disorder" or "dysthymia." People with PDD are usually gloomy all day and find it difficult to enjoy life. Most people with PDD may experience MDD as a co-occurring condition. Some may also have MDD prior to the onset of PDD.

CAUSES AND RISK FACTORS OF PERSISTENT DEPRESSIVE DISORDER
Anyone can experience PDD at any age. It is still unclear what causes PDD. As with other types of depression, PDD risk may be elevated by certain factors, including the following:
- **Brain chemical imbalance.** Serotonin is a neurotransmitter that regulates feelings and emotions in the brain. It is a natural mood booster. Low levels of serotonin can cause PDD.
- **Adverse life events and trauma.** Chronic stress and traumatic life events such as job loss, problems with relationships, and the death of a loved one can all trigger PDD.
- **Family history.** People with close family members with PDD are at increased risk of developing this condition. Hormonal changes during or after pregnancy may

trigger PDD symptoms in genetically predisposed people.

In addition to the above factors, having a medical history of chronic illnesses or other mental health disorders can also increase the likelihood of developing PDD.

SYMPTOMS OF PERSISTENT DEPRESSIVE DISORDER

Persistent depressive disorder is a mild and long-lasting form of MDD. So they have many symptoms overlapping with clinical depression. The symptoms include:
- feeling depressed for most of the day
- feeling worthless and isolated
- losing interest in day-to-day activities
- problems falling and staying asleep
- inability to concentrate and make decisions

COMPLICATIONS OF PERSISTENT DEPRESSIVE DISORDER

Sometimes, people with PDD also develop MDD, and when these two types of depression overlap, it causes double depression, a severe form of depression that combines the chronicity of PDD and the severity of MDD. Although double depression is a poorly studied phenomenon, experts say that the same factors that raise the risk of PDD or MDD appear to be involved in this too. Experts also believe that people with double depression are at a higher risk for heart disease, suicide, and other adverse health impacts of mental disorders than those with other types of depression.

DIAGNOSIS OF PERSISTENT DEPRESSIVE DISORDER

There are no direct tests for PDD. The most important component of diagnosis is a psychological evaluation. If you think you have PDD, it is important to talk to your primary health-care provider. Your primary care provider will perform a physical examination and also order laboratory tests to eliminate other medical conditions with similar symptoms. You will be referred to a mental

Persistent Depressive Disorder (Dysthymic Disorder)

health professional for further assessment and treatment based on the test results.

TREATMENT FOR PERSISTENT DEPRESSIVE DISORDER
Medications, talk therapy, and counseling are the most commonly used treatment approaches for PDD:
- **Medications**. PDDs are treated with antidepressant medications such as selective serotonin reuptake inhibitors (SSRIs), tricyclic antidepressants (TCAs), and serotonin norepinephrine reuptake inhibitors (SNRIs). These medications may need to be taken for several weeks as prescribed by the health-care provider.
- **Talk therapy**. Psychotherapy or talk therapy is a powerful treatment that involves one-on-one or group sessions with the therapist. The therapist helps the patients reflect on their thoughts and actions, learn new problem-solving techniques, and stick to their treatment plan.
- **Counseling**. This type of treatment is usually offered by a psychologist or licensed therapist who is experienced in treating mental health disorders. They help patients with PDD manage their stress and maintain a healthy lifestyle.

The treatment regimen for PDD usually combines medication, psychotherapy, and counseling.

LIVING WITH PERSISTENT DEPRESSIVE DISORDER
Embracing a healthy lifestyle increases the chances of the medication or therapy being effective and helps you feel better. Some of the lifestyle changes that help people in coping with PDD symptoms include the following:
- **Eating healthy**. Research has shown that a nutritious diet comprising fruit, veggies, whole grain, nuts, seeds, and lean protein (such as Greek yogurt and fish) can significantly improve physical health and emotional well-being.

- **Reducing alcohol consumption.** Excessive drinking can worsen existing mental health disorders. Cutting down on alcohol improves your mood, increases your energy, and helps you stay focused.
- **Exercising regularly.** Physical activity increases endorphin levels in the body, which helps in mood upliftment and reducing stress.
- **Improving the quality of sleep.** Getting proper sleep is vital for the brain to regulate our emotions. Practice a regular bedtime routine, follow proper screen time, and avoid using caffeine and alcohol just before hitting the bed.
- **Spending time on favorite activities.** This includes watching your favorite television program, reading books, trying new recipes, painting, and so on. Spending quality time with family and friends helps strengthen relationships.
- **Practicing mindfulness and meditation.** Both mindfulness and meditation techniques help relax your mind and relieve stress. This helps in boosting mental health and quality of life.

References

"An Overview of Persistent Depressive Disorder (Dysthymia)," Verywell Mind, May 23, 2022. Available online. URL: www.verywellmind.com/what-is-dysthymia-dysthymic-disorder-1066954#toc-coping-with-persistent-depressive-disorder-dysthymia. Accessed May 5, 2023.

"How Does It Feel to Live with Persistent Depressive Disorder (Dysthymia)?" *Psych Central,* April 6, 2022. Available online. URL: https://psychcentral.com/depression/depression-and-dysthymia-what-it-feels-like. Accessed May 5, 2023.

"Persistent Depressive Disorder (PDD)," Cleveland Clinic, March 8, 2021. Available online. URL: https://my.clevelandclinic.org/health/diseases/9292-persistent-depressive-disorder-pdd. Accessed May 5, 2023.

Persistent Depressive Disorder (Dysthymic Disorder)

"Persistent Depressive Disorder (PDD)," Healthline, October 21, 2021. Available online. URL: www.healthline.com/health/dysthymia#outlook. Accessed May 5, 2023.

"Persistent Depressive Disorder (PDD)," Mayo Clinic, December 2, 2022. Available online. URL: www.mayoclinic.org/diseases-conditions/persistentdepressive-disorder/symptoms-causes/syc-20350929. Accessed May 5, 2023.

Chapter 10 | **Psychotic Depression**

WHAT IS PSYCHOTIC DEPRESSION?
Psychotic depression is a form of depression with psychosis, such as delusions (false beliefs) and/or hallucinations (hearing or seeing things that are not there).[1]

WHAT IS PSYCHOSIS?
The word psychosis is used to describe conditions that affect the mind, where there has been some loss of contact with reality. When someone becomes ill in this way, it is called a "psychotic episode." During a period of psychosis, a person's thoughts and perceptions are disturbed, and the individual may have difficulty understanding what is real and what is not.

Who Develops Psychosis?
Psychosis can affect people from all walks of life. Psychosis often begins when a person is in his or her late teens to mid-20s. There are about 100,000 new cases of psychosis each year in the United States.

---

[1] "Living Well with Major Depressive Disorder," Substance Abuse and Mental Health Services Administration (SAMHSA), September 27, 2022. Available online. URL: www.samhsa.gov/serious-mental-illness/major-depression. Accessed March 27, 2023.

What Are the Signs and Symptoms of Psychosis?

Typically, a person will show changes in his or her behavior before psychosis develops. Behavioral warning signs for psychosis include the following:

- a sudden drop in grades or job performance
- trouble thinking clearly or concentrating
- suspiciousness, paranoid ideas, or uneasiness with others
- withdrawing socially, spending a lot more time alone than usual
- unusual, overly intense new ideas, strange feelings, or no feelings at all
- decline in self-care or personal hygiene
- difficulty telling reality from fantasy
- confused speech or trouble communicating

Symptoms of psychosis include delusions (false beliefs) and hallucinations (seeing or hearing things that others do not see or hear). Other symptoms include incoherent or nonsense speech and behavior that is inappropriate for the situation. A person in a psychotic episode may also experience depression, anxiety, sleep problems, social withdrawal, lack of motivation, and difficulty functioning overall.

Someone experiencing any of the symptoms on this list should consult a mental health professional.

What Causes Psychosis?

There is no one specific cause of psychosis. Psychosis may be a symptom of a mental illness, such as schizophrenia or bipolar disorder. However, a person may experience psychosis and never be diagnosed with schizophrenia or any other mental disorder. There are other causes, such as sleep deprivation, general medical conditions, certain prescription medications, and the misuse of alcohol or other drugs, such as marijuana. A mental illness, such as schizophrenia, is typically diagnosed by excluding all of these other causes of psychosis. To receive a thorough assessment and accurate diagnosis, visit a qualified health-care professional (such as a psychologist, psychiatrist, or social worker).

How Is Psychosis Treated?

Studies have shown that it is common for a person to have psychotic symptoms for more than a year before receiving treatment. Reducing this duration of untreated psychosis is critical because early treatment often means a better recovery. A qualified psychologist, psychiatrist, or social worker will be able to make a diagnosis and help develop a treatment plan.

People with psychosis may behave in confusing and unpredictable ways and may become threatening or violent. However, people with psychotic symptoms are more likely to harm themselves than someone else. If you notice these changes in behavior and they begin to intensify or do not go away, it is important to seek help.

Research supports a variety of treatments for early psychosis, especially coordinated specialty care. In 2008, the National Institute of Mental Health (NIMH) launched the research initiative, Recovery After an Initial Schizophrenia Episode (RAISE) project. RAISE studied coordinated specialty care treatments and the best ways to intervene after people begin to experience psychotic symptoms and to help them return to a path toward productive, independent lives. Coordinated specialty care involves the following components:

- Individual or group psychotherapy is typically based on principles of cognitive-behavioral therapy. This therapy is tailored to each patient's needs and emphasizes resilience training, illness and wellness management, and building coping skills.
- Family support and education teach family members about psychosis, coping, communication, and problem-solving skills. Family members who are informed and involved are more prepared to help loved ones through the recovery process.
- Medication management (also called "pharmacotherapy") helps reduce psychosis symptoms.

Medication selection and dosing are tailored to patients with early psychosis and their individual needs. Like all medications, antipsychotic drugs have risks and benefits. Patients should talk with their health-care providers about side effects, medication costs, and dosage preferences (daily pill or monthly injection).
- Supported employment and education services help patients return to work or school and achieve their personal goals. Emphasis is on rapid placement in a work or school setting, combined with coaching and support, to ensure success.
- Case management helps patients with problem-solving. The case manager may offer solutions to address practical problems and coordinate social services across multiple areas of need.

Individuals with psychosis should be involved in their treatment planning. Their needs and goals should drive their treatment programs, which will help them stay engaged throughout the recovery process.

It is important to find a mental health professional who is trained in psychosis treatment and who makes the patient feel comfortable.[2]

---

[2] "Understanding Psychosis," National Institute of Mental Health (NIMH), December 22, 2016. Available online. URL: www.nimh.nih.gov/health/publications/understanding-psychosis. Accessed March 27, 2023.

Chapter 11 | Seasonal Affective Disorder

WHAT IS SEASONAL AFFECTIVE DISORDER?
Many people go through short periods of time where they feel sad or not like their usual selves. Sometimes, these mood changes begin and end when the seasons change. People may start to feel "down" when the days get shorter in the fall and winter (also known as "winter blues") and begin to feel better in the spring, with longer daylight hours.

In some cases, these mood changes are more serious and can affect how a person feels, thinks, and handles daily activities. If you have noticed significant changes in your mood and behavior whenever the seasons change, you may be suffering from seasonal affective disorder (SAD), a type of depression.

In most cases, SAD symptoms start in the late fall or early winter and go away during the spring and summer; this is known as "winter-pattern SAD" or "winter depression." Some people may experience depressive episodes during the spring and summer months; this is known as "summer-pattern SAD" or "summer depression" and is less common.

WHAT ARE THE SIGNS AND SYMPTOMS OF SEASONAL AFFECTIVE DISORDER?
Seasonal affective disorder is not considered a separate disorder but is a type of depression characterized by its recurrent seasonal pattern, with symptoms lasting about four to five months per year. Therefore, the signs and symptoms of SAD include those associated with major depression and some specific symptoms that differ for

winter- and summer-pattern SAD. Not every person with SAD will experience all of the symptoms listed below.

Symptoms of major depression may include:
- feeling depressed most of the day, nearly every day
- losing interest in activities you once enjoyed
- experiencing changes in appetite or weight
- having problems with sleep
- feeling sluggish or agitated
- having low energy
- feeling hopeless or worthless
- having difficulty concentrating
- having frequent thoughts of death or suicide

For winter-pattern SAD, additional specific symptoms may include:
- oversleeping (hypersomnia)
- overeating, particularly with a craving for carbohydrates
- weight gain
- social withdrawal (feeling such as "hibernating")

Specific symptoms for summer-pattern SAD may include:
- trouble sleeping (insomnia)
- poor appetite, leading to weight loss
- restlessness and agitation
- anxiety
- episodes of violent behavior

WHO DEVELOPS SEASONAL AFFECTIVE DISORDER?

Millions of American adults may suffer from SAD although many may not know they have the condition. SAD occurs much more often in women than in men, and it is more common in those living farther north, where there are shorter daylight hours in the winter. For example, people living in Alaska or New England may be more likely to develop SAD than people living in Florida. In most cases, SAD begins in young adulthood.

Seasonal Affective Disorder

SAD is more common in people with major depressive disorder or bipolar disorder, especially bipolar II disorder, which is associated with recurrent depressive and hypomanic episodes (less severe than the full-blown manic episodes typical of bipolar I disorder). Additionally, people with SAD tend to have other mental disorders, such as attention deficit hyperactivity disorder (ADHD), an eating disorder, an anxiety disorder, or a panic disorder.

SAD sometimes runs in families. SAD is more common in people who have relatives with other mental illnesses, such as major depression or schizophrenia.

WHAT CAUSES SEASONAL AFFECTIVE DISORDER?

Scientists do not fully understand what causes SAD. Research indicates that people with SAD may have reduced activity of the brain chemical (neurotransmitter) serotonin, which helps regulate mood. Research also suggests that sunlight controls the levels of molecules that help maintain normal serotonin levels, but in people with SAD, this regulation does not function properly, resulting in decreased serotonin levels in the winter.

Other findings suggest that people with SAD produce too much melatonin—a hormone that is central to maintaining the normal sleep–wake cycle. Overproduction of melatonin can increase sleepiness.

Both serotonin and melatonin help maintain the body's daily rhythm that is tied to the seasonal night–day cycle. In people with SAD, the changes in serotonin and melatonin levels disrupt the normal daily rhythms. As a result, they can no longer adjust to the seasonal changes in day length, leading to sleep, mood, and behavior changes.

Deficits in vitamin D may exacerbate these problems because vitamin D is believed to promote serotonin activity. In addition to vitamin D consumed with diet, the body produces vitamin D when exposed to sunlight on the skin. With less daylight in the winter, people with SAD may have lower vitamin D levels, which may further hinder serotonin activity.

Negative thoughts and feelings about the winter and its associated limitations and stresses are common among people with

SAD (as well as others). It is unclear whether these are "causes" or "effects" of the mood disorder, but they can be a useful focus of treatment.

HOW IS SEASONAL AFFECTIVE DISORDER DIAGNOSED?

If you think you may be suffering from SAD, talk to your healthcare provider or a mental health specialist about your concerns. They may have you fill out specific questionnaires to determine if your symptoms meet the criteria for SAD.

To be diagnosed with SAD, a person must meet the following criteria:
- They must have symptoms of major depression or the more specific symptoms listed above.
- The depressive episodes must occur during specific seasons (i.e., only during the winter months or the summer months) for at least two consecutive years. However, not all people with SAD experience symptoms every year.
- The episodes must be much more frequent than other depressive episodes that the person may have had at other times of the year during their lifetime.

HOW IS SEASONAL AFFECTIVE DISORDER TREATED?

Treatments are available that can help many people with SAD. They fall into four main categories that may be used alone or in combination:
- light therapy
- psychotherapy
- antidepressant medications
- vitamin D

CAN SEASONAL AFFECTIVE DISORDER BE PREVENTED?

Because the timing of the onset of winter-pattern SAD is so predictable, people with a history of SAD might benefit from starting the treatments mentioned above before the fall to help prevent or

Seasonal Affective Disorder

reduce depression. To date, very few studies have investigated this question, and existing studies have found no convincing evidence that starting light therapy or psychotherapy ahead of time could prevent the onset of depression. Only preventive treatment with the antidepressant bupropion prevented SAD in study participants, but it also had a higher risk of side effects. Therefore, people with SAD should discuss with their health-care providers if they want to initiate treatment early to prevent depressive episodes.[1]

---

[1] "Seasonal Affective Disorder," National Institute of Mental Health (NIMH), March 29, 2016. Available online. URL: www.nimh.nih.gov/health/publications/seasonal-affective-disorder. Accessed March 2, 2023.

Part 3 | Who Develops Depression?

Chapter 12 | Women and Depression

Women are twice as likely as men to be diagnosed with depression. It is more than twice as common for African American, Hispanic, and White women to have depression compared to Asian American women. Depression is also more common in women whose families live below the federal poverty line.

WHAT CAUSES DEPRESSION IN WOMEN?
There is no single cause of depression. Also, different types of depression may have different causes. There are many reasons why a woman may have depression:
- **Family history**. Women with a family history of depression may be more at risk. But depression can also happen in women who do not have a family history of depression.
- **Brain changes**. The brains of people with depression look and function differently from those of people who do not have depression.
- **Chemistry**. In someone who has depression, parts of the brain that manage mood, thoughts, sleep, appetite, and behavior may not have the right balance of chemicals.
- **Hormone levels**. Changes in the female hormones estrogen and progesterone during the menstrual cycle, pregnancy, postpartum period, perimenopause, or menopause may all raise a woman's risk for depression.

Having a miscarriage can also put a woman at a higher risk for depression.
- **Stress.** Serious and stressful life events, or the combination of several stressful events, such as trauma, the loss of a loved one, a bad relationship, work responsibilities, caring for children and aging parents, abuse, and poverty, may trigger depression in some people.
- **Medical problems.** Dealing with a serious health problem, such as stroke, heart attack, or cancer, can lead to depression. Research shows that people who have a serious illness and depression are more likely to have more serious types of both conditions. Some medical illnesses, such as Parkinson disease (PD), hypothyroidism, and stroke, can cause changes in the brain that can trigger depression.
- **Pain.** Women who feel emotional or physical pain for long periods are much more likely to develop depression. The pain can come from a chronic (long-term) health problem, accident, or trauma such as sexual assault or abuse.

WHAT ARE THE SYMPTOMS OF DEPRESSION IN WOMEN?

Not all people with depression have the same symptoms. Some people might have only a few symptoms, while others may have many. How often symptoms happen, how long they last, and how severe they are may be different for each person.

If you have any of the following symptoms for at least two weeks, talk to a doctor, nurse, or mental health professional:
- feeling sad, "down," or empty, including crying often
- feeling hopeless, helpless, worthless, or useless
- loss of interest in hobbies and activities that you once enjoyed
- decreased energy
- difficulty staying focused, remembering, or making decisions
- sleeplessness, early morning awakening, or oversleeping and not wanting to get up

- lack of appetite, leading to weight loss, or eating to feel better, leading to weight gain
- thoughts of hurting yourself
- thoughts of death or suicide
- feeling easily annoyed, bothered, or angered
- constant physical symptoms that do not get better with treatment, such as headaches, upset stomach, and pain that does not go away[1]

WHAT ARE THE DIFFERENT TYPES OF DEPRESSION IN WOMEN?

Pregnancy, the postpartum period, perimenopause, and the menstrual cycle are all associated with dramatic physical and hormonal changes. Certain types of depression can occur at different stages of a woman's life.

Premenstrual Dysphoric Disorder

Premenstrual syndrome (PMS) refers to "moodiness and irritability" in the weeks before menstruation. It is quite common, and the symptoms are usually mild. But there is a less common, more severe form of PMS called "premenstrual dysphoric disorder" (PMDD). PMDD is a serious condition with disabling symptoms such as irritability, anger, depressed mood, sadness, suicidal thoughts, appetite changes, bloating, breast tenderness, and joint or muscle pain.

Perinatal Depression

Being pregnant is not easy. Pregnant women commonly deal with morning sickness, weight gain, and mood swings. Caring for a newborn is challenging, too. Many new moms experience the "baby blues"—a term used to describe mild mood changes and feelings of worry, unhappiness, and exhaustion that many women sometimes experience in the first two weeks after having a baby. These feelings usually last a week or two and then go away as a new mom adjusts to having a newborn.

---

[1] Office on Women's Health (OWH), "Depression," U.S. Department of Health and Human Services (HHS), February 17, 2021. Available online. URL: www.womenshealth.gov/mental-health/mental-health-conditions/depression. Accessed March 10, 2023.

Perinatal depression is a mood disorder that can affect women during pregnancy and after childbirth and is much more serious than the "baby blues." The word "perinatal" refers to the time before and after the birth of a child. Perinatal depression includes depression that begins during pregnancy (called "prenatal depression") and depression that begins after the baby is born (called "postpartum depression"). Mothers with perinatal depression experience feelings of extreme sadness, anxiety, and fatigue that may make it difficult for them to carry out daily tasks, including caring for themselves, their new child, or others.

If you think you have perinatal depression, you should talk to your health-care provider or trained mental health-care professional. If you see any signs of depression in a loved one during her pregnancy or after the child is born, encourage her to see a health-care provider or visit a clinic.

Perimenopausal Depression

Perimenopause (the transition into menopause) is a normal phase in a woman's life that can sometimes be challenging. If you are going through perimenopause, you might be experiencing abnormal periods, problems sleeping, mood swings, and hot flashes. Although these symptoms are common, feeling depressed is not. If you are struggling with irritability, anxiety, sadness, or loss of enjoyment at the time of the menopause transition, you may be experiencing perimenopausal depression.

Depression Affects Each Woman Differently

Not every woman who is depressed experiences every symptom. Some women experience only a few symptoms. Others have many. The severity and frequency of symptoms, and how long they last, will vary depending on the individual and the severity of the illness.[2]

---

[2] Office on Women's Health (OWH), "Depression in Women: 5 Things You Should Know," U.S. Department of Health and Human Services (HHS), 2020. Available online. URL: www.nimh.nih.gov/health/publications/depression-in-women. Accessed March 10, 2023.

HOW IS DEPRESSION LINKED TO OTHER HEALTH PROBLEMS IN WOMEN?

Depression is linked to many health problems in women, including the following:

- **Heart disease.** People with heart disease are about twice as likely to have depression as people who do not have heart disease.
- **Obesity.** Studies show that 43 percent of adults with depression have obesity. Women, especially White women, with depression are more likely to have obesity than women without depression. Women with depression are also more likely than men with depression to have obesity.
- **Cancer.** Up to one in four people with cancer may also experience depression. More women with cancer than men with cancer experience depression.

HOW IS DEPRESSION DIAGNOSED IN WOMEN?

Talk to your doctor or nurse if you have symptoms of depression. Certain medicines and some health problems (such as viruses or a thyroid disorder) can cause the same symptoms as depression. Sometimes, depression can be part of another mental health condition.

Diagnosis of depression includes a mental health professional asking questions about your life, emotions, struggles, and symptoms. The doctor, nurse, or mental health professional may order lab tests on a sample of your blood or urine and do a regular checkup to rule out other problems that could be causing your symptoms.

HOW IS DEPRESSION TREATED IN WOMEN?

Your doctor or mental health professional may treat depression with therapy, medicine, or a combination of the two. Your doctor or nurse may refer you to a mental health specialist for therapy.

Some people with milder forms of depression get better after a few months of therapy. People with moderate-to-severe depression might need therapy and a type of medicine called an "antidepressant." Antidepressants change the levels of certain chemicals in your brain. It may take several weeks for antidepressants to work. There are different types of antidepressant medicines, and some work better than others for certain people. Some people get better only with both treatments—therapy and antidepressants.

Having depression can make some people more likely to turn to drugs or alcohol to cope. But drugs or alcohol can make your mental health condition worse and can affect how antidepressants work. Talk to your therapist or doctor or nurse about any alcohol or drug use.

Does Exercise Help Treat Depression?

For some people, yes. Researchers think that exercise may work better than no treatment at all to treat depression. They also think that regular exercise can lower your risk of getting depression and help many depression symptoms get better. Researchers do not know whether exercise works as well as therapy or medicine to treat depression. People with depression often find it very difficult to exercise, even though they know it will help make them feel better. Walking is a good way to begin exercising if you have not exercised recently.

Are There Other Natural or Complementary Treatments for Depression?

Researchers are studying natural and complementary treatments (add-on treatments to medicine or therapy) for depression. Currently, none of the natural or complementary treatments are proven to work as well as medicine and therapy for depression. However, natural or complementary treatments that have little or no risk, such as exercise, meditation, or relaxation training, may help improve your depression symptoms and usually will not make them worse.

Will Treatment for Depression Affect My Chances of Getting Pregnant?

Maybe. Some medicines, such as some types of antidepressants, may make it more difficult for you to get pregnant, but more research is needed. Talk to your doctor about other treatments for depression that do not involve medicine if you are trying to get pregnant. For example, a type of talk therapy called "cognitive-behavioral therapy" (CBT) helps women with depression. This type of therapy has little to no risk for women trying to get pregnant. During CBT, you work with a mental health professional to explore why you are depressed and train yourself to replace negative thoughts with positive ones. Certain mental health-care professionals specialize in depression related to infertility.

Women who are already taking an antidepressant and who are trying to get pregnant should talk to their doctor or nurse about the risks and benefits of stopping the medicine.[3]

---

[3] See footnote [1].

Chapter 13 | Depression and Mental Health during Reproductive Transitions in Women

Chapter Contents
Section 13.1—Depression and Anxiety Associated with the Menstrual Cycle: Premenstrual Syndrome 75
Section 13.2—Premenstrual Dysphoric Disorder........................ 81
Section 13.3—Depression during Pregnancy: Risk Factors, Signs, and Symptoms 84
Section 13.4—Postpartum Depression... 86
Section 13.5—What Is the Link between Menopause and Depression? 96

Section 13.1 | Depression and Anxiety Associated with the Menstrual Cycle: Premenstrual Syndrome

WHAT IS PREMENSTRUAL SYNDROME?

Premenstrual syndrome (PMS) is a combination of physical and emotional symptoms that many women get after ovulation and before the start of their menstrual period. Researchers think that PMS happens in the days after ovulation because estrogen and progesterone levels begin falling dramatically if you are not pregnant. PMS symptoms go away within a few days after a woman's period starts as hormone levels begin rising again.

Some women get their periods without any signs of PMS or only very mild symptoms. For others, PMS symptoms may be so severe that it makes it hard to do everyday activities such as going to work or school. Severe PMS symptoms may be a sign of premenstrual dysphoric disorder (PMDD). PMS goes away when you no longer get a period, such as after menopause. After pregnancy, PMS might come back, but you might have different PMS symptoms.

WHO GETS PREMENSTRUAL SYNDROME?

As many as three in four women say they get PMS symptoms at some point in their lifetime. For most women, PMS symptoms are mild.

Less than 5 percent of women of childbearing age get a more severe form of PMS, called "PMDD." PMS may happen more often in women who:
- have high levels of stress
- have a family history of depression
- have a personal history of either postpartum depression or depression

DOES PREMENSTRUAL SYNDROME CHANGE WITH AGE?

Yes. PMS symptoms may get worse as you reach your late 30s or 40s and approach menopause and are in the transition to menopause, called "perimenopause."

This is especially true for women whose moods are sensitive to changing hormone levels during the menstrual cycle. In the years leading up to menopause, your hormone levels also go up and down in an unpredictable way as your body slowly transitions to menopause. You may get the same mood changes, or they may get worse.

PMS stops after menopause when you no longer get a period.

WHAT ARE THE SYMPTOMS OF PREMENSTRUAL SYNDROME?

Premenstrual syndrome symptoms are different for every woman. You may get physical symptoms, such as bloating or gassiness, or emotional symptoms, such as sadness, or both. Your symptoms may also change throughout your life.

Physical Symptoms
- swollen or tender breasts
- constipation or diarrhea
- bloating or a gassy feeling
- cramping
- headache or backache
- clumsiness
- lower tolerance for noise or light

Emotional or Mental Symptoms
- irritability or hostile behavior
- feeling tired
- sleep problems (sleeping too much or too little)
- appetite changes or food cravings
- trouble with concentration or memory
- tension or anxiety
- depression, feelings of sadness, or crying spells
- mood swings
- less interest in sex

Talk to your doctor or nurse if your symptoms bother you or affect your daily life.

WHAT CAUSES PREMENSTRUAL SYNDROME?
Researchers do not know exactly what causes PMS. Changes in hormone levels during the menstrual cycle may play a role. These changing hormone levels may affect some women more than others.

HOW IS PREMENSTRUAL SYNDROME DIAGNOSED?
There is no single test for PMS. Your doctor will talk with you about your symptoms, including when they happen and how much they affect your life.

You probably have PMS if you have symptoms that:
- happen in the five days before your period for at least three menstrual cycles in a row
- end within four days after your period starts
- keep you from enjoying or doing some of your normal activities

Keep track of which PMS symptoms you have and how severe they are for a few months. Write down your symptoms each day on a calendar or with an app on your phone. Take this information with you when you see your doctor.

HOW DOES PREMENSTRUAL SYNDROME AFFECT OTHER HEALTH PROBLEMS?
About half of women who need relief from PMS also have another health problem, which may get worse in the time before their menstrual period. These health problems share many symptoms with PMS and include the following.

Depression and Anxiety Disorders
These are the most common conditions that overlap with PMS. Depression and anxiety symptoms are similar to PMS and may get worse before or during your period.

Myalgic Encephalomyelitis/Chronic Fatigue Syndrome
Some women report that their symptoms often get worse right before their period. Research shows that women with myalgic

encephalomyelitis/chronic fatigue syndrome (ME/CFS) may also be more likely to have heavy menstrual bleeding and early or premature menopause.

Irritable Bowel Syndrome
Irritable bowel syndrome (IBS) causes cramping, bloating, and gas. Your IBS symptoms may get worse right before your period.

Bladder Pain Syndrome
Women with bladder pain syndrome (BPS) are more likely to have painful cramps during PMS.

PMS may also worsen some health problems, such as asthma, allergies, and migraines.

WHAT CAN YOU DO AT HOME TO RELIEVE PREMENSTRUAL SYNDROME SYMPTOMS?
These tips will help you be healthier in general and may relieve some of your PMS symptoms:
- **Get regular aerobic physical activity throughout the month.** Exercise can help with symptoms such as depression, difficulty concentrating, and fatigue.
- **Choose healthy foods most of the time.** Avoiding foods and drinks with caffeine, salt, and sugar in the two weeks before your period may lessen many PMS symptoms.
- **Get enough sleep.** Try to get about eight hours of sleep each night. Lack of sleep is linked to depression and anxiety and can make PMS symptoms such as moodiness worse.
- **Find healthy ways to cope with stress.** Talk to your friends or write in a journal. Some women also find yoga, massage, or meditation helpful.
- **Do not smoke.** In one large study, women who smoked reported more PMS symptoms and worse PMS symptoms than women who did not smoke.

WHAT MEDICINES CAN TREAT PREMENSTRUAL SYNDROME SYMPTOMS?

Over-the-counter (OTC) and prescription medicines can help treat some PMS symptoms.

You can buy OTC pain relievers in most stores that may help lessen physical symptoms, such as cramps, headaches, backaches, and breast tenderness. These include the following:
- ibuprofen
- naproxen
- aspirin

Some women find that taking an OTC pain reliever right before their period starts reduces the amount of pain and bleeding they have during their period. Prescription medicines may help if OTC pain medicines do not work.
- Hormonal birth control may help with the physical symptoms of PMS, but it may make other symptoms worse. You may need to try several different types of birth control before you find one that helps your symptoms.
- Antidepressants can help relieve the emotional symptoms of PMS for some women when other medicines do not help.

Selective serotonin reuptake inhibitors (SSRIs) are the most common type of antidepressant used to treat PMS.
- Diuretics (water pills) may reduce symptoms of bloating and breast tenderness.
- Antianxiety medicine may help reduce feelings of anxiousness.

All medicines have risks. Talk to your doctor or nurse about the benefits and risks.

SHOULD YOU TAKE VITAMINS OR MINERALS TO TREAT PREMENSTRUAL SYNDROME SYMPTOMS?

Maybe. Studies show that certain vitamins and minerals may help relieve some PMS symptoms. The U.S. Food and Drug

Administration (FDA) does not regulate vitamins or minerals and herbal supplements in the same way they regulate medicines. Talk to your doctor before taking any supplements.

Studies have found benefits for the following:
- **Calcium.** Studies show that calcium can help reduce some PMS symptoms, such as fatigue, cravings, and depression. Calcium is found in foods such as milk, cheese, and yogurt. Some foods, such as orange juice, cereal, and bread, have calcium added (fortified). You can also take a calcium supplement.
- **Vitamin B$_6$.** It may help with PMS symptoms, including moodiness, irritability, forgetfulness, bloating, and anxiety. Vitamin B$_6$ can be found in foods such as fish, poultry, potatoes, fruit (except for citrus fruits), and fortified cereals. You can also take it as a dietary supplement.

Studies have found mixed results for the following:
- **Magnesium.** It may help relieve some PMS symptoms, including migraines. If you get menstrual migraines, talk to your doctor about whether you need more magnesium. Magnesium is found in green, leafy vegetables such as spinach, as well as in nuts, whole grains, and fortified cereals. You can also take a supplement.
- **Polyunsaturated fatty acids.** Studies show that taking a supplement with 1–2 grams of polyunsaturated fatty acids (omega-3 and omega-6) may help reduce cramps and other PMS symptoms. Good sources of polyunsaturated fatty acids include flaxseed, nuts, fish, and green leafy vegetables.

WHAT COMPLEMENTARY OR ALTERNATIVE MEDICINES MAY HELP RELIEVE PREMENSTRUAL SYNDROME SYMPTOMS?

Some women report relief from their PMS symptoms with yoga or meditation. Others say herbal supplements help relieve symptoms. Talk with your doctor or nurse before taking any of these supplements. They may interact with other medicines you take, making your other medicine not work or causing dangerous side effects. The FDA does not regulate herbal supplements at the same level that it regulates medicines.

Some research studies show relief from PMS symptoms with these herbal supplements, but other studies do not. Many herbal supplements should not be used with other medicines. Some herbal supplements women use to ease PMS symptoms include the following:

- **Black cohosh.** The underground stems and roots of black cohosh are used fresh or dried to make tea, capsules, pills, or liquid extracts. Black cohosh is most often used to help treat menopausal symptoms, and some women use it to help relieve PMS symptoms.
- **Chasteberry.** Dried ripe chasteberry is used to prepare liquid extracts or pills that some women take to relieve PMS symptoms. Women taking hormonal birth control or hormone therapy for menopausal symptoms should not take chasteberry.
- **Evening primrose oil.** The oil is taken from the plant's seeds and put into capsules. Some women report that the pill helps relieve PMS symptoms, but the research results are mixed.[1]

Section 13.2 | Premenstrual Dysphoric Disorder

WHAT IS PREMENSTRUAL DYSPHORIC DISORDER?

Premenstrual dysphoric disorder (PMDD) is a condition similar to premenstrual syndrome (PMS) that also happens a week or two before your period starts as hormone levels begin to fall after

---

[1] Office on Women's Health (OWH), "Premenstrual Syndrome (PMS)," U.S. Department of Health and Human Services (HHS), February 22, 2021. Available online. URL: www.womenshealth.gov/menstrual-cycle/premenstrual-syndrome. Accessed March 9, 2023.

ovulation. PMDD causes more severe symptoms than PMS, including severe depression, irritability, and tension.

WHO GETS PREMENSTRUAL DYSPHORIC DISORDER?
Premenstrual dysphoric disorder affects up to 5 percent of women of childbearing age. Many women with PMDD may also have anxiety or depression.

WHAT ARE THE SYMPTOMS OF PREMENSTRUAL DYSPHORIC DISORDER?
Symptoms of PMDD include the following:
- lasting irritability or anger that may affect other people
- feelings of sadness or despair or even thoughts of suicide
- feelings of tension or anxiety
- panic attacks
- mood swings or crying often
- lack of interest in daily activities and relationships
- trouble thinking or focusing
- tiredness or low energy
- food cravings or binge eating
- trouble sleeping
- feeling out of control
- physical symptoms, such as cramps, bloating, breast tenderness, headaches, and joint or muscle pain

WHAT CAUSES PREMENSTRUAL DYSPHORIC DISORDER?
Researchers do not know for sure what causes PMDD. Hormonal changes throughout the menstrual cycle may play a role. A brain chemical called "serotonin" may also play a role in PMDD. Serotonin levels change throughout the menstrual cycle. Some women may be more sensitive to these changes.

HOW IS PREMENSTRUAL DYSPHORIC DISORDER DIAGNOSED?
Your doctor will talk to you about your health history and do a physical examination. You will need to keep a calendar or diary of your symptoms to help your doctor diagnose PMDD.

You must have five or more PMDD symptoms, including one mood-related symptom, to be diagnosed with PMDD.

HOW IS PREMENSTRUAL DYSPHORIC DISORDER TREATED?
Treatments for PMDD include the following:
- **Antidepressants called "selective serotonin reuptake inhibitors" (SSRIs).** SSRIs change serotonin levels in the brain. The U.S. Food and Drug Administration (FDA) approved three SSRIs to treat PMDD:
  - sertraline
  - fluoxetine
  - paroxetine HCI
- **Birth control pills.** The FDA has approved a birth control pill containing drospirenone and ethinyl estradiol to treat PMDD.
- **Over-the-counter (OTC) pain relievers.** These medicines may help relieve physical symptoms, such as cramps, joint pain, headaches, backaches, and breast tenderness. These include the following:
  - ibuprofen
  - naproxen
  - aspirin
- **Stress management.** It involves relaxation techniques and spending time on activities you enjoy.

Making healthy changes, such as eating a healthy combination of foods across the food groups, cutting back on salty and sugary foods, and getting more physical activity, may also help relieve some PMDD symptoms. But PMDD can be serious enough that some women should go to a doctor or nurse to discuss treatment options. And, if you are thinking of hurting yourself or others, call 911 immediately.[2]

---

[2] Office on Women's Health (OWH), "Premenstrual Dysphoric Disorder (PMDD)," U.S. Department of Health and Human Services (HHS), February 22, 2021. Available online. URL: www.womenshealth.gov/menstrual-cycle/premenstrual-syndrome/premenstrual-dysphoric-disorder-pmdd. Accessed March 9, 2023.

Section 13.3 | Depression during Pregnancy: Risk Factors, Signs, and Symptoms

MENTAL HEALTH WHILE PLANNING A PREGNANCY

If you are considering or planning a pregnancy, it is a great time to take stock of your mental health. When planning a pregnancy, it is important to remember that improving your well-being and lowering your stress increase the likelihood of a healthy pregnancy and healthy baby. The sooner you can prevent or address any mental health challenges, the better outcome you are likely to have. It is never too soon or too late to take care of your mental health. In therapy, you may discover tools that will help you through other events and life stages, including the often-difficult postpartum phase (the first year after giving birth) and early parenthood.

If you are pregnant or planning a pregnancy, talk with your health-care provider about your mental health history and any symptoms you may be experiencing. Do not stop taking any prescribed medicines without first consulting your provider, as doing so could be harmful to you or your baby.

Are you planning a pregnancy and interested in improving your mental health? Complete the following checklist for preconception mental health planning.

Checklist for Preconception Mental Health Planning

- Are you sometimes anxious in a way you think is disproportionate to circumstances?
- Have you felt sad, down, or depressed?
- Do you wish you could handle anger differently?
- Have you experienced very stressful or traumatic situations in the past that still affect you?
- Do you sometimes use alcohol, cigarettes, cannabis, or other substances in an attempt to relax or cope?
- If you have a partner, do you want to improve the way you and your partner communicate or share household responsibilities?

Depression and Mental Health during Reproductive Transitions in Women

- Do you feel confident that you can manage most stress without feeling overwhelmed?
- If you have been diagnosed with a mental health condition, have you spoken with a mental health clinician about how the symptoms could affect pregnancy or how pregnancy could affect your condition?
- If you are taking medication for mental health, have you spoken with a doctor, nurse, or pharmacist about the pros and cons of continuing the medication while pregnant?

If you answered yes to any of questions one to six or no to any of questions seven to nine, consider speaking with your primary care provider or mental health clinician about treatment options for preconception mental health.[3]

MISCARRIAGE AND MENTAL HEALTH

A miscarriage is the loss of a pregnancy before 20 weeks. Grieving a loss after expecting to bring a life into the world can be especially difficult. Often, nothing else in a woman's experience has prepared her for this. Other people may not know how to be supportive, so it may be difficult to talk about this loss.

There is a wide range of emotional reactions to miscarriage. Many women feel as though the baby is still inside, dream about pregnancy or about the baby, and think about the baby a great deal. Some women become depressed or anxious. Some blame themselves for the miscarriage. Women with partners may find that miscarriage makes them feel closer to their partners or creates tension in the relationship.

While depression or anxiety is normal after a miscarriage, it can be distressing and make it difficult to function at times. If you have had a miscarriage and are experiencing these reactions, consider speaking with your primary care provider or mental health clinician about counseling and other treatment options.[4]

---

[3] "Mental Health While Planning a Pregnancy," U.S. Department of Veterans Affairs (VA), November 30, 2022. Available online. URL: www.mentalhealth.va.gov/women-vets/reproductive-mental-health/pregnancy-planning.asp. Accessed April 26, 2023.

[4] "Miscarriage and Mental Health," U.S. Department of Veterans Affairs (VA), November 30, 2022. Available online. URL: www.mentalhealth.va.gov/women-vets/reproductive-mental-health/miscarriage.asp. Accessed April 26, 2023.

ECTOPIC PREGNANCY AND MENTAL HEALTH

During an ectopic pregnancy, a fertilized egg implants itself somewhere outside the uterus, such as in a fallopian tube. A woman with an ectopic pregnancy may experience typical pregnancy symptoms at first, such as a missed period, breast tenderness, and nausea, along with having a positive pregnancy test. When it becomes clear that the pregnancy is ectopic, it is treated as a medical emergency. Because it is so unexpected and urgent, the process of diagnosis and treatment can be stressful and sometimes traumatic.

Individuals differ widely in their long-term reactions to ectopic pregnancy loss. Some women experience prolonged grief, anxiety, depression, posttraumatic symptoms, and suicidality. Others, especially if they have good support and counseling, can experience a deepened sense of meaning and spirituality. This can include, for example, living more in the moment and finding meaning in helping others.

If you have had an ectopic pregnancy and are feeling distressed, consider speaking with your primary care provider or mental health clinician about counseling and other treatment options.[5]

Section 13.4 | Postpartum Depression

WHAT IS POSTPARTUM DEPRESSION?

"Postpartum" means the time after childbirth. Most women get the "baby blues" or feel sad or empty within a few days of giving birth. For many women, the baby blues go away in three to five days. If your baby blues do not go away or you feel sad, hopeless, or empty for longer than two weeks, you may have postpartum depression. Feeling hopeless or empty after childbirth is not a regular or expected part of being a mother.

---

[5] "Ectopic Pregnancy and Mental Health," U.S. Department of Veterans Affairs (VA), November 30, 2022. Available online. URL: www.mentalhealth.va.gov/women-vets/reproductive-mental-health/ectopic-pregnancy.asp. Accessed April 26, 2023.

Postpartum depression is a serious mental illness that involves the brain and affects your behavior and physical health. If you have depression, then sad, flat, or empty feelings do not go away and can interfere with your day-to-day life. You might feel unconnected to your baby as if you are not the baby's mother, or you might not love or care for the baby. These feelings can be mild to severe.

How Common Is Postpartum Depression?

Depression is a common problem after pregnancy. One in nine new mothers has postpartum depression.

What Causes Postpartum Depression?

Hormonal changes may trigger symptoms of postpartum depression. When you are pregnant, levels of the female hormones estrogen and progesterone are the highest they will ever be. In the first 24 hours after childbirth, hormone levels quickly drop back to normal prepregnancy levels. Researchers think this sudden change in hormone levels may lead to depression. This is similar to hormone changes before a woman's period but involves much more extreme swings in hormone levels.

Levels of thyroid hormones may also drop after giving birth. The thyroid is a small gland in the neck that helps regulate how your body uses and stores energy from food. Low levels of thyroid hormones can cause symptoms of depression. A simple blood test can tell whether this condition is causing your symptoms. If so, your doctor can prescribe thyroid medicine.

Other feelings may contribute to postpartum depression. Many new mothers say they feel:
- tired after labor and delivery
- tired from a lack of sleep or broken sleep
- overwhelmed with a new baby
- doubts about their ability to be a good mother
- stress from changes in work and home routines
- an unrealistic need to be a perfect mom
- grief about the loss of who they were before having the baby

- less attractive
- a lack of free time

These feelings are common among new mothers. But postpartum depression is a serious health condition and can be treated. Postpartum depression is not a regular or expected part of being a new mother.

Are Some Women More at Risk of Postpartum Depression?

Yes. You may be more at risk of postpartum depression if you:
- have a personal history of depression or bipolar disorder
- have a family history of depression or bipolar disorder
- do not have support from family and friends
- were depressed during pregnancy
- had problems with a previous pregnancy or birth
- have relationship or money problems
- are younger than 20
- have alcohol, use illegal drugs, or have some other problem with drugs
- have a baby with special needs
- have difficulty breastfeeding
- had an unplanned or unwanted pregnancy

The U.S. Preventive Services Task Force (USPSTF) recommends that doctors look for and ask about symptoms of depression during and after pregnancy, regardless of a woman's risk of depression.

Symptoms of Postpartum Depression

Some normal changes after pregnancy can cause symptoms similar to those of depression. Many mothers feel overwhelmed when a new baby comes home. But if you have any of the following symptoms of depression for more than two weeks, call your doctor, nurse, or midwife:
- feeling restless or moody
- feeling sad, hopeless, or overwhelmed
- crying a lot

- having thoughts of hurting the baby
- having thoughts of hurting yourself
- not having any interest in the baby, not feeling connected to the baby, or feeling as if your baby is someone else's baby
- having no energy or motivation
- eating too little or too much
- sleeping too little or too much
- having trouble focusing or making decisions
- having memory problems
- feeling worthless, guilty, or like a bad mother
- losing interest or pleasure in activities you used to enjoy
- withdrawing from friends and family
- having headaches, aches and pains, or stomach problems that do not go away

Some women do not tell anyone about their symptoms. New mothers may feel embarrassed, ashamed, or guilty about feeling depressed when they are supposed to be happy. They may also worry they will be seen as bad mothers. Any woman can become depressed during pregnancy or after having a baby. It does not mean you are a bad mom. You and your baby do not have to suffer. There is help. Your doctor can help you figure out whether your symptoms are caused by depression or something else.

What Should You Do If You Have Symptoms of Postpartum Depression?

Call your doctor, nurse, midwife, or pediatrician if:
- your baby blues do not go away after two weeks
- symptoms of depression get more and more intense
- symptoms of depression begin within one year of delivery and last more than two weeks
- it is difficult to work or get things done at home
- you cannot care for yourself or your baby (e.g., eating, sleeping, bathing)
- you have thoughts about hurting yourself or your baby

Depression Sourcebook, Sixth Edition

Ask your partner or a loved one to call for you if necessary. Your doctor, nurse, or midwife can ask you questions to test for depression. They can also refer you to a mental health professional for help and treatment.

What Can You Do at Home to Feel Better while Seeing a Doctor for Postpartum Depression?

Here are some ways to begin feeling better or getting more rest, in addition to talking to a health-care professional:

- Rest as much as you can. Sleep when the baby is sleeping.
- Do not try to do too much or to do everything by yourself. Ask your partner, family, and friends for help.
- Make time to go out, visit friends, or spend time alone with your partner.
- Talk about your feelings with your partner, supportive family members, and friends.
- Talk with other mothers so that you can learn from their experiences. Join a support group. Ask your doctor or nurse about groups in your area.
- Do not make any major life changes right after giving birth. More major life changes in addition to a new baby can cause unneeded stress. Sometimes, big changes cannot be avoided. When that happens, try to arrange support and help in your new situation ahead of time.

Having a partner, a friend, or another caregiver who can help take care of the baby while you are depressed can also help. If you are feeling depressed during pregnancy or after having a baby, do not suffer alone. Tell a loved one and call your doctor right away.

How Is Postpartum Depression Treated?

The common types of treatment for postpartum depression are as follows:

- **Therapy.** During therapy, you talk to a therapist, psychologist, or social worker to learn strategies to change how depression makes you think, feel, and act.

- **Medicine.** There are different types of medicines for postpartum depression. All of them must be prescribed by your doctor or nurse. The most common type is antidepressants. Antidepressants can help relieve symptoms of depression, and some can be taken while you are breastfeeding. Antidepressants may take several weeks to start working.

  The U.S. Food and Drug Administration (FDA) has also approved a medicine called "brexanolone" to treat postpartum depression in adult women. Brexanolone is given by a doctor or nurse through an IV for two and a half days (60 hours). Because of the risk of side effects, this medicine can only be given in a clinic or office while you are under the care of a doctor or nurse. Brexanolone may not be safe to take while pregnant or breastfeeding.

  Another type of medicine called "esketamine" can treat depression and is given as a nasal (nose) spray in a doctor's office or clinic. Esketamine can hurt an unborn baby. You should not take esketamine if you are pregnant or breastfeeding.
- **Electroconvulsive therapy (ECT).** This can be used in extreme cases to treat postpartum depression.

These treatments can be used alone or together. Talk with your doctor or nurse about the benefits and risks of taking medicine to treat depression when you are pregnant or breastfeeding.

Having depression can affect your baby. Getting treatment is important for you and your baby. Taking medicines for depression or going to therapy does not make you a bad mother or a failure. Getting help is a sign of strength.

What Can Happen If Postpartum Depression Is Not Treated?

Untreated postpartum depression can affect your ability to parent. You may:
- not have enough energy
- have trouble focusing on the baby's needs and your own needs

- feel moody
- not be able to care for your baby
- have a higher risk of attempting suicide

Feeling like a bad mother can make depression worse. It is important to reach out for help if you feel depressed.

Researchers believe postpartum depression in a mother can affect her child throughout childhood, causing:
- delays in language development and problems learning
- problems with mother–child bonding
- behavior problems
- more crying or agitation
- shorter height and a higher risk of obesity in preschoolers
- problems dealing with stress and adjusting to school and other social situations

WHAT IS POSTPARTUM PSYCHOSIS?

Postpartum psychosis is rare. It happens in up to 4 new mothers out of every 1,000 births. It usually begins in the first two weeks after childbirth. It is a medical emergency. Women who have bipolar disorder or another mental health condition called "schizoaffective disorder" have a higher risk of postpartum psychosis. Symptoms may include:
- seeing or hearing things that are not there
- feeling confused most of the time
- having rapid mood swings within several minutes (e.g., crying hysterically, then laughing a lot, followed by extreme sadness)
- trying to hurt yourself or your baby
- paranoia (thinking that others are focused on harming you)
- restlessness or agitation
- behaving recklessly or in a way that is not normal for you[6]

[6] Office on Women's Health (OWH), "Postpartum Depression," U.S. Department of Health and Human Services (HHS), February 17, 2021. Available online. URL: www.womenshealth.gov/mental-health/mental-health-conditions/postpartum-depression. Accessed March 13, 2023.

Depression and Mental Health during Reproductive Transitions in Women

POSTPARTUM DEPRESSION MAY LAST FOR YEARS

Many women develop symptoms of postpartum depression after giving birth. These include anxiety, sadness, difficulty sleeping, exhaustion, or disturbing thoughts.

Postpartum depression can make it difficult for new mothers to take care of themselves and their babies. But many women do not recognize its symptoms or do not know that treatments are available.

Current guidelines recommend that pediatricians screen mothers for postpartum depression at their children's well visits for up to six months after birth. Using pediatrician visits in this way may help identify more women with the condition and guide them to resources and treatment.

Postpartum depression is not the same for everyone. Researchers have found many differences in symptoms between individual women, as well as how early it starts and how long it lasts.

To better understand the different trajectories for postpartum depression, a research team led by Dr. Diane Putnick from the *Eunice Kennedy Shriver* National Institute of Child Health and Human Development (NICHD) of the National Institute of Health (NIH) used data from a study that tracked more than 4,500 women and their children for three years after birth.

The study asked women about symptoms of postpartum depression four months and one, two, and three years after birth. The researchers also looked at factors that might influence the length or severity of postpartum depression. These included age, race, education, marital status, gestational diabetes or high blood pressure, and preexisting mental health conditions. Results were published on November 1, 2020, in *Pediatrics*.

The women's experiences with postpartum depression fell into four main trajectories. In the most common, women had levels of symptoms that remained low over time. Almost three-quarters of the participants fell into this category.

A second group, making up 8 percent of participants, had low levels of symptoms at four months after birth that grew worse over time. Another 13 percent had moderate symptoms that decreased over time. And about 5 percent experienced high levels of depressive symptoms that stayed higher than the other groups, even years after giving birth.

Women with a previous mood disorder diagnosis and those who experienced gestational diabetes were the most likely to fall into the group with persistently high symptoms. Women with persistently high symptoms were also more likely to be younger and have less education.

More work is needed to better understand the factors that influence the trajectory of postpartum depression for different women. Improved screening could eventually help doctors identify more women who are struggling with the condition.

"Our study indicates that six months may not be long enough to gauge depressive symptoms," Dr. Putnick says. "These long-term data are key to improving our understanding of mom's mental health, which we know is critical to her child's well-being and development."[7]

DEPRESSION DURING PREGNANCY IS ASSOCIATED WITH DEVELOPMENTAL DELAYS IN CHILDREN

Depression during pregnancy is associated with developmental delays in children although the reason for this association is not known. Breastfeeding is known to promote children's cognitive development; however, women who experience depression during pregnancy may be less likely to breastfeed or may breastfeed for a shorter time, compared to mothers without depression. Women with depression during pregnancy are more likely to be depressed after giving birth. Mothers with postnatal depression may interact less with their infants, which could also potentially affect cognitive development.

For the current study, researchers sought to determine mediators—factors that help explain an association—for developmental delays that may follow depression in pregnancy. Potential mediators were gestational age (the week of pregnancy a child was born),

---

[7] *NIH News in Health*, "Postpartum Depression May Last for Years," National Institutes of Health (NIH), November 10, 2020. Available online. URL: www.nih.gov/news-events/nih-research-matters/postpartum-depression-may-last-years. Accessed March 23, 2023.

whether maternal depression continued after birth, and breastfeeding history.

The researchers analyzed questionnaire data and medical records from 3,450 children and their mothers who took part in a larger study.

Results

Children of mothers with depression during pregnancy were more likely to have developmental delays if their mothers had more symptoms of depression after pregnancy and if they breastfed for a shorter time. For example, children of mothers with depression in pregnancy were 5 percent more likely to have a developmental delay if their mothers discontinued breastfeeding one month earlier and 16 percent more likely to have a developmental delay if their mothers scored one point higher on a depression screening test after pregnancy. A child's gestational age at birth did not increase the risk of developmental delay because women in the study with depression during pregnancy were no more likely to give birth early than women without depression.

Significance

The findings suggest that physicians may wish to offer treatment to women experiencing depression during pregnancy and after birth. Physicians may also wish to counsel women with depression during pregnancy and after birth on the benefits of breastfeeding and provide them with strategies to overcome barriers to breastfeeding.[8]

---

[8] "Science Update: Postpartum Depression, Reduced Breastfeeding May Help Account for Developmental Delays Seen in Children Born to Women with Depression during Pregnancy," *Eunice Kennedy Shriver* National Institute of Child Health and Human Development (NICHD), January 17, 2023. Available online. URL: www.nichd.nih.gov/newsroom/news/011723-depression-pregnancy. Accessed March 23, 2023.

Section 13.5 | What Is the Link between Menopause and Depression?

As women transition into menopause, they may experience changes in their menstrual cycles, hot flashes, night sweats, vaginal dryness, urinary changes, and other physical symptoms. This transition into menopause is called "perimenopause." Perimenopause begins when menstrual cycles first change and ends a year after the last menstrual cycle when a woman enters menopause. During perimenopause, a woman's risk of feeling depressed is double what it is before or after. Women may also experience increased anxiety. This is due in part to fluctuating hormones and midlife stress. Many women experience major life changes in middle age, such as retirement, children leaving home, divorce, widowhood, caring for elderly parents, and coping with chronic medical concerns in themselves and loved ones.[9]

DEPRESSION AND ANXIETY: A SYMPTOM OF MENOPAUSE

Your risk for depression and anxiety is higher during the time around menopause. This may be caused by changing hormones, menopausal symptoms, or both. You may experience sadness or depression over the loss of fertility or the changes in your body. If you have symptoms of depression or anxiety, see your doctor. Your doctor may recommend therapy or medicine or both to treat depression or anxiety.[10]

DO YOU THINK YOU MIGHT HAVE DEPRESSION OR ANXIETY AFFECTED BY MENOPAUSE OR PERIMENOPAUSE?
Checklist for Depression or Anxiety Related to Menopause or Perimenopause

- Is there a recent change in how often you have periods?
  - Is there a recent change in how many days you bleed?

---

[9] "Menopause and Mental Health," U.S. Department of Veterans Affairs (VA), November 30, 2022. Available online. URL: www.mentalhealth.va.gov/women-vets/reproductive-mental-health/menopause.asp. Accessed March 27, 2023.
[10] Office on Women's Health (OWH), "Menopause Symptoms and Relief," U.S. Department of Health and Human Services (HHS), February 22, 2021. Available online. URL: www.womenshealth.gov/menopause/menopause-symptoms-and-relief. Accessed March 27, 2023.

Depression and Mental Health during Reproductive Transitions in Women

- Has your period recently become very heavy?
- Do you have any of these symptoms?
  - hot flashes
  - night sweats
  - increased difficulty sleeping
  - increased fatigue
  - irritability
  - anxiety
  - depressed mood
  - crying spells
  - increased urination
  - leaking urine
  - dry or itchy vagina
  - pain during sexual intercourse

If you answered yes to at least three questions, consider speaking with your primary care provider or mental health clinician about assessment and treatment options.[11]

WHAT YOU CAN DO

- **Sleep.** Try to get enough sleep. Most adults need between seven and eight hours of sleep each night. Lack of sleep is linked to depression.
- **Exercise.** Get at least 30 minutes of physical activity on most days of the week. Exercise is proven to help with depression.
- **Limit alcohol.** Limit how much alcohol you drink, if any. A moderate amount of alcohol for women is one drink a day and no more than seven drinks in a week. Drinking more than four drinks at a time is considered binge drinking.
- **Lower stress.** Set limits for how much you take on. Look for positive ways to unwind and ease daily stress. Try relaxation techniques, reading a book, spending some quiet time outdoors, or other healthy ways to unwind.[12]

---

[11] See footnote [9].
[12] See footnote [10].

Chapter 14 | Depression in Children and Adolescents

Chapter Contents
Section 14.1—Understanding Depression in Children............. 101
Section 14.2—Teen Depression: More than
 Just Moodiness 103

Section 14.1 | Understanding Depression in Children

Occasionally being sad or feeling hopeless is a part of every child's life. However, some children feel sad or uninterested in things that they used to enjoy or feel helpless or hopeless in situations they are able to change. When children feel persistent sadness and hopelessness, they may be diagnosed with depression.

Examples of behaviors often seen in children with depression include:
- feeling sad, hopeless, or irritable a lot of the time
- not wanting to do or enjoy doing fun things
- showing changes in eating patterns—eating a lot more or a lot less than usual
- showing changes in sleep patterns—sleeping a lot more or a lot less than normal
- showing changes in energy—being tired and sluggish or tense and restless a lot of the time
- having a hard time paying attention
- feeling worthless, useless, or guilty
- showing self-injury and self-destructive behavior

Extreme depression can lead a child to think about suicide or plan for suicide. Some children may not talk about their helpless and hopeless thoughts and may not appear sad. Depression might also cause a child to make trouble or act unmotivated, causing others not to notice that the child is depressed or to incorrectly label the child as a troublemaker or lazy.

MANAGING SYMPTOMS: STAYING HEALTHY

Being healthy is important for all children and can be especially important for children with depression. In addition to getting the right treatment, leading a healthy lifestyle can play a role in managing symptoms of depression. Here are some healthy behaviors that may help:
- having a healthy eating plan centered on fruits, vegetables, whole grains, legumes (e.g., beans, peas, and lentils), lean protein sources, and nuts and seeds

- participating in physical activity for at least 60 minutes each day
- getting the recommended amount of sleep each night based on age
- practicing mindfulness or relaxation techniques

TREATMENT FOR DEPRESSION IN CHILDREN

The first step to treatment is to talk with a health-care provider such as your child's primary care provider, or a mental health specialist, about getting an evaluation. Some of the signs and symptoms of depression in children could be caused by other conditions, such as trauma. Specific symptoms such as having a hard time focusing could be a sign of attention deficit hyperactivity disorder (ADHD). It is important to get a careful evaluation to get the best diagnosis and treatment. Consultation with a health provider can help determine if medication should be part of the treatment. A mental health professional can develop a therapy plan that works best for the child and family. Behavior therapy includes child therapy, family therapy, or a combination of both. The school can also be included in the treatment plan. For very young children, involving parents in treatment is key. Cognitive-behavioral therapy (CBT) is one form of therapy that is used to treat depression, particularly in older children. It helps the child change negative thoughts into more positive, effective ways of thinking, leading to more effective behavior.

Treatments can also include a variety of ways to help the child feel less stressed and be healthier, such as nutritious food, physical activity, sufficient sleep, predictable routines, and social support.

PREVENTION OF DEPRESSION IN CHILDREN

It is not known exactly why some children develop depression. Many factors may play a role, including biology and temperament. But it is also known that some children are more likely to develop depression when they experience trauma or stress, when they are maltreated, when they are bullied or rejected by other children, or when their own parents have depression.

Although these factors appear to increase the risk of depression, there are ways to decrease the chance that children experience them.[1]

Section 14.2 | Teen Depression: More than Just Moodiness

WHAT IS DEPRESSION IN TEENS?

Depression in teens (aged 13–17) is a serious medical illness. It is more than just a feeling of being sad or "blue" for a few days. It is an intense feeling of sadness, hopelessness, and anger or frustration that lasts much longer. These feelings make it hard for you to function normally and do your usual activities. You may also have trouble focusing and have no motivation or energy. Depression can make you feel like it is hard to enjoy life or even get through the day.

WHAT CAUSES DEPRESSION IN TEENS?

Many factors may play a role in depression, including the following:
- genetics, as depression can run in families
- brain biology and chemistry
- hormonal changes
- stressful childhood events such as trauma, the death of a loved one, bullying, and abuse

WHICH TEENS ARE AT RISK OF DEPRESSION?

Depression can happen at any age but often begins in the teens or early adulthood. Certain teens are at a higher risk of depression, such as those who:
- have other mental health conditions, such as anxiety, eating disorders, and substance use

---

[1] "Anxiety and Depression in Children," Centers for Disease Control and Prevention (CDC), March 8, 2023. Available online. URL: www.cdc.gov/childrensmentalhealth/depression.html. Accessed March 9, 2023.

- have other diseases, such as diabetes, cancer, and heart disease
- have family members with mental illness
- have a dysfunctional family/family conflict
- have problems with friends or other kids at school
- have learning disabilities or attention deficit hyperactivity disorder (ADHD)
- have had trauma in childhood
- have low self-esteem, a pessimistic outlook, or poor coping skills
- are members of the lesbian, gay, bisexual, transgender, queer or questioning, intersex, asexual, and more (LGBTQIA+) community, especially when their families are not supportive

WHAT ARE THE SYMPTOMS OF DEPRESSION IN TEENS?

If you have depression, you have one or more of these symptoms most of the time:
- sadness
- feeling of emptiness
- hopelessness
- being angry, irritable, or frustrated, even at minor things

You may also have other symptoms, such as:
- no longer caring about things you used to enjoy
- changes in weight, such as losing weight when you are not dieting or gaining weight from eating too much
- changes in sleep, such as having trouble falling asleep or staying asleep or sleeping much more than usual
- feeling restless or having trouble sitting still
- feeling very tired or not having energy
- feeling worthless or very guilty
- having trouble concentrating, remembering information, or making decisions
- thinking about dying or suicide

HOW IS DEPRESSION IN TEENS DIAGNOSED?
If you think you might be depressed, tell someone that you trust, such as your:
- parents or guardian
- teacher or counselor
- doctor

The next step is to see your doctor for a checkup. Your doctor can first make sure that you do not have another health problem that is causing your depression. To do this, you may have a physical exam and lab tests.

If you do not have another health problem, you will get a psychological evaluation. Your doctor may do it, or you may be referred to a mental health professional to get one. You may be asked about things such as:
- your thoughts and feelings
- how you are doing at school
- any changes in your eating, sleeping, or energy level
- whether you are suicidal
- whether you use alcohol or drugs

HOW IS DEPRESSION IN TEENS TREATED?
Effective treatments for depression in teens include talk therapy or a combination of talk therapy and medicines.

Talk Therapy
Talk therapy, also called "psychotherapy" or "counseling," can help you understand and manage your moods and feelings. It involves going to see a therapist, such as a psychiatrist, a psychologist, a social worker, or a counselor. You can talk out your emotions to someone who understands and supports you. You can also learn how to stop thinking negatively and start to look at the positives in life. This will help you build confidence and feel better about yourself.

There are many different types of talk therapy. Certain types have been shown to help teens deal with depression, including the following:
- **Cognitive-behavioral therapy (CBT).** This helps you identify and change negative and unhelpful thoughts. It also helps you build coping skills and change behavioral patterns.
- **Interpersonal therapy (IPT).** This focuses on improving your relationships. It helps you understand and work through troubled relationships that may contribute to your depression. IPT may help you change behaviors that are causing problems. You also explore major issues that may add to your depression, such as grief or life changes.

Medicines

In some cases, your doctor will suggest medicines along with talk therapy. There are a few antidepressants that have been widely studied and proven to help teens. If you are taking medicine for depression, it is important to see your doctor regularly.

It is also important to know that it will take some time for you to get relief from antidepressants:
- It can take three to four weeks until an antidepressant takes effect.
- You may have to try more than one antidepressant to find one that works for you.
- It can also take some time to find the right dose of an antidepressant.

In some cases, teenagers may have an increase in suicidal thoughts or behavior when taking antidepressants. This risk is higher in the first few weeks after starting the medicine and when the dose is changed. Make sure to tell your parents or guardian if you start feeling worse or have thoughts of hurting yourself.

You should not stop taking the antidepressants on your own. You need to work with your doctor to slowly and safely decrease the dose before you stop.

Depression in Children and Adolescents

Programs for Severe Depression
Some teens who have severe depression or are at risk of hurting themselves may need more intensive treatment. They may go into a psychiatric hospital or do a day program. Both offer counseling, group discussions, and activities with mental health professionals and other patients. Day programs may be full- or half-day, and they often last for several weeks.[2]

HOW DO YOU GET HELP FOR DEPRESSION?
- Talk to a trusted adult (such as your parent or guardian, teacher, or school counselor) about how you have been feeling.
- Ask your doctor about options for professional help.
- Try to spend time with friends or family, even if you do not feel like you want to.
- Stay active and exercise, even if it is just going for a walk. Physical activity releases chemicals, such as endorphins, in your brain that can help you feel better.
- Try to keep a regular sleep schedule.
- Eat healthy foods.[3]

---

[2] MedlinePlus, "Teen Depression," National Institutes of Health (NIH), December 14, 2022. Available online. URL: https://medlineplus.gov/teendepression.html. Accessed March 10, 2023.
[3] "Teen Depression: More than Just Moodiness," National Institute of Mental Health (NIMH), June 26, 2015. Available online. URL: www.nimh.nih.gov/health/publications/teen-depression. Accessed March 10, 2023.

Chapter 15 | Men and Depression

Men and women both experience depression, but their symptoms can be very different. Because men who are depressed may appear to be angry or aggressive instead of sad, their families, friends, and even their doctors may not always recognize anger or aggression as depression symptoms. In addition, men are less likely than women to recognize, talk about, and seek treatment for depression. Yet depression affects a large number of men.

Depression affects the ability to feel, think, and handle daily activities. Also known as "major depressive disorder" (MDD) or "clinical depression," a man must have symptoms for at least two weeks to be diagnosed with depression.

WHAT CAUSES DEPRESSION IN MEN?

Depression is one of the most common mental disorders in the United States. Research suggests that depression is caused by a combination of risk factors, including the following:

- **Genetic factors**. Men with a family history of depression may be more likely to develop it than those whose family members do not have the illness.
- **Environmental stress**. Financial problems, loss of a loved one, a difficult relationship, major life changes, work problems, or any stressful situation may trigger depression in some men.
- **Illness**. Depression can occur with other serious medical illnesses, such as diabetes, cancer, heart disease, or Parkinson disease (PD). Depression

can make these conditions worse and vice versa. Sometimes, medications taken for these illnesses may cause side effects that trigger or worsen depression.

WHAT ARE THE SIGNS AND SYMPTOMS OF DEPRESSION IN MEN?

Different men have different symptoms, but some common depression symptoms include:
- anger, irritability, or aggressiveness
- feeling anxious, restless, or "on the edge"
- loss of interest in work, family, or once pleasurable activities
- problems with sexual desire and performance
- feeling sad, "empty," flat, or hopeless
- not being able to concentrate or remember details
- feeling very tired, not being able to sleep, or sleeping too much
- overeating or not wanting to eat at all
- thoughts of suicide or suicide attempts
- physical aches or pains, headaches, cramps, or digestive problems
- inability to meet the responsibilities of work, caring for family, or other important activities
- engaging in high-risk activities
- a need for alcohol or drugs
- withdrawing from family and friends or becoming isolated

Not every man who is depressed experiences every symptom. Some men experience only a few symptoms, while others may experience many.

WHAT ARE THE DIFFERENT TYPES OF DEPRESSION THAT AFFECT MEN?

The most common types of depression are as follows:
- **Major depression.** These depressive symptoms interfere with a man's ability to work, sleep, study, eat,

and enjoy most aspects of life. An episode of major depression may occur only once in a person's lifetime. But it is common for a person to have several episodes. Special forms (subtypes) of major depression include the following:
- **Psychotic depression.** It is severe depression associated with delusions (false, fixed beliefs) or hallucinations (hearing or seeing things that are not really there). These psychotic symptoms are depression-themed. For example, a man may believe he is sick or poor when he is not, or he may hear voices that are not real that say that he is worthless.
- **Seasonal affective disorder (SAD).** It is characterized by depression symptoms that appear every year during the winter months when there is less natural sunlight.
- **Persistent depressive disorder.** This is also called "dysthymia." Depressive symptoms last a long time (two years or longer) but are less severe than those of major depression.
- **Minor depression.** This type of depression is similar to major depression and persistent depressive disorder, but symptoms are less severe and may not last as long.
- **Bipolar disorder.** This type of disorder is different from depression, but a person with bipolar disorder experiences episodes of extreme low moods (depression) or extreme high moods (called "mania").

HOW DOES DEPRESSION IN MEN DIFFER FROM THAT IN WOMEN?

Both men and women get depression, but their willingness to talk about their feelings may be very different. This is one of the reasons that depression symptoms for men and women may be very different as well.

For example, some men with depression hide their emotions and may seem to be angry, irritable, or aggressive, while many women seem sad or express sadness. Men with depression may feel very tired and lose interest in work, family, or hobbies. They may be more likely to have difficulty sleeping than women who have depression. Sometimes, mental health symptoms appear to be physical issues. For example, a racing heart, tightening chest, ongoing headaches, or digestive issues can be signs of a mental health problem. Many men are more likely to see their doctor about physical symptoms than emotional symptoms.

Some men may turn to drugs or alcohol to try to cope with their emotional symptoms. Also, while women with depression are more likely to attempt suicide, men are more likely to die by suicide because they tend to use more lethal methods. Depression can affect any man at any age. With the right treatment, most men with depression can get better and gain back their interest in work, family, and hobbies.

HOW IS DEPRESSION IN MEN TREATED?

Men often avoid addressing their feelings, and in many cases, friends and family members are the first to recognize that their loved one is depressed. It is important that friends and family support their loved one and encourage him to visit a doctor or mental health professional for an evaluation. A health professional can do an exam or lab tests to rule out other conditions that may have symptoms that are like those of depression. He or she can also tell if certain medications are affecting the depression.

The doctor needs to get a complete history of symptoms, such as when they started, how long they have lasted, how bad they are, whether they have occurred before, and, if so, how they were treated. It is important that the man seeking help be open and honest about any efforts at "self-medication" with alcohol, nonprescribed drugs, gambling, or high-risk activities. A complete history should include information about a family history of depression or other mental disorders.

After a diagnosis, depression is usually treated with medications or psychotherapy, or a combination of the two. The increasingly popular "collaborative care" approach combines physical and behavioral health care. Collaborative care involves a team of health-care providers and managers, including a primary care doctor and specialists.

Medication

Medications called "antidepressants" can work well to treat depression, but they can take several weeks to be effective. Often with medication, symptoms such as sleep, appetite, and concentration problems improve before mood lifts, so it is important to give medication a chance before deciding whether it is effective or not.

Antidepressants can have side effects, including:
- headache
- nausea or feeling sick to your stomach
- difficulty sleeping and nervousness
- agitation or restlessness
- sexual problems

Most side effects lessen over time, but it is important to talk with your doctor about any side effects that you may have. Starting antidepressant medication at a low dose and gradually increasing it to a full therapeutic dose may help minimize adverse effects.

It is important to know that although antidepressants can be safe and effective for many people, they may present serious risks to some young adults. A "black box" warning—the most serious type of warning that a prescription drug can have—has been added to the labels of antidepressant medications to warn people that antidepressants may cause some young people to have suicidal thoughts or may increase the risk for suicide attempts. This is especially true for those who become agitated when they first start taking the medication and before it begins to work. Anyone taking antidepressants should be monitored closely, especially when they first start taking them.

For most people, though, the risks of untreated depression far outweigh those of taking antidepressant medications under a doctor's supervision. Careful monitoring by a health professional will also minimize any potential risks.

For reasons that are not well understood, many people respond better to some antidepressants than to others. If one does not respond to one medication, his or her doctor may suggest trying another. Sometimes, a medication may be only partially effective. In that case, another medication might be added to help make the antidepressant more effective.

If you begin taking antidepressants, do not stop taking them without the help of a doctor. Sometimes, people take antidepressants to feel better and then stop taking the medication on their own, and the depression returns. When it is time to stop the medication, usually after a course of 6–12 months, the doctor will help you slowly and safely decrease your dose. Stopping them abruptly can cause withdrawal symptoms.

Some people who relapse back into depression after stopping an antidepressant benefit from staying on medication for additional months or years.

Psychotherapy

Several types of psychotherapy or "talk therapy" can help treat depression. Some therapies are just as effective as medications for certain types of depression. Therapy helps by teaching new ways of thinking and behaving and changing habits that may be contributing to depression. Therapy can also help men understand and work through difficult situations or relationships that may be causing their depression or making it worse. Cognitive-behavioral therapy (CBT), interpersonal therapy (IPT), and problem-solving therapy are examples of evidence-based talk therapy treatments for depression. Treatment for depression should be personalized. Some men might try therapy first and add antidepressant medication later if it is needed. Others might start treatment with both medication and psychotherapy.

HOW CAN YOU HELP YOURSELF IF YOU ARE DEPRESSED?

As you continue treatment, gradually you will start to feel better. Remember that if you are taking an antidepressant, it may take several weeks for it to start working. Try to do things that you used to enjoy before you had depression. Go easy on yourself.

Other things that may help include:
- spending time with other people and talking with a friend or relative about your feelings
- increasing your level of physical activity (Regular exercise can help people with mild-to-moderate

depression and may be one part of a treatment plan for those with severe depression. Talk with your healthcare professional about what kind of exercise is right for you.)
- breaking up large tasks into small ones and tackling what you can as you can (Do not try to do too many things at once.)
- delaying important decisions until you feel better (Discuss decisions with others who know you well.)
- keeping stable daily routines (e.g., eating and going to bed at the same time every day)
- avoiding alcohol

HOW CAN YOU HELP A LOVED ONE WHO IS DEPRESSED?

It is important to remember that a person with depression cannot simply "snap out of it." It is also important to know that he may not recognize the symptoms and may not want to get professional treatment.

If you think someone has depression, you can support him by finding a doctor or mental health professional and then helping him make an appointment. Even men who have trouble recognizing that they are depressed may agree to seek help for physical symptoms, such as feeling tired or run down. They may be willing to talk with their regular health professional about a new difficulty they are having at work or losing interest in doing things they usually enjoy. Talking with a primary care provider may be a good first step toward learning about and treating possible depression.

Other ways to help include:
- offering him support, understanding, patience, and encouragement
- listening carefully and talking with him
- never ignoring comments about suicide and alerting his therapist or doctor
- helping him increase his level of physical and social activity by inviting him out for hikes, games, and other events (If he says "no," keep trying, but do not push him to take on too much too soon.)

Depression Sourcebook, Sixth Edition

- encouraging him to report any concerns about medications to his health-care provider
- ensuring that he gets to his doctor's appointments
- reminding him that with time and treatment, the depression will lift

WHERE CAN YOU GO FOR HELP?

If you are unsure of where to go for help, ask your family doctor or health-care provider. You can also find resources online, including the website of the National Institute of Mental Health (NIMH) at www.nimh.nih.gov/FindHelp or check with your insurance carrier to find someone who participates in your plan. Hospital doctors can help in an emergency.[1]

---

[1] "Men and Depression," National Institute of Mental Health (NIMH), January 2017. Available online. URL: www.nimh.nih.gov/health/publications/men-and-depression. Accessed March 10, 2023.

Chapter 16 | Depression in Older Adults

Depression is a common problem among older adults, but clinical depression is not a normal part of aging. In fact, studies show that most older adults feel satisfied with their lives, despite having more illnesses or physical problems, than younger people. However, if you have experienced depression as a younger person, you may be more likely to have depression as an older adult.

Depression is serious, and treatments are available to help. For most people, depression gets better with treatment. Counseling, medicine, or other forms of treatment can help. You do not need to suffer—help and treatment options are available. Talk with your doctor if you think you might have depression.

WHAT ARE THE RISK FACTORS FOR DEPRESSION IN OLDER ADULTS?

There are many things that may be risk factors for depression. For some people, changes in the brain can affect mood and result in depression. Others may experience depression after a major life event, such as a medical diagnosis or a loved one's death. Sometimes, those under a lot of stress—especially people who care for loved ones with a serious illness or disability—can feel depressed. Others may become depressed for no clear reason.

Research has shown that the following factors are related to the risk of depression but do not necessarily cause depression:
- medical conditions, such as stroke or cancer
- genes (People who have a family history of depression may be at a higher risk.)

- stress, including caregiver stress
- sleep problems
- social isolation and loneliness
- lack of exercise or physical activity
- functional limitations that make engaging in activities of daily living difficult
- addiction and/or alcoholism—included in substance-induced depressive disorder

WHAT ARE THE SIGNS AND SYMPTOMS OF DEPRESSION IN OLDER ADULTS?

Depression in older adults may be difficult to recognize because older people may have different symptoms compared with younger people. For some older adults with depression, sadness is not their main symptom. They could instead be feeling more numbness or a lack of interest in activities. They may not be as willing to talk about their feelings.

The following is a list of common symptoms. Still, because people experience depression differently, there may be symptoms that are not on this list:

- persistent sad, anxious, or "empty" mood
- feelings of hopelessness, guilt, worthlessness, or helplessness
- irritability, restlessness, or having trouble sitting still
- loss of interest in once pleasurable activities, including sex
- decreased energy or fatigue
- moving or talking more slowly
- difficulty concentrating, remembering, or making decisions
- difficulty sleeping, waking up too early in the morning, or oversleeping
- eating more or less than usual, usually with unplanned weight gain or loss
- thoughts of death or suicide or suicide attempts

If you have several of these signs and symptoms and they last for more than two weeks, talk with your doctor. These could be signs of depression or another health condition. Do not ignore the warning signs. If left untreated, serious depression may lead to death by suicide.

If you are a health-care provider of an older person, ask how they are feeling during their visits. Research has shown that intervening during primary care visits is highly effective in reducing suicide later in life. If you are a family member or friend, watch for clues. Listen carefully if someone of any age says they feel depressed, sad, or empty for long periods of time. That person may really be asking for help.

WHAT ARE THE DIFFERENT TYPES OF DEPRESSION THAT AFFECT OLDER ADULTS?

There are several types of depression that older adults may experience:
- **Major depressive disorder (MDD).** This type of depression includes symptoms lasting at least two weeks that interfere with a person's ability to perform daily tasks.
- **Persistent depressive disorder (dysthymia).** A depressed mood lasts more than two years, but the person may still be able to perform daily tasks, unlike someone with MDD.
- **Substance-/medication-induced depressive disorder.** It is a depression related to the use of substances, such as alcohol or pain medication.
- **Depressive disorder due to a medical condition.** This type of depression is related to a separate illness, such as heart disease or multiple sclerosis.

Other forms of depression include psychotic depression, postmenopausal depression, and seasonal affective disorder (SAD).

SUPPORTING FRIENDS AND FAMILY WITH DEPRESSION

Depression is a medical condition that requires treatment from a doctor. While family and friends can help by offering support in finding treatment, they cannot treat a person's depression.

As a friend or family member of a person with depression, here are a few things you can do:
- Encourage the person to seek medical treatment and stick with the treatment plan the doctor prescribes.
- Help set up medical appointments or accompany the person to the doctor's office or a support group.
- Participate in activities the person likes to do.
- Ask if the person wants to go for a walk or a bike ride. Physical activity can be great for boosting mood.

HOW IS DEPRESSION IN OLDER ADULTS TREATED?

Depression, even severe depression, can be treated. It is important to seek treatment as soon as you begin noticing signs. If you think you may have depression, start by making an appointment to see your doctor or health-care provider.

Certain medications or medical conditions can sometimes cause the same symptoms as depression. A doctor can rule out these possibilities through a physical exam, learning about your health and personal history, and lab tests. If a doctor finds there is no medical condition that is causing the depression, he or she may suggest a psychological evaluation and refer you to a mental health professional such as a psychologist to perform this test. This evaluation will help determine a diagnosis and a treatment plan.

Common forms of treatment for depression include the following:
- **Psychotherapy, counseling, or "talk therapy."** This can help a person identify and change troubling emotions, thoughts, and behavior. It may be done with a psychologist, licensed clinical social worker (LCSW), psychiatrist, or other licensed mental health-care professional. Examples of approaches specific to the treatment of depression include cognitive-behavioral therapy (CBT) and interpersonal therapy (IPT).
- **Medications for depression.** This may balance hormones that affect mood, such as serotonin. There are many different types of commonly used antidepressant medications. Selective serotonin

Depression in Older Adults

reuptake inhibitors (SSRIs) are antidepressants commonly prescribed to older adults. A psychiatrist, mental health nurse practitioner, or primary care physician can prescribe and help monitor medications and potential side effects.

- **Electroconvulsive therapy (ECT).** During this therapy, electrodes are placed on a person's head to enable a safe, mild electric current to pass through the brain. This type of therapy is usually considered only if a person's illness has not improved with other treatments.
- **Repetitive transcranial magnetic stimulation (rTMS).** This uses magnets to activate the brain. rTMS does not require anesthesia and targets only specific regions of the brain to help reduce side effects such as fatigue, nausea, or memory loss that could happen with ECT.

Treatment, particularly a combination of psychotherapy and medications, has been shown to be effective for older adults. However, not all medications or therapies will be right for everyone. Treatment choices differ for each person, and sometimes, multiple treatments must be tried in order to find one that works. It is important to tell your doctor if your current treatment plan is not working and to keep trying to find something that does.

Some people may try complementary health approaches, such as yoga, to improve well-being and cope with stress. However, there is little evidence to suggest that these approaches, on their own, can successfully treat depression. While they can be used in combination with other treatments prescribed by a person's doctor, they should not replace medical treatment. Talk with your doctor about what treatment(s) might be good to try.

Do not avoid getting help because you do not know how much treatment will cost. Treatment for depression is usually covered by private insurance and Medicare. Also, some community mental health centers may offer treatment based on a person's ability to pay.

CAN DEPRESSION IN OLDER ADULTS BE PREVENTED?

Many people wonder if depression can be prevented and how they may be able to lower their risk of depression. Although most cases of depression cannot be prevented, healthy lifestyle changes can have long-term benefits for your mental health.

Here are a few steps you can take:
- Be physically active and eat a healthy, balanced diet. This may help avoid illnesses that can bring on disability or depression. Some diets—including the low-sodium DASH diet—have been shown to reduce the risk of depression.
- Get seven to nine hours of sleep each night.
- Stay in touch with friends and family.
- Participate in activities you enjoy.
- Let friends, family, and your physician know when you are experiencing symptoms of depression.[1]

---

[1] National Institute on Aging (NIA), "Depression and Older Adults," National Institutes of Health (NIH), July 7, 2021. Available online. URL: www.nia.nih.gov/health/depression-and-older-adults. Accessed March 2, 2023.

Chapter 17 | Depression in Racial and Ethnic Minorities

MENTAL AND BEHAVIORAL HEALTH IN AFRICAN AMERICANS
- In 2020, suicide was the third leading cause of death for Blacks or African Americans aged 15–24.
- The death rate from suicide for Black or African American men was four times greater than that for African American women, in 2018.
- The overall suicide rate for Black or African Americans was 60 percent lower than that of the non-Hispanic White population, in 2018.
- Black females in grades 9–12 were 60 percent more likely to attempt suicide in 2019 than non-Hispanic White females of the same age.
- The poverty level affects mental health status. Black or African Americans living below the poverty level, as compared to those over twice the poverty level, are twice as likely to report serious psychological distress.

Tables 17.1–17.4 show the percentage of African American adults aged 18 and above who took medications or underwent treatment for psychological distress or depression.

Depression Sourcebook, Sixth Edition

Mental Health Status

Table 17.1. Serious Psychological Distress in the Past Year among Adults 18 Years of Age and Over, Percentage, 2019

Non-Hispanic Black	Non-Hispanic White	Non-Hispanic Black/Non-Hispanic White Ratio
11.9%	12.7%	0.9

(Source: Substance Abuse and Mental Health Services Administration (SAMHSA), 2022. Results from the 2019 National Survey on Drug Use and Health: Mental Health Detailed Tables. Table 10.43B (www.samhsa.gov/data/report/2019-nsduh-detailed-tables).)

Access to Health Care

Table 17.2. Percentage of Adults Aged 18 and Over Who Received Mental Health Services* in the Past Year, 2020

Non-Hispanic Black	Non-Hispanic White	Non-Hispanic Black/Non-Hispanic White Ratio
37.1%	51.8%	0.6

*For any mental illness
(Source: Substance Abuse and Mental Health Services Administration (SAMHSA), 2022. Results from the 2020 National Survey on Drug Use and Health: Mental Health Detailed Tables. Table 8.17B (www.samhsa.gov/data/report/2020-nsduh-detailed-tables).)

Table 17.3. Percentage of Adults Aged 18 and Over Who Received Prescription Medications for Mental Health Services*, 2020

Non-Hispanic Black	Non-Hispanic White	Non-Hispanic Black/Non-Hispanic White Ratio
27.5%	44.5%	0.4

*Prescription for any mental illness
(Source: Substance Abuse and Mental Health Services Administration (SAMHSA), 2022. Results from the 2020 National Survey on Drug Use and Health: Mental Health Detailed Tables. Table 8.21B (www.samhsa.gov/data/report/2020-nsduh-detailed-tables).)

Depression in Racial and Ethnic Minorities

Table 17.4. Percentage of Adults Aged 18 and Over with a Past Year Major Depressive Episode Who Received Treatment for Depression, 2019[1]

Non-Hispanic Black	Non-Hispanic White	Non-Hispanic Black/Non-Hispanic White Ratio
59.6%	70.2%	0.8

(Source: Substance Abuse and Mental Health Services Administration (SAMHSA), 2022. Results from the 2019 National Survey on Drug Use and Health: Mental Health Detailed Tables. Table 8.39B (www.samhsa.gov/data/report/2019-nsduh-detailed-tables).)

MENTAL AND BEHAVIORAL HEALTH IN AMERICAN INDIANS/ALASKA NATIVES

- In 2019, suicide was the second leading cause of death for American Indian/Alaska Natives between the ages of 10 and 34.
- American Indian/Alaska Natives are 60 percent more likely to experience the feeling that everything is an effort, all or most of the time, than non-Hispanic Whites.
- The overall death rate from suicide for American Indian/Alaska Native adults is about 20 percent higher than that for the non-Hispanic White population.
- In 2019, adolescent American Indian/Alaska Native females aged 15–19 had a death rate that was five times higher than non-Hispanic White females in the same age group.

Tables 17.5–17.8 show the percentage of American Indian/Alaska Native adults aged 18 and above who took medications or underwent treatment for psychological distress or depression.

---

[1] Office of Minority Health (OMH), "Mental and Behavioral Health–African Americans," U.S. Department of Health and Human Services (HHS), February 17, 2023. Available online. URL: www.minorityhealth.hhs.gov/omh/browse.aspx?lvl=4&lvlid=24. Accessed March 3, 2023.

Mental Health Status

Table 17.5. Serious Psychological Distress in the Past Year among Adults 18 Years of Age and Over, Percentage, 2019

American Indian/Alaska Native*	Non-Hispanic White	American Indian/Alaska Native/Non-Hispanic White Ratio
11.6%	12.7%	0.9

*All data in the above surveys relate to non-Hispanic American Indians/Alaska Natives.
(Source: Substance Abuse and Mental Health Services Administration (SAMHSA), 2020. Results from the 2019 National Survey on Drug Use and Health: Mental Health Detailed Tables. Table 10.43B (www.samhsa.gov/data/report/2019-nsduh-detailed-tables).)

Access to Health Care

Table 17.6. Percentage of Adults Aged 18 and Over Who Received Mental Health Services in the Past Year, 2019

American Indian/Alaska Native*	Non-Hispanic White	American Indian/Alaska Native/Non-Hispanic White Ratio
13.9%	19.8%	0.7

*All data in the above surveys relate to non-Hispanic American Indians/Alaska Natives.
(Source: Substance Abuse and Mental Health Services Administration (SAMHSA), 2020. Results from the 2019 National Survey on Drug Use and Health: Mental Health Detailed Tables. Table 8.17B (www.samhsa.gov/data/report/2019-nsduh-detailed-tables).)

Table 17.7. Percentage of Adults Aged 18 and Over Who Received Prescription Medications for Mental Health Services, 2019

American Indian/Alaska Native*	Non-Hispanic White	American Indian/Alaska Native/Non-Hispanic White Ratio
11.1%	16.6%	0.7

*All data in the above surveys relate to non-Hispanic American Indians/Alaska Natives.
(Source: Substance Abuse and Mental Health Services Administration (SAMHSA), 2020. Results from the 2019 National Survey on Drug Use and Health: Mental Health Detailed Tables. Table 8.21B (www.samhsa.gov/data/report/2019-nsduh-detailed-tables).)

Depression in Racial and Ethnic Minorities

Table 17.8. Percentage of Adults Aged 18 and Over with a Past Year Major Depressive Episode Who Received Treatment for Depression, 2019[2]

American Indian/Alaska Native	Non-Hispanic White	American Indian/Alaska Native/Non-Hispanic White Ratio
—	70.2%	—

(Source: Substance Abuse and Mental Health Services Administration (SAMHSA), 2020. Results from the 2019 National Survey on Drug Use and Health: Mental Health Detailed Tables. Table 8.39B (www.samhsa.gov/data/report/2019-nsduh-detailed-tables).)

MENTAL AND BEHAVIORAL HEALTH IN ASIAN AMERICANS

- Suicide was the leading cause of death for Asian/Pacific Islanders aged 15–24 in 2019.
- Asian American males in grades 9–12 were 30 percent more likely to consider attempting suicide than non-Hispanic White male students, in 2019.
  - Southeast Asian refugees are at risk for posttraumatic stress disorder (PTSD) associated with trauma experienced before and after immigration to the United States. One study found that 70 percent of Southeast Asian refugees receiving mental health care were diagnosed with PTSD.
  - The overall suicide rate for Asians is less than half that of the non-Hispanic White population.

Tables 17.9–17.12 show the percentage of Asian American adults aged 18 and above who took medications or underwent treatment for psychological distress or depression.

---

[2] Office of Minority Health (OMH), "Mental and Behavioral Health–American Indians/Alaska Natives," U.S. Department of Health and Human Services (HHS), May 19, 2021. Available online. URL: www.minorityhealth.hhs.gov/omh/browse.aspx?lvl=4&lvlid=39. Accessed March 3, 2023.

Depression Sourcebook, Sixth Edition

Mental Health Status

Table 17.9. Serious Psychological Distress in the Past Year among Adults 18 Years of Age and Over, Percentage, 2019

Asian*	Non-Hispanic White	Asian/Non-Hispanic White Ratio
9.0%	12.7%	0.6

*All data in the above surveys relate to non-Hispanic Asians.
(Source: Substance Abuse and Mental Health Services Administration (SAMHSA), 2020. Results from the 2019 National Survey on Drug Use and Health: Mental Health Detailed Tables. Table 10.43B (www.samhsa.gov/data/report/2019-nsduh-detailed-tables).)

Access to Health Care

Table 17.10. Percentage of Adults Aged 18 and Over Who Received Mental Health Services in the Past Year, 2019

Asian	Non-Hispanic White	Asian/Non-Hispanic White Ratio
7.0%	19.8%	0.3

(Source: Substance Abuse and Mental Health Services Administration (SAMHSA), 2020. Results from the 2019 National Survey on Drug Use and Health: Mental Health Detailed Tables. Table 8.17B (www.samhsa.gov/data/report/2019-nsduh-detailed-tables).)

Table 17.11. Percentage of Adults Aged 18 and Over Who Received Prescription Medications for Mental Health Services, 2019

Asian	Non-Hispanic White	Asian/Non-Hispanic White Ratio
4.8%	16.6%	0.2

(Source: Substance Abuse and Mental Health Services Administration (SAMHSA), 2020. Results from the 2019 National Survey on Drug Use and Health: Mental Health Detailed Tables. Table 8.21B (www.samhsa.gov/data/report/2019-nsduh-detailed-tables).)

Table 17.12. Percentage of Adults Aged 18 and Over with a Past Year Major Depressive Episode Who Received Treatment for Depression, 2019[3]

Asian	Non-Hispanic White	Asian/Non-Hispanic White Ratio
51.7%	70.2%	0.6

(Source: Substance Abuse and Mental Health Services Administration (SAMHSA), 2020. Results from the 2019 National Survey on Drug Use and Health: Mental Health Detailed Tables. Table 8.39B (www.samhsa.gov/data/report/2019-nsduh-detailed-tables).)

---

[3] Office of Minority Health (OMH), "Mental and Behavioral Health–Asian Americans," U.S. Department of Health and Human Services (HHS), May 19, 2021. Available online. URL: https://minorityhealth.hhs.gov/omh/browse.aspx?lvl=4&lvlid=54. Accessed March 3, 2023.

Depression in Racial and Ethnic Minorities

MENTAL AND BEHAVIORAL HEALTH IN HISPANICS

- In 2019, suicide was the second leading cause of death for Hispanics aged 15–34.
- Suicide attempts for Hispanic girls in grades 9–12 were 30 percent higher than those for non-Hispanic White girls in the same age group, in 2019.
- The poverty level affects mental health status. Hispanics living below the poverty level, as compared to Hispanics over twice the poverty level, are twice as likely to report serious psychological distress.

Tables 17.13–17.16 show the percentage of Hispanic adults aged 18 and above who took medications or underwent treatment for psychological distress or depression.

Mental Health Status

Table 17.13. Serious Psychological Distress in the Past Year among Adults 18 Years of Age and Over, Percentage, 2019

Hispanic	Non-Hispanic White	Hispanic/Non-Hispanic White Ratio
58.0%	70.2	0.8

(Source: Substance Abuse and Mental Health Services Administration (SAMHSA), 2020. Results from the 2019 National Survey on Drug Use and Health: Mental Health Detailed Tables. Table 10.43B (www.samhsa.gov/data/report/2019-nsduh-detailed-tables).)

Access to Health Care

Table 17.14. Percentage of Adults Aged 18 and Over Who Received Mental Health Services in the Past Year, 2019

Hispanic	Non-Hispanic White	Hispanic/Non-Hispanic White Ratio
9.7%	19.8%	0.5

(Source: Substance Abuse and Mental Health Services Administration (SAMHSA), 2020. Results from the 2019 National Survey on Drug Use and Health: Mental Health Detailed Tables. Table 8.17B (www.samhsa.gov/data/report/2019-nsduh-detailed-tables).)

Table 17.15. Percentage of Adults Aged 18 and Over Who Received Prescription Medications for Mental Health Services, 2019

Hispanic	Non-Hispanic White	Hispanic/Non-Hispanic White Ratio
7.3%	16.6%	0.4

(Source: Substance Abuse and Mental Health Services Administration (SAMHSA), 2020. Results from the 2019 National Survey on Drug Use and Health: Mental Health Detailed Tables. Table 8.37B (www.samhsa.gov/data/report/2019-nsduh-detailed-tables).)

Table 17.16. Percentage of Adults Aged 18 and Over with a Past Year Major Depressive Episode Who Received Treatment for Depression, 2019[4]

Hispanic	Non-Hispanic White	Hispanic/Non-Hispanic White Ratio
58.0%	70.2%	0.8

(Source: Substance Abuse and Mental Health Services Administration (SAMHSA), 2020. Results from the 2019 National Survey on Drug Use and Health: Mental Health Detailed Tables. Table 8.39B (www.samhsa.gov/data/report/2019-nsduh-detailed-tables).)

AFRICAN AMERICANS AND LATINOS ARE MORE LIKELY TO BE AT RISK OF DEPRESSION THAN WHITES

A study published in the May 2018 issue of *Preventive Medicine* shows that African Americans and Latinos are significantly more likely to experience serious depression than Whites, but chronic stress does not seem to explain these differences. Dr. Eliseo J. Pérez-Stable, director of the National Institute on Minority Health and Health Disparities (NIMHD), was the senior author of the study, which also found that African Americans and Latinos were more likely to have higher levels of chronic stress and more unhealthy behaviors. The NIMHD is part of the National Institutes of Health.

To examine the relationship between unhealthy behaviors, chronic stress, and risk of depression by race and ethnicity, researchers used data collected from 12,272 participants aged 40–70 years from 2005 to 2012. These data were part of the National Health

---

[4] Office of Minority Health (OMH), "Mental and Behavioral Health–Hispanics," U.S. Department of Health and Human Services (HHS), May 20, 2021. Available online. URL: https://minorityhealth.hhs.gov/omh/browse.aspx?lvl=4&lvlid=69. Accessed March 3, 2023.

and Nutrition Examination Survey (NHANES), a nationally representative health interview and examination survey of U.S. adults. This age range population was selected for this study to capture the effects of chronic stress over the lifetime of the participants.

"Understanding the social and behavioral complexities associated with depression and unhealthy behaviors by race/ethnicity can help us understand how to best improve overall health," said Dr. Pérez-Stable.

The unhealthy behaviors examined were current cigarette smoking, excessive or binge drinking, insufficient exercise, and a fair or poor diet. The researchers measured chronic stress using 10 objective biological measures, including blood pressure, body mass index, and total cholesterol. The researchers assessed the risk of depression using results from the Patient Health Questionnaire 9 (PHQ-9).

Chronic stress during adulthood may be an important factor in depression. This effect may be worse among racial and ethnic minorities due to the stress experienced from social and economic inequalities, but the relationships between race/ethnicity, stress, behavior, and depression are not well understood. A theoretical framework called the "environmental affordances model" has been proposed to explain how chronic stress and risk behaviors interact to affect health. This model proposes, for example, that engaging in unhealthy behaviors actually reduces the effects of chronic stress on depression in African Americans.

The investigators designed this research to gain a better understanding of the relationship between chronic stress and the chance of depression by race and ethnicity. The study asked whether unhealthy behaviors (current smoking, excessive or binge drinking, insufficient exercise, and fair or poor diet) reduce the chance of depression due to chronic stress in African Americans but increase the chance of depression due to chronic stress in Latinos, compared with Whites.

On average, Latinos and African Americans had more chronic stress, more unhealthy behaviors, and more chance of depression. However, the study found that engaging in more unhealthy behaviors was strongly associated with a greater chance of depression only in African Americans and Whites.

The study also found that for all three groups:
- the level of chronic stress did not affect the relationship between unhealthy behavior and the chance of depression
- unhealthy behaviors did not alter the association between stress and the chance of depression
- more education offered more protection against depression

Contrary to previous research, this study found that in all three racial/ethnic groups, chronic stress levels were inversely related to excessive or binge drinking (i.e., more stress, less excess drinking). This study also found no evidence—as some previous research has suggested—that African Americans engage in unhealthy behaviors as a way to cope with chronic stress and reduce depression or that unhealthy behaviors interact with chronic stress in Latinos to increase depression.[5]

---

[5] News and Events, "African Americans and Latinos Are More Likely to Be at Risk for Depression than Whites," National Institutes of Health (NIH), May 24, 2018. Available online. URL: www.nih.gov/news-events/news-releases/african-americans-latinos-are-more-likely-be-risk-depression-whites. Accessed March 27, 2023.

Chapter 18 | Depression and Mental Health Challenges in Sexually Diverse and Gender-Diverse Populations

Most lesbian, gay, bisexual, and transgender (LGBT) youth are happy and thrive during their adolescent years. Having a school that creates a safe and supportive learning environment for all students and having caring and accepting parents are especially important. Positive environments can help all youth achieve good grades and maintain good mental and physical health. However, some LGBT youth are more likely than their heterosexual peers to experience negative health and life outcomes.

For youth to thrive in schools and communities, they need to feel socially, emotionally, and physically safe and supported. A positive school climate has been associated with decreased depression, suicidal feelings, substance use, and unexcused school absences among LGBT students.[1]

---

[1] "LGBTQ+ Youth," Centers for Disease Control and Prevention (CDC), February 23, 2023. Available online. URL: www.cdc.gov/lgbthealth/youth.htm. Accessed March 22, 2023.

MENTAL HEALTH CHALLENGES IN GAY AND BISEXUAL MEN

The majority of gay and bisexual men have and maintain good mental health, even though research has shown that they are at a greater risk of mental health problems. Like everyone else, the majority of gay and bisexual men are able to cope successfully if connected to the right resources.

However, ongoing homophobia, stigma (negative and usually unfair beliefs), and discrimination (treating a person or group of people unfairly) can have negative effects on their health. Research also shows that compared to other men, gay and bisexual men have higher chances of having:

- major depression
- bipolar disorder
- generalized anxiety disorder

Gay and bisexual men may also face other health threats that usually happen along with mental health problems. These include more use of illegal drugs and a greater risk of suicide. Gay and bisexual men are more likely than other men to have tried to commit suicide as well as to have succeeded at suicide. Human immunodeficiency virus (HIV) is another issue that has had a huge impact on the mental health of gay and bisexual men. It affects men who are living with HIV, those who are at high risk but HIV-negative, and loved ones of those living with or who have died from HIV.

Revealing Sexual Orientation

Keeping your sexual orientation hidden from others (being "in the closet") and fear of having your sexual orientation disclosed (being "outed") can add to the stress of being gay or bisexual. In general, research has shown that gay and bisexual men who are open about their sexual orientation with others have better health outcomes than gay and bisexual men who do not. However, being "out" in some settings and to people who react negatively can add to the stress experienced by gay and bisexual men and can lead to poorer mental health and discrimination.[2]

---

[2] "Mental Health," Centers for Disease Control and Prevention (CDC), February 29, 2016. Available online. URL: www.cdc.gov/msmhealth/mental-health.htm. Accessed March 3, 2023.

HOUSEHOLD PULSE SURVEY AND MENTAL HEALTH

Regardless of age, LGBT adults have consistently reported higher rates of symptoms of both anxiety and depression than non-LGBT adults during the COVID-19 pandemic, according to a new analysis of the U.S. Census Bureau's experimental Household Pulse Survey (HPS).

The HPS provides insight into respondents' mental health and well-being.

Since the HPS began in April 2020, it has asked two questions related to symptoms of anxiety and two questions about symptoms of depression.

In July 2021, it added questions about sexual orientation and gender identity (SOGI).

This analysis relies on data from two different collection phases of the survey to assess the pandemic's mental health toll on U.S. adults 18 years and older:

- **Phase 3.2.** July 21–October 20, 2021 (approximately 6.2 million invitations sent, 382,908 responses, response rate of 6.1%)
- **Phase 3.5.** June 1–August 8, 2022 (approximately 3.1 million invitations sent, 167,931 responses, response rate of 5.3%)

The reason these collection cycles were selected are as follows: Phase 3.2 was the first one to include SOGI questions, and Phase 3.5 covered a period about a year later and further from the onset of the COVID-19 pandemic.

Mental Health Challenges and Age

LGBT respondents to the HPS are younger on average than non-LGBT respondents. Approximately 40 percent of LGBT respondents in Phase 3.5 were between ages 18 and 29, compared with only about 13 percent of non-LGBT respondents (see Figure 18.1).

Conversely, adults aged 65 and older made up only about 7 percent of LGBT respondents but nearly a quarter of non-LGBT respondents.

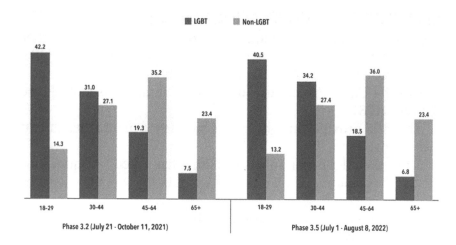

Figure 18.1. Percentage of U.S. Adults by Age and LGBT Status

U.S. Census Bureau, Household Pulse Survey Public Use Files, 2021–2022

According to the survey, younger respondents, whether they are LGBT or non-LGBT, struggled more with both anxiety and depression symptoms, but younger LGBT respondents struggled the most (see Figure 18.2).

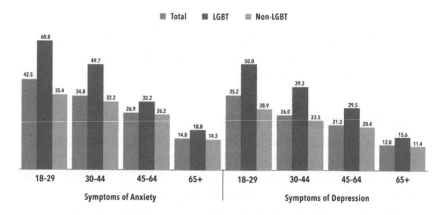

Figure 18.2. Percentage of U.S. Adults with Symptoms of Anxiety and Depression by Age and LGBT Status: June 1–August 8, 2022

U.S. Census Bureau, Household Pulse Survey Public Use Files, 2022

Sexually Diverse and Gender-Diverse Populations

In Phase 3.5, about 35 percent of non-LGBT respondents aged 18–29 reported symptoms of anxiety, compared with 61 percent of LGBT respondents in this age group.

In contrast, only about 14 percent of non-LGBT and 19 percent of LGBT respondents aged 65 and up reported anxiety symptoms.

LGBT respondents reported higher levels of anxiety symptoms than non-LGBT respondents in all age groups.

The survey's findings were similar for those who reported symptoms of depression. Half of LGBT respondents aged 18–29 reported symptoms of depression, compared with about 29 percent of non-LGBT respondents in this age group.

Depression symptoms also declined with age—about 16 percent of LGBT respondents and 11 percent of non-LGBT respondents aged 65 and older in this group reported feeling depressed.

LGBT adults reported higher levels of anxiety and depression symptoms than non-LGBT respondents in both Phases 3.2 and 3.5 of the survey, indicating the persistence of these disparities over time, even multiple years into the COVID-19 pandemic.

As Figure 18.3 illustrates, younger LGBT respondents (about 60%) in both phases were more likely to report anxiety symptoms than older LGBT respondents.

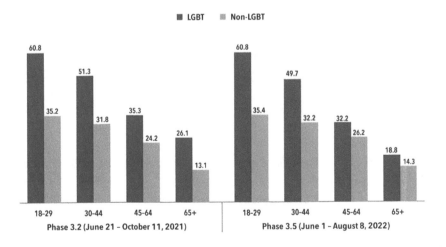

Figure 18.3. Percentage of U.S. Adults with Symptoms of Anxiety by Age and LGBT Status

U.S. Census Bureau, Household Pulse Survey Public Use Files, 2021–2022

Depression Sourcebook, Sixth Edition

Anxiety symptoms among LGBT respondents 65 and older abated somewhat as the pandemic progressed: About 26 percent reported anxiety symptoms in Phase 3.2, compared to only 19 percent in Phase 3.5.

Figure 18.4 shows results for depression symptoms. In both phases of the survey, at least half of young LGBT respondents reported depression symptoms, but the share of those 65 and older with depression symptoms decreased from about a quarter during Phase 3.2 to about 16 percent during Phase 3.5.

Taken together, these findings reveal how symptoms of anxiety and depression vary across age groups by LGBT status and over time.

Younger adults, especially LGBT adults, were the most susceptible to both conditions. Conversely, older, non-LGBT adults were less likely to report either anxiety or depression symptoms.[3]

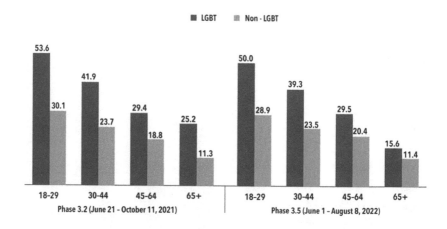

Figure 18.4. Percentage of U.S. Adults with Symptoms of Depression by Age and LGBT Status

U.S. Census Bureau, Household Pulse Survey Public Use Files, 2021–2022

---

[3] "Mental Health Struggles Higher among LGBT Adults than Non-LGBT Adults in All Age Groups," United States Census Bureau, December 14, 2022. Available online. URL: www.census.gov/library/stories/2022/12/lgbt-adults-report-anxiety-depression-at-all-ages.html. Accessed March 3, 2023.

Sexually Diverse and Gender-Diverse Populations

KEYS TO MAINTAINING GOOD MENTAL HEALTH IN LGBT YOUTH
What Schools Can Do

Schools can implement evidence-based policies, procedures, and activities designed to promote a healthy environment for all youth, including LGBT students. For example, research has shown that in schools with LGBT support groups (such as gay–straight alliances), LGBT students were less likely to experience threats of violence, miss school because they felt unsafe, or attempt suicide than those students in schools without LGBT support groups. A recent study found that LGBT students had fewer suicidal thoughts and attempts when schools had gay–straight alliances and policies prohibiting the expression of homophobia in place for three or more years.

To help promote health and safety among LGBT youth, schools can implement the following policies and practices:

- Encourage respect for all students and prohibit bullying, harassment, and violence against all students.
- Identify "safe spaces," such as counselors' offices or designated classrooms, where LGBT youth can receive support from administrators, teachers, or other school staff.
- Encourage student-led and student-organized school clubs that promote a safe, welcoming, and accepting school environment (e.g., gay–straight alliances or gender and sexuality alliances, which are school clubs open to youth of all sexual orientations and genders).
- Ensure that health curricula or educational materials include HIV, other sexually transmitted disease (STD), and pregnancy prevention information that is relevant to LGBT youth (such as ensuring that curricula or materials use language and terminology).
- Provide training to school staff on how to create safe and supportive school environments for all students, regardless of sexual orientation or gender identity, and encourage staff to attend the training.
- Facilitate access to community-based providers who have experience providing health services, including HIV/STD testing and counseling, social services, and psychological services to LGBT youth.

What Parents Can Do

Positive parenting practices, such as having honest and open conversations, can help reduce teen health risk behaviors. How parents engage with their LGBT teen can have a tremendous impact on their adolescent's current and future mental and physical health. Supportive and accepting parents can help youth cope with the challenges of being an LGBT teen. On the other hand, unsupportive parents who react negatively to learning that their daughter or son is LGBT can make it harder for their teen to thrive. Parental rejection has been linked to depression, use of drugs and alcohol, and risky sexual behavior among teens.

To be supportive, parents should talk openly and supportively with their teens about any problems or concerns. It is also important for parents to watch for behaviors that might indicate their teen is a victim of bullying or violence or that their teen may be victimizing others. If bullying, violence, or depression is suspected, parents should take immediate action, working with school personnel and other adults in the community.

WAYS PARENTS CAN INFLUENCE THE HEALTH OF THEIR LGBT YOUTH

More research is needed to better understand the associations between parenting and the health of LGBT youth. The following are research-based steps parents can take to support the health and well-being of their LGBT teen:

- **Talk and listen.** Parents who talk with and listen to their teen in a way that invites an open discussion about sexual orientation can help their teen feel loved and supported. Parents should have honest conversations with their teens about sex and how to avoid risky behaviors and unsafe situations.
- **Provide support.** Parents who take time to come to terms with how they feel about their teen's sexual orientation will be more able to respond calmly and use respectful language. Parents should develop common goals with their teen, including being healthy and doing well in school.

Sexually Diverse and Gender-Diverse Populations

- **Stay involved.** Parents who make an effort to know their teen's friends and know what their teen is doing can help their teen stay safe and feel cared about.
- **Be proactive.** Parents can access many organizations and online information resources to learn more about how they can support their LGBT teen, other family members, and their teen's friends.[4]

---

[4] See footnote [1].

Chapter 19 | Workplace Stress and Depression

WORKPLACE STRESS: UNDERSTANDING THE PROBLEM

Stress can increase loneliness, isolation, uncertainty, grief, fear, and other mental health challenges and can be harmful to our health. The amount and type of stress experienced vary from person to person due to many factors, including those experienced at work.

While there are many things in life that induce stress, work can be one of those factors. Workplace stress and poor mental health can negatively affect workers through their job performance and productivity, as well as their engagement with others at work. It can also impact workers' physical health, given that stress can be a risk factor for various cardiovascular diseases. However, workplaces can also be a key place for resources, solutions, and activities designed to improve our mental health and well-being.

Work has always presented various stresses. Workers are constantly dealing with new stressors introduced to the workplace, and in some instances, these stressors have amplified other issues at work. More than 80 percent of U.S. workers have reported experiencing workplace stress, and more than 50 percent believe their stress related to work impacts their life at home.

Workplace stressors may include:
- concerns about job security (e.g., potential layoffs, reductions in assigned hours)
- lack of access to the tools and equipment needed to perform work safely
- fear of employer retaliation

- facing confrontations from customers, patients, coworkers, supervisors, or employers
- adapting to new or different workspace and schedule or work rules
- having to learn new or different tasks or take on more responsibilities
- having to work more frequent or extended shifts or being unable to take adequate breaks
- physically demanding work
- learning new communication tools and dealing with technical difficulties
- blurring of work–life boundaries, making it hard for workers to disconnect from the office
- finding ways to work while simultaneously caring for children, including overseeing online schooling or juggling other caregiving responsibilities while trying to work, such as caring for sick, elderly, or disabled household members
- concerns about work performance and productivity
- concerns about the safety of using public transit as a commuting option

These, and many other, work-related stressors can take a toll on a person's sense of well-being and negatively impact their mental health. For some, these stressors can contribute to serious problems, such as the development or exacerbation of mental health challenges (e.g., anxiety disorder, depression disorder, or substance use disorders). Psychologists and psychiatrists are sounding the alarm about a mental health crisis forming, and data supporting their concerns have started to emerge. As one example, survey results from the Centers for Disease Control and Prevention (CDC) suggest that about 40 percent of U.S. adults were experiencing negative mental or behavioral health effects in June 2020, including symptoms of anxiety disorder or depressive disorder, trauma-related symptoms, new or increased substance use, or suicidal thoughts. An article published by the National Safety Council in August 2020 detailing a spike in opioid overdoses further highlights the need for more mental health resources.

Workplace Stress and Depression

Because of many potential stressors workers may be experiencing, a comprehensive approach is needed to address stressors throughout the community, and employers can be part of the solution. More than 85 percent of employees surveyed in 2021 by the American Psychological Association reported that actions from their employer would help their mental health. The goal is to find ways to alleviate or remove stressors in the workplace to the greatest extent possible, build coping and resilience supports, and ensure that people who need help know where to turn.[1]

MENTAL HEALTH IN THE WORKPLACE
Mental Health Issues Affect Businesses and Their Employees
Poor mental health and stress can negatively affect employees in the following ways:
- job performance and productivity
- engagement with one's work
- communication with coworkers
- physical capability and daily functioning

Mental illnesses, such as depression, are associated with higher rates of disability and unemployment.
- Depression interferes with a person's ability to complete physical job tasks about 20 percent of the time and reduces cognitive performance about 35 percent of the time.
- Only 57 percent of employees who report moderate depression and 40 percent of those who report severe depression receive treatment to control depression symptoms.

Even after taking other health risks—such as smoking and obesity—into account, employees at high risk of depression had the highest health-care costs during the three years after an initial health risk assessment.

---

[1] "Workplace Stress - Understanding the Problem," Occupational Safety and Health Administration (OSHA), October 25, 2022. Available online. URL: www.osha.gov/workplace-stress/understanding-the-problem. Accessed March 29, 2023.

STRATEGIES FOR MANAGING MENTAL HEALTH AND STRESS IN THE WORKPLACE

What Can Health-Care Providers Do?

- Ask patients about any depression or anxiety and recommend screenings, treatment, and services as appropriate.
- Include clinical psychologists, social workers, physical and occupational therapists, and other allied health professionals as part of core treatment teams to provide comprehensive, holistic care.

What Can Federal and State Governments Do?

- Provide tool kits and materials for organizations and employers delivering mental health and stress management education.
- Provide courses, guidance, and decision-making tools to help people manage their mental health and well-being.
- Collect data on workers' well-being and conduct prevention and biomedical research to guide ongoing public health innovations.
- Promote strategies designed to reach people in underserved communities, such as the use of community health workers to help patients access mental health and substance abuse prevention services from local community groups (e.g., churches and community centers).

What Can Employers Do?

- Make mental health self-assessment tools available to all employees.
- Offer free or subsidized clinical screenings for depression from a qualified mental health professional, followed by directed feedback and clinical referral when appropriate.
- Offer health insurance with no or low out-of-pocket costs for depression medications and mental health counseling.

Workplace Stress and Depression

- Provide free or subsidized lifestyle coaching, counseling, or self-management programs.
- Distribute materials, such as brochures, flyers, and videos, to all employees about the signs and symptoms of poor mental health and opportunities for treatment.
- Host seminars or workshops that address depression and stress management techniques, such as mindfulness, breathing exercises, and meditation, to help employees reduce anxiety and stress and improve focus and motivation.
- Create and maintain dedicated, quiet spaces for relaxation activities.
- Provide managers with training to help them recognize the signs and symptoms of stress and depression in team members and encourage them to seek help from qualified mental health professionals.
- Give employees opportunities to participate in decisions about issues that affect job stress.

What Can Employees Do?
- Encourage employers to offer mental health and stress management education and programs that meet their needs and interests if they are not already in place.
- Participate in employer-sponsored programs and activities to learn skills and get the support they need to improve their mental health.
- Serve as dedicated wellness champions and participate in training on topics such as financial planning and how to manage unacceptable behaviors and attitudes in the workplace as a way to help others when appropriate.
- Share personal experiences with others to help reduce stigma, when appropriate.
- Be open-minded about the experiences and feelings of colleagues. Respond with empathy, offer peer support, and encourage others to seek help.
- Adopt behaviors that promote stress management and mental health.

- Eat healthy, well-balanced meals, exercise regularly, and get seven to eight hours of sleep a night.
- Take part in activities that promote stress management and relaxation, such as yoga, meditation, mindfulness, or tai chi.
- Build and nurture real-life, face-to-face social connections.
- Take the time to reflect on positive experiences and express happiness and gratitude.
- Set and work toward personal, wellness, and work-related goals and ask for help when it is needed.[2]

---

[2] "Mental Health in the Workplace," Centers for Disease Control and Prevention (CDC), April 10, 2019. Available online. URL: www.cdc.gov/workplacehealthpromotion/tools-resources/workplace-health/mental-health/index.html. Accessed March 29, 2023.

Chapter 20 | Depression and Mental Health in Correctional Facilities

Inmates often view depression as a personal weakness, and they can be reluctant to discuss their feelings because of the stigma associated with a mental health problem. Clinicians, nursing staff, and social work staff can help alleviate the stress felt by inmates diagnosed with depression by emphasizing that depression is a common and highly treatable medical condition.[1]

As corrections staff across the United States struggle to keep up with the rapid influx of new inmates while maintaining a secure environment, their efforts are increasingly hampered by the presence of individuals with serious mental illnesses who are entering corrections facilities in growing numbers. Numerous studies show that jail detainees have a significantly higher rate of serious mental illness (e.g., bipolar disorder, major depression, schizophrenia, and other psychoses) than the general population. One pair of studies reported that approximately 6 percent of men and 15 percent of women who were admitted to Chicago's Cook County jail displayed severe symptoms of mental illness and required treatment.

Many serious mental illnesses are chronic and are subject to exacerbation and relapse. The stress of incarceration can worsen symptoms in persons with preexisting mental disorders, leading to acute psychiatric disturbances, including harm to self or others;

---

[1] "Management of Major Depressive Disorder," Federal Bureau of Prisons (BOP), May 2014. Available online. URL: www.bop.gov/resources/pdfs/depression.pdf. Accessed March 16, 2023.

inmates with histories of severe mental illness may present an even greater risk. Moreover, several studies have shown that inmates with psychiatric impairment may exhibit more serious and more numerous adjustment and disciplinary problems (such as refusal to leave one's cell or destruction of property) during incarceration than unimpaired inmates.

Prisons and jails have a substantial legal obligation to provide health and mental health care for inmates. Case law and statutes have not provided a clear definition of what constitutes adequate mental health care. The American Psychiatric Association (APA) has, however, recommended that all corrections facilities provide at minimum mental health screening, referral, and evaluation; crisis intervention and short-term treatment (most often medication); and discharge and prerelease planning. A national survey of 1,706 U.S. jails reported that 83 percent of them provide some form of initial screening for mental health treatment needs. Still, screening procedures are highly variable; they may consist of anything from one or two questions about previous treatment to a detailed, structured mental status examination. One result of this variability is apparent in data that showed fully 63 percent of inmates who were found to have acute mental symptoms through independently administered testing were missed by routine screening performed by jail staff and remained untreated.

Clearly, there is a pressing need to develop valid and reliable procedures to screen incoming detainees for signs and symptoms of acute psychiatric disturbance and disorder.

Researchers funded by the National Institute of Justice (NIJ) have created and tested two brief mental health screening tools and found that they are likely to work well in correctional settings. These tools are the Correctional Mental Health Screen (CMHS) and the Brief Jail Mental Health Screen (BJMHS).

- **CMHS**. The CMHS uses separate questionnaires for men and women. The version for women (CMHS–W) consists of eight yes/no questions, and the version for men (CMHS–M) contains 12 yes/no questions about current and lifetime indications of serious mental disorder. Six questions regarding symptoms and history of mental illness are the same on both questionnaires; the remaining questions are unique to each gender screen. Each screen takes about three to five minutes to administer. It is recommended that male inmates who answer six or more questions with "yes" and female inmates who answer five or more questions with "yes" be referred for further evaluation.

- **BJMHS.** The BJMHS has eight yes/no questions, takes about two to three minutes, and requires minimal training to administer. It asks six questions about current mental disorders plus two questions about the history of hospitalization and medication for mental or emotional problems. Inmates who answer "yes" to two or more questions about current symptoms or answer "yes" to either of the other two questions are referred for further evaluation. Instructions for administering the screen appear on the back of the form. Corrections classification officers, intake staff, or nursing staff can administer the screen without specialized mental health training but may receive brief informal training before administration.

CRITERIA FOR DETECTING MENTAL ILLNESS IN JAILS

When inmates enter a corrections facility, the staff's first task is to separate out those who may be at significant risk for suicide, acute psychotic breakdown, or complications from recent substance abuse from those who are merely experiencing varying degrees of distress usually associated with arrest, conviction, and detention.

Effective mental health triage in the corrections setting can be viewed as a three-stage process: routine, systematic, and universal mental health screening performed by corrections staff during the intake or classification stage to identify those inmates who may need closer monitoring and mental health assessment for a severe mental disorder; a more in-depth assessment by trained mental health personnel conducted within 24 hours of a positive screen; and a full-scale psychiatric evaluation when an inmate's degree of acute disturbances warrants it.

Screening is the crucial part of the process because it is the primary means by which staff can determine which inmates require more specialized mental health assessment or evaluation, as well as treatment. Unless inmates are identified as potentially needing mental health treatment, they will not receive it.

Screening, however, is the weak link and, as already noted, varies considerably. Until now, there were no valid, standardized tools available that could be recommended for adoption nationwide.

A valid standard screen needs to be brief because corrections classification staff have only a limited amount of time to spend with any one inmate. It also needs to provide explicit decision criteria because the mental health training and experience of corrections staff are likely to be relatively low. Corrections staff traditionally are confident in their ability to discern overtly psychotic symptoms but are considerably more uncertain about identifying less obvious—though equally serious—signs and symptoms of depression. Thus, they need a tool that can provide them with the basis for a clear decision ("refer" or "do not refer").

A useful jail mental health screen also needs to exhibit a low false-negative rate—that is, it would not miss many inmates who have a serious mental disorder because the potential consequences of not treating an inmate with a serious mental illness could be grave. On the other hand, it must have a low false-positive rate too because mental health resources in corrections settings are scarce, and burdening trained mental health staff with the need to assess many people who do not have a serious mental illness is an inefficient use of their time. Thus, an effective mental health screening tool would have a high degree of predictive validity, in that most of the people who are flagged by it as being "positive" should, on further assessment, be found to have a treatable serious mental illness.[2]

---

[2] "A Journey Toward Health and Hope," Office of Justice Programs (OJP), May 2007. Available online. URL: www.ojp.gov/pdffiles1/nij/216152.pdf. Accessed March 16, 2023.

Part 4 | Risk Factors for Depression: Genetics, Trauma, and More

Chapter 21 | Factors That Affect Depression Risk

Chapter Contents
Section 21.1—Genetic and Environmental
　　　　　　Risk Factors... 157
Section 21.2—Probing the Depression–
　　　　　　Rumination Cycle 161

Section 21.1 | Genetic and Environmental Risk Factors

The exact cause of depression is unknown. It may be caused by a combination of genetic, biological, environmental, and psychological factors. Everyone is different, but the following factors may increase a person's chances of becoming depressed:
- having blood relatives who have had depression
- experiencing traumatic or stressful events, such as physical or sexual abuse, the death of a loved one, or financial problems
- going through a major life change, even if it was planned
- having a medical problem, such as cancer, stroke, or chronic pain
- taking certain medications
- using alcohol or drugs

Talk to your doctor if you have questions about whether your medications might be making you feel depressed.[1]

CAUSES OF DEPRESSION

Depression is known to run in families, suggesting that genetic factors contribute to the risk of developing this disease. However, research into the genetics of depression is in its early stages, and very little is known for certain about the genetic basis of the disease. Studies suggest that variations in many genes, each with a small effect, combine to increase the risk of developing depression.

Genetic Factors

Determining the genetic risk factors for depression is challenging for several reasons. It is possible that what is currently considered to be a single disease called "depression" is actually multiple disorders

---

[1] "Mental Health Conditions: Depression and Anxiety," Centers for Disease Control and Prevention (CDC), September 14, 2022. Available online. URL: www.cdc.gov/tobacco/campaign/tips/diseases/depression-anxiety.html. Accessed March 7, 2023.

with similar signs and symptoms; these disorders could have different genetic risk factors. The genetic variations related to depression may also be somewhat different between men and women. Researchers suspect that studies with many more people will be required to pinpoint the genetic variations that influence the risk of depression.

The genes thought to be associated with depression have diverse functions in the brain. Some of these genes may control the production (synthesis), transport, and activity of chemicals called "neurotransmitters," which relay chemical signals that allow nerve cells (neurons) to communicate with one another. Other genes that may influence the risk of depression are involved in the growth, maturation, and maintenance of neurons, as well as the ability of the connections between neurons (synapses) to change and adapt over time in response to experience, a characteristic known as "synaptic plasticity."

Nongenetic Factors

Nongenetic (environmental) factors also play critical roles in a person's risk of developing depression. The disorder can be triggered by substance abuse, certain medications, or stressful life events (such as divorce or the death of a loved one). Other risk factors include difficulties in relationships or social isolation, unemployment, financial problems, and childhood abuse or neglect. Some physical illnesses, such as cancer, thyroid disease, and chronic pain, are also associated with an increased risk of developing depression. It is likely that environmental conditions interact with genetic factors to determine the overall risk of developing this disease.[2]

A STUDY ON RISK AND PROTECTIVE FACTORS

Depression is a common, serious mood disorder. Everyone feels sad or lonely sometimes. But, if you have depression, these feelings go on for long periods of time. You may feel hopeless or pessimistic,

---

[2] MedlinePlus, "Depression," National Institutes of Health (NIH), April 1, 2018. Available online. URL: https://medlineplus.gov/genetics/condition/depression/#genes. Accessed March 7, 2023.

Factors That Affect Depression Risk

feel irritable, or have decreased energy or fatigue. You might stop enjoying your hobbies and normal activities and have difficulty concentrating, remembering things, or making decisions.

Experiencing trauma early in life and having certain genes can put you at a higher risk of depression. But there are actions that can help protect against depression, such as eating a healthy diet and getting enough sleep and physical activity.

A research team led by Dr. Karmel W. Choi, a clinical and research fellow at Massachusetts General Hospital, and Jordan W. Smoller, M.D., Sc.D., who is a professor of psychiatry at Harvard University, analyzed 106 factors in people's daily lives to see whether they could find other factors that affect depression risk. The work was funded in part by the National Institute of Mental Health (NIMH) of the National Institutes of Health (NIH). Results were published on August 14, 2020, in the *American Journal of Psychiatry*.

The team applied a novel, two-stage approach to identify factors that can affect the risk of developing depression. In the first stage, they screened a wide range of lifestyle and environmental factors for links with depression in more than 112,000 older British adults. They looked at behaviors and social factors that people are able to change, including exercise, sleep, television and computer use, diet, social activities, and social support. Environmental factors included how much green space and noise or air pollution the people lived around. Depression was assessed in the participants at a follow-up survey about six to eight years later.

The researchers found 18 factors linked with lower chances of depression and 11 with higher chances. Those that showed the greatest protection included confiding in others, sleep duration, engaging in exercises such as swimming or cycling, a faster walking pace, being part of a sports club or gym, and eating cereal. Factors that had the highest associations with depression were daytime napping; how much time people spend using the computer, watching television, or using a cell phone; and eating a healthy diet inconsistently.

To find out which actions might be most helpful for people at high risk of depression, researchers divided the participants into three groups: those with genetic risk factors for depression, those who experienced early-life trauma, and those without these known risk factors for depression.

For people with genetic risk factors for depression, frequency of confiding in others and sleep duration were the most protective. How much time they spent on the computer and how much salt they consumed showed the highest increase in risk of depression.

For those who experienced traumatic life events, the frequency of confiding in others, engaging in exercises such as swimming or cycling, and sleep duration showed the most protective effects. The factor that most increased the risk of depression was how much television they watched.

For the second stage of the study, the team used a method called "Mendelian randomization" to narrow down the list to those factors with a causal connection to depression risk. Confiding in others appeared to have the strongest protective effect on depression across all three groups. Visiting with family and friends also appeared to have a protective effect, suggesting that social interactions may be key to reducing the risk of depression. Television use increased the risk the most.

"Depression takes an enormous toll on individuals, families, and society, yet we still know very little about how to prevent it," Dr. Smoller says. "We've shown that it's now possible to address these questions of broad public health significance through a large-scale, data-based approach that wasn't available even a few years ago. We hope this work will motivate further efforts to develop actionable strategies for preventing depression."

More research is needed to determine how the factors identified in this study might contribute to depression. Controlled clinical trials will be needed to test whether changing these factors can help prevent depression.[3]

---

[3] "Factors That Affect Depression Risk," National Institutes of Health (NIH), September 1, 2020. Available online. URL: www.nih.gov/news-events/nih-research-matters/factors-affect-depression-risk. Accessed March 7, 2023.

Factors That Affect Depression Risk

Section 21.2 | Probing the Depression–Rumination Cycle

Rumination is a thought process in which people obsessively focus on negative experiences and replay them over and over in their minds. It is derived from the Latin word "ruminari" or "rumen," which means the digestive system of animals that chew their cud. People who ruminate tend to chew over unpleasant situations repeatedly or brood about troubling issues constantly. Although self-reflection and analysis of past experiences can be helpful in problem-solving, rumination rarely offers new insights or leads to a better understanding of a situation. Instead, people who ruminate focus so intensely on negative feelings that they lose perspective and become unable to experience positive feelings, which can cause anxiety and depression.

RUMINATION AND DEPRESSION

Research has found links between rumination and several mental health conditions, including depression, anxiety, posttraumatic stress disorder (PTSD), substance abuse, and eating disorders. For instance, studies indicate that people who ruminate are four times more likely than other people to develop major depression. Rumination intensifies the negative feelings associated with depression, such as hopelessness, inadequacy, and worthlessness. In addition, rumination destroys self-confidence and creates uncertainty that makes people doubt their own judgment and avoid taking positive steps toward finding solutions to problems.

Rumination also reduces the level of social support available to help with personal problems. Research has shown that ruminators seek help more often than other people. Yet their persistently negative outlook and tendency to dwell on unpleasantness can create social friction and drive friends and relatives away. After a while, people being asked for support become frustrated and respond less compassionately, perhaps telling the ruminator to just forget about whatever they are obsessing over and move on with their life. The ruminator may interpret this response as rejection or abandonment, which then provides another negative experience for them to ruminate about. In this way, rumination and depression can become locked in a self-reinforcing cycle.

RUMINATION TRIGGERS

Many of the triggers for rumination are similar to those for depression. In women, grief, sadness, and regret often serve as triggers for depressive rumination. In men, anger and resentment are the most common emotions that trigger rumination. Rumination is often associated with traumatic or stressful life events, such as losing a job, experiencing the death of a loved one, or having an illness or accident.

People who are prone to rumination often share some basic personality characteristics. Many ruminators are perfectionists who struggle to cope with less-than-perfect results. Many ruminators also tend to exhibit neuroticism and place an excessive value on interpersonal relationships. Finally, ruminators are likely to feel as if they face constant sources of pressure or stress that are beyond their control. Most do not view their rumination as part of the problem but rather as a means of gaining the necessary insight to deal with their problems.

BREAKING THE RUMINATION CYCLE

Since rumination and depression can become linked in a self-perpetuating cycle, finding ways to stop ruminating can also help lighten symptoms of depression. Although depression is a medical condition that cannot be simply willed away, some people experience improvements in mood when they utilize techniques to avoid ruminating on negative thoughts and feelings. Some suggested methods of stopping or preventing rumination include the following:

- **Healthy distraction**. With practice, many ruminators can learn to recognize when they become focused on negative thoughts and experiences and employ various methods to distract themselves. Possible distraction techniques include doing chores such as vacuuming or mowing the lawn, watching a movie, taking a nap, or

Factors That Affect Depression Risk

engaging in meditation or prayer. It may also be helpful to imagine a soothing image, such as a slowly rotating fan, a babbling brook, or the details of a childhood bedroom or yard. Practicing mindfulness is another valuable distraction tool. When negative thoughts about past events intrude upon the enjoyment of the present, it may be helpful to redirect thoughts toward the immediate moment by carefully recognizing and considering what each sense is experiencing. Research has shown that distraction techniques can help reduce the time ruminators spend dwelling on and discussing negative events, which can also help improve the quality of their relationships.

- **Positive thinking.** The rumination–depression cycle works by activating neural networks in the brain that are attuned to negative thoughts and emotions. One bad memory of a negative outcome triggers additional memories of negative experiences, which leads to anxiety, self-doubt, and depression. With practice, however, many people can develop the skill of deliberately shifting their focus away from these neural networks and activating memories of positive experiences. Interrupting rumination and shifting to a network of positive thoughts can be difficult for people with depression. Some tips for accessing positive memories include asking family and friends for help and encouragement in remembering good times; listening to music associated with happy times and good moods; looking at photographs or videos of joyful experiences and trying to remember the sounds, smells, and other sensations; and physically going to a place connected with positive outcomes and states of mind. Accessing a positive neural network can provide a change of perspective and reveal new approaches to dealing with problems.
- **Planning.** Depressive ruminators tend to become immobilized by negative thoughts and feel incapable

of moving forward. They envision terrible outcomes and become afraid to try because they might fail. Breaking the cycle requires letting go of unattainable goals and things that are beyond one's control or ability to change. It may be helpful to break down a seemingly big problem into smaller, actionable pieces. Then, instead of focusing on the big problem, it may be possible to plan a series of small steps toward solving each part of the problem. Making a plan of action and achieving small goals can help increase self-confidence and decrease feelings of inadequacy and hopelessness. To avoid becoming paralyzed by inaction, it is important to view inevitable mistakes and failures as opportunities for learning and personal growth.

- **Containment**. Of course, it is not possible to keep negative thoughts at bay all of the time. But there are proven techniques for containing those thoughts, reducing their power, and preventing them from turning into harmful rumination. One way to eliminate the power of negative thoughts and insecurities is to identify and confront them directly. Keeping a journal of emotions and triggers can help clarify the source of negative thoughts. Once the underlying fear has been identified, the next step is to envision the worst-case scenario. Someone who panics at the thought of speaking in front of an audience, for instance, could picture forgetting a speech and looking foolish. In most cases, confronting the worst-case scenario helps people realize that they are resilient enough to handle it. To avoid ruminating, it may be helpful to contain negative thoughts by scheduling 15–30 minutes of worry time per day to dwell upon them. This method makes it easier to dismiss negative thoughts when they intrude at other times.
- **Therapy**. Seeing a professional counselor may be helpful for people whose rumination interferes with their enjoyment of life. Mental health professionals

can offer support, encouragement, and additional techniques and guidance to help people break out of the rumination–depression cycle and improve their mood, confidence, and self-esteem.

References

Chand, Suma. "Uplift Your Mood: Stop Ruminating," Anxiety and Depression Association of America (ADAA), 2016. Available online. URL: www.adaa.org/blog/uplift-your-mood-stop-ruminating. Accessed April 25, 2023.

Feiner, Lauren. "Eight Tips to Help Stop Ruminating," *Psych Central*, February 16, 2014. Available online. URL: http://psychcentral.com/blog/archives/2014/02/16/8-tips-to-help-stop-ruminating/. Accessed April 25, 2023.

Law, Bridget Murray. "Probing the Depression-Rumination Cycle," *APA Monitor*, November 2005, p. 38. Available online. URL: www.apa.org/monitor/nov05/cycle.aspx. Accessed April 25, 2023.

Wehrenberg, Margaret. "Rumination: A Problem in Anxiety and Depression," *Psychology Today*, April 20, 2016. Available online. URL: www.psychologytoday.com/blog/depression-management-techniques/201604/rumination-problem-in-anxiety-and-depression. Accessed April 25, 2023.

Chapter 22 | Stress as a Risk Factor for Depression

Chapter Contents
Section 22.1—Stress and Your Health 169
Section 22.2—Caregiver Stress: A Risk Factor
　　　　　　　for Depression 172
Section 22.3—Parenting Stress and Mental Health:
　　　　　　　A Strong Connection 177

Section 22.1 | **Stress and Your Health**

Stress is a normal part of life. But, if your stress does not go away or keeps getting worse, you may need help. Over time, stress can lead to serious problems such as depression or anxiety.

WHAT ARE THE SIGNS OF STRESS?
When you are under stress, you may feel:
- worried
- angry
- irritable
- depressed
- unable to focus

Stress also affects your body. Physical signs of stress include the following:
- headaches
- trouble sleeping or sleeping too much
- upset stomach
- weight gain or loss
- tense muscles

Stress can also lead to a weakened immune system (the system in the body that fights infections), which could make you more likely to get sick.

WHAT CAUSES STRESS?
Stress is how the body reacts to a challenge or demand.
Change is often a cause of stress. Even positive changes, such as having a baby or getting a job promotion, can be stressful.
Stress can be short- or long-term.
Common causes of short-term stress are as follows:
- needing to do a lot in a short amount of time
- having a lot of small problems in the same day, such as getting stuck in a traffic jam or running late

- getting ready for a work or school presentation
- having an argument

Common causes of long-term stress are as follows:
- having problems at work or at home
- having money problems
- having a long-term illness
- taking care of someone with an illness
- dealing with the death of a loved one

STRATEGIES FOR MANAGING STRESS

Over time, long-term stress can lead to health problems. Managing stress can help you:
- sleep better
- control your weight
- have less muscle tension
- be in a better mood
- get along better with family and friends

Plan and Prepare

You cannot always avoid stress, but you can take steps to deal with stress in a positive way. Follow these tips for preventing and managing stress.

Being prepared and feeling in control of your situation might help lower your stress.

Plan Your Time

Think ahead about how you are going to use your time. Write a to-do list and figure out what is most important—then do that thing first. Be realistic about how long each task will take.

Prepare Yourself

Prepare ahead for stressful events such as a hard conversation with a loved one. You can:
- picture what the room will look like and what you will say

Stress as a Risk Factor for Depression

- think about different ways the conversation could go—and how you could respond
- have a plan for ending the conversation early if you need time to think

CONSULT YOUR DOCTOR
You may make an appointment with your health-care provider:
- If you are feeling down or hopeless, talk with your doctor about depression.
- If you are feeling anxious, find out how to get help for anxiety.
- If you have lived through a traumatic event (such as a major accident, crime, or natural disaster), find out about treatment for posttraumatic stress disorder (PTSD).

A mental health professional (such as a psychologist or social worker) can help treat these conditions with talk therapy (called "psychotherapy") or medicine.

PRACTICE RELAXATION TECHNIQUES
Stress causes tension in your muscles. Try stretching or taking a hot shower to help you relax. Deep breathing and meditation can also help relax your muscles and clear your mind.

GET ACTIVE
Regular physical activity can help prevent and manage stress. It can also help relax your muscles and improve your mood. So get active:
- Aim for 150 minutes a week of moderate-intensity aerobic activity—try going for a bike ride or taking a walk.
- Do strengthening activities—such as push-ups or lifting weights—at least two days a week.

Remember, any amount of physical activity is better than none!

FOOD AND ALCOHOL

Give your body plenty of energy by eating healthy—including vegetables, fruits, grains, and proteins. Get tips for healthy eating. Avoid using alcohol or other drugs to manage stress. If you choose to drink, drink only in moderation. This means:
- one drink or less in a day for women
- two drinks or less in a day for men

GET SUPPORT

Talk to your friends and family if you are feeling stressed. They may be able to help. Finally, keep in mind that lots of people need help dealing with stress—it is nothing to be ashamed of.[1]

Section 22.2 | Caregiver Stress: A Risk Factor for Depression

WHO IS A CAREGIVER?

A caregiver is anyone who provides care for another person in need, such as a child, aging parent, husband or wife, relative, friend, or neighbor. A caregiver also may be a paid professional who provides care in the home or at a place that is not the person's home.

People who are not paid to give care are called "informal caregivers" or "family caregivers." This chapter focuses on family caregivers who provide care on a regular basis for a loved one with an injury, an illness such as dementia, or a disability. The family caregiver often has to manage the person's daily life. This can include helping with daily tasks such as bathing, eating, or taking medicine. It can also include arranging activities and making health and financial decisions. Most caregivers are women. And nearly three in five family caregivers have paid jobs in addition to their caregiving.

---

[1] Office of Disease Prevention and Health Promotion (ODPHP), "Manage Stress," U.S. Department of Health and Human Services (HHS), July 20, 2022. Available online. URL: health.gov/myhealthfinder/health-conditions/heart-health/manage-stress#the-basics_3. Accessed March 2, 2023.

Stress as a Risk Factor for Depression

WHO GETS CAREGIVER STRESS?

Anyone can get caregiver stress, but more women caregivers say they have stress and other health problems than men caregivers. And some women have a higher risk for health problems from caregiver stress, including those who do the following:

- **Care for a loved one who needs constant medical care and supervision.** Caregivers of people with Alzheimer disease (AD) or dementia are more likely to have health problems and to be depressed than caregivers of people with conditions that do not require constant care.
- **Care for a spouse.** Women who are caregivers of spouses are more likely to have high blood pressure, diabetes, and high cholesterol and are twice as likely to have heart disease as women who provide care for others, such as parents or children.

Women caregivers may also be less likely to get regular screenings, and they may not get enough sleep or regular physical activity.

WHAT ARE THE SIGNS AND SYMPTOMS OF CAREGIVER STRESS?

Caregiver stress can take many forms. For instance, you may feel frustrated and angry one minute and helpless the next. You may make mistakes when giving medicines. Or you may turn to unhealthy behaviors such as smoking or drinking too much alcohol.

Other signs and symptoms include:
- feeling overwhelmed
- feeling alone, isolated, or deserted by others
- sleeping too much or too little
- gaining or losing a lot of weight
- feeling tired most of the time
- losing interest in activities you used to enjoy
- becoming easily irritated or angered
- feeling worried or sad often
- having headaches or body aches often

Talk to your doctor about your symptoms and ways to relieve stress. Also, let others give you a break. Reach out to family, friends, or a local resource.

HOW DOES CAREGIVER STRESS AFFECT YOUR HEALTH?

Some stress can be good for you, as it helps you cope and respond to a change or challenge. But long-term stress of any kind, including caregiver stress, can lead to serious health problems.

The following are some of the ways stress affects caregivers:

- **Depression and anxiety.** Women who are caregivers are more likely than men to develop symptoms of anxiety and depression. Anxiety and depression also raise your risk for other health problems, such as heart disease and stroke.
- **Weak immune system.** Stressed caregivers may have weaker immune systems than noncaregivers and spend more days sick with the cold or flu. A weak immune system can also make vaccines such as flu shots less effective. Also, it may take longer to recover from surgery.
- **Obesity.** Stress causes weight gain in more women than men. Obesity raises your risk for other health problems, including heart disease, stroke, and diabetes.
- **Higher risk of chronic diseases.** High levels of stress, especially when combined with depression, can raise your risk of health problems, such as heart disease, cancer, diabetes, or arthritis.
- **Problems with short-term memory or paying attention.** Caregivers of spouses with AD are at a higher risk for problems with short-term memory and focusing.

Caregivers also report symptoms of stress more often than people who are not caregivers.

WHAT CAN YOU DO TO PREVENT OR RELIEVE CAREGIVER STRESS?

Taking steps to relieve caregiver stress helps prevent health problems. Also, taking care of yourself helps you take better care of your loved one and enjoy the rewards of caregiving.

Here are some tips to help you prevent or manage caregiver stress:

- **Learn ways to better help your loved one.** Some hospitals offer classes that can teach you how to care for

someone with an injury or illness. To find these classes, ask your doctor or call your local Area Agency on Aging (AAA).
- **Find caregiving resources in your community to help you.** Many communities have adult day-care services or respite services to give primary caregivers a break from their caregiving duties.
- **Ask for and accept help.** Make a list of ways others can help you. Let helpers choose what they would like to do. For instance, someone might sit with the person you care for while you do an errand. Someone else might pick up groceries for you.
- **Join a support group for caregivers.** You can find a general caregiver support group or a group with caregivers who care for someone with the same illness or disability as your loved one. You can share stories, pick up caregiving tips, and get support from others who face the same challenges as you do.
- **Get organized.** Make to-do lists and set a daily routine.
- **Take time for yourself.** Stay in touch with family and friends and do things you enjoy with your loved ones.
- **Take care of your health.** Find time to be physically active on most days of the week, choose healthy foods, and get enough sleep.
- **See your doctor for regular checkups.** Make sure to tell your doctor or nurse you are a caregiver. Also, tell them about any symptoms of depression or sickness you may have.

If you work outside the home and are feeling overwhelmed, consider taking a break from your job. Under the federal Family and Medical Leave Act (FMLA), eligible employees can take up to 12 weeks of unpaid leave per year to care for relatives. Ask your human resources office about your options.

WHAT CAREGIVING SERVICES CAN YOU FIND IN YOUR COMMUNITY?

Caregiving services include:
- meal delivery
- home health-care services, such as nursing or physical therapy
- nonmedical home care services, such as housekeeping, cooking, or companionship
- making changes to your home, such as installing ramps or modified bathtubs
- legal and financial counseling
- respite care, which is a substitute caregiving (Someone comes to your home, or you may take your loved one to an adult day-care center or day hospital.)

The National Eldercare Locator, a service of the U.S. Administration on Aging (AOA), can help you find caregiving services in your area. You can also contact your local AAA.

HOW CAN YOU PAY FOR HOME HEALTH-CARE AND OTHER CAREGIVING SERVICES?

Medicare, Medicaid, and private insurance companies will cover some costs of home health care. Other costs you will have to pay for yourself.
- If the person who needs care has insurance, check with the person's insurance provider to find out what is included in the plan.
- If the person who needs care has Medicare, find out what home health services are covered.
- If the person who needs care has Medicaid, coverage of home health services varies between states. Check with your state's Medicaid program to learn what the benefits are.

If you or the person who needs caregiving also needs health insurance, learn about the services covered under Marketplace plans at Healthcare.gov.[2]

---

[2] Office on Women's Health (OWH), "Caregiver Stress," U.S. Department of Health and Human Services (HHS), January 6, 2023. Available online. URL: www.womenshealth.gov/a-z-topics/caregiver-stress. Accessed March 13, 2023.

Stress as a Risk Factor for Depression

Section 22.3 | **Parenting Stress and Mental Health: A Strong Connection**

Parental burnout is characterized by "an overwhelming exhaustion related to one's parental role, an emotional distancing from one's children, and a sense of parental ineffectiveness." It can lead to more serious consequences such as escape ideation and neglect. Parental burnout can come as a result of many stressors—small and large—such as behavioral problems and sibling fights where the parent feels they have no more resources to help resolve these issues and become detached from their children.

Parental burnout is common even in normal circumstances. Kids can pick up on parental stress, especially infants. When children start feeling the stress of a parent, they get stressed themselves and, depending on their age, will manifest their stress and anxiety in various ways. Infants manifest stress by crying and being generally fussy. Older children may lash out, hitting or throwing objects, while others may "shut down." Some child development experts claim that parents' levels of chronic stress can seriously impact a child's development. Not to mention, when kids act out due to anxiety and stress, this can then lead to more stress for you, becoming a vicious cycle!

The first thing all parents must know is that they are not alone. Feeling overwhelmed happens to all parents at one time or another, and everyone is doing the best they can right now. The trick is to learn how to manage stressors and remain the best parent you can be. Below are some tips and resources to help relieve stress and, hopefully, help bring joy back to parenting.

- **Create a routine.** Although schedules can be hard to maintain depending on the age of your children, establishing even one routine can help set up your home for success. According to the American Academy of Pediatrics (AAP), creating healthy and consistent routines can promote more calm in the house. Even simple things such as keeping morning and bedtime routines can improve a sense of order.

- **Some screen time is okay.** While common advice is to try to limit screen time, do not feel guilty about using it if you need to do some work or to regroup while your child is occupied. You can also use screen time to bond with your children. Carving out time to watch a movie or documentary together not only can promote conversation but also can relieve stress.
- **Plan time to get active together.** A great way to relieve stress is to exercise, stretch, or move around in general. If you feel your stress level beginning to rise, take a break together! Take a brisk walk, put on some music and dance to your favorite tunes, or do some yoga or stretching. Deep breathing also relieves anxiety. Remember, it is okay to stop what you are doing, close your eyes for a few moments, and take a couple of deep breaths.
- **Go easy on yourself and practice self-care.** During stressful times, it is understandable that you may slip up on some chores. It is okay to order out food or do a simple meal. It is okay to take a longer shower than normal just to get a few minutes alone. Maybe you are a night owl; give yourself time after everyone has gone to bed to relax, meditate, or do yoga—whatever relaxes you. Wake up before everyone else and have some "me" time. Things are stressful right now, and your priority should be self-care for you and your children.
- **Do not be afraid to get outside support.** Although you may not be able to see your family and friends, they are only a phone call away. Do not be afraid to call someone you love and say you are having a hard time. It is also okay to seek professional help. There are many virtual therapy options out there, and some are even offering free or reduced prices right now to help support those in need but cannot afford the typical fees. One option is BetterHelp (www.betterhelp.com/thoughtfulhuman/), which is currently offering the first month free for anyone who needs to talk to a licensed therapist.

Stress as a Risk Factor for Depression

- **Make time to play with your kids.** Making time to play with your kids is always important, no matter the age. However, in times when their routines are off and kids may not fully understand what is happening, it is especially important to set aside time for play. Children often act out as a way to get attention from the adults in their lives. Give them that special time by finding activities to do together to engage in all sorts of play. While kids benefit from a schedule and structure, they equally benefit from unstructured playtime to be creative and stimulate their cognitive skills.

Parenting can be difficult. And it is especially hard when your normal routine has changed, and you are having to balance more responsibility at home. The most important thing you can do is self-care. You cannot take care of others if you are not well yourself. Just continue to look for ways to do the best you can and remember you are not alone.[3]

---

[3] "Parental Burnout: It Is Real and It Is Manageable," National Responsible Fatherhood Clearinghouse (NRFC), August 13, 2020. Available online. URL: www.fatherhood.gov/dadtalk-blog/parental-burnout-its-real-and-its-manageable. Accessed April 13, 2023.

Chapter 23 | Trauma as a Risk Factor for Depression

Chapter Contents
Section 23.1—Depression, Trauma, and Posttraumatic
 Stress Disorder... 183
Section 23.2—Adverse Childhood Experiences.......................... 185

Chapter 23 | Trauma as a Risk Factor

Section 23.1 | Depression, Trauma, and Posttraumatic Stress Disorder

Depression is a common problem that can occur following trauma. It involves feelings of sadness or low mood that last more than just a few days. Unlike a blue mood that comes and goes, depression is longer lasting. Depression can get in the way of daily life and make it hard to function. It can affect your eating and sleeping, how you think, and how you feel about yourself.

HOW COMMON IS DEPRESSION FOLLOWING TRAUMA?

Depression is more than just feeling sad. Most people with depression feel down or sad more days than not for at least two weeks. Or they find they no longer enjoy or have an interest in things anymore. If you have depression, you may notice that you are sleeping and eating a lot more or less than you used to. You may find it hard to stay focused. You may feel down on yourself or hopeless. With more severe depression, you may think about hurting or killing yourself.

HOW ARE DEPRESSION AND TRAUMA RELATED?

Depression can sometimes seem to come from out of the blue. It can also be caused by a stressful event such as a divorce or trauma. Trouble coping with painful experiences or losses often leads to depression. For example, veterans returning from a war zone may have painful memories and feelings of guilt or regret about their war experiences. They may have been injured or lost friends. Disaster survivors may have lost a loved one or a home or have been injured. Survivors of violence or abuse may feel like they can no longer trust other people. These kinds of experiences can lead to both depression and posttraumatic stress disorder (PTSD).

Many symptoms of depression overlap with the symptoms of PTSD. For example, with both depression and PTSD, you may have trouble sleeping or keeping your mind focused. You may not feel pleasure or interest in things you used to enjoy. You may not want to be with other people as much. Both PTSD and depression may involve greater irritability. It is quite possible to have both depression and PTSD at the same time.

WHAT COULD YOU DO ABOUT FEELINGS OF DEPRESSION?

Depression can make you feel worn out, worthless, helpless, hopeless, and sad. These feelings can make you feel as though you are never going to feel better. You may even think that you should just give up. Some symptoms of depression, such as being tired or not having the desire to do anything, can also get in the way of your treatment.

It is very important for you to know that these negative thoughts and feelings are part of depression. If you think you might be depressed, you should seek help in spite of these feelings. You can expect them to change as treatment begins working. In the meantime, here is a list of things you can do that may improve your mood:

- Talk with your doctor or health-care provider.
- Talk with your family and friends.
- Spend more time with others and get support from them. Do not close yourself off.
- Take part in activities that might make you feel better. Do the things you used to enjoy before you began feeling depressed. Even if you do not feel like it, try doing some of these things. Chances are you will feel better after you do.
- Engage in mild exercise.
- Set realistic goals for yourself.
- Break up goals and tasks into smaller ones that you can manage.

HOW IS DEPRESSION TREATED?

Depression is common in those who have PTSD. The symptoms of depression can make it hard to function and may also get in the way of your treatment.

There are many treatment options for depression. You should be assessed by a health-care professional who can decide which type

Trauma as a Risk Factor for Depression

of treatment is best for you. In many cases, milder forms of depression are treated by counseling or therapy. More severe depression is treated with medicines or with both therapy and medicine.

Research has shown that certain types of therapy and medicine are effective for both depression and PTSD. Since the symptoms of PTSD and depression can overlap, treatment that helps with PTSD may also result in improvement of depression. Cognitive-behavioral therapy (CBT) is a type of therapy that is proven effective for both problems. CBT can help patients change negative styles of thinking and acting that can lead to both depression and PTSD. A type of medicine that is effective for both depression and PTSD is a selective serotonin reuptake inhibitor (SSRI).[1]

Section 23.2 | Adverse Childhood Experiences

WHAT ARE ADVERSE CHILDHOOD EXPERIENCES?

Adverse childhood experiences (ACEs) are potentially traumatic events that occur in childhood (0–17 years), for example:
- experiencing violence, abuse, or neglect
- witnessing violence in the home or community
- having a family member attempt or die by suicide

Also included are aspects of the child's environment that can undermine their sense of safety, stability, and bonding, such as growing up in a household with:
- substance use problems
- mental health problems
- instability due to parental separation or household members being in jail or prison

---

[1] National Center for Posttraumatic Stress Disorder (NCPTSD), "Depression, Trauma, and PTSD," U.S. Department of Veterans Affairs (VA), September 22, 2022. Available online. URL: www.ptsd.va.gov/understand/related/depression_trauma.asp. Accessed March 3, 2023.

Please note the examples above are not a complete list of adverse experiences. Many other traumatic experiences could impact health and well-being.

ACEs are linked to chronic health problems, mental illness, and substance use problems in adolescence and adulthood. ACEs can also negatively impact education, job opportunities, and earning potential. However, ACEs can be prevented.

HOW BIG IS THE PROBLEM?

- Adverse childhood experiences are common. About 61 percent of adults surveyed across 25 states reported they had experienced at least one type of ACE before the age of 18, and nearly one in six reported they had experienced four or more types of ACEs.
- Preventing ACEs could potentially reduce many health conditions. For example, by preventing ACEs, up to 1.9 million heart disease cases and 21 million depression cases could have been potentially avoided.
- Some children are at a greater risk than others. Women and several racial/ethnic minority groups were at a greater risk of experiencing four or more types of ACEs.
- ACEs are costly. The economic and social costs to families, communities, and society total hundreds of billions of dollars each year. A 10 percent reduction in ACEs in North America could equate to annual savings of $56 billion.

WHAT ARE THE CONSEQUENCES?

ACEs can have lasting, negative effects on health, well-being, as well as life opportunities such as education and job potential. These experiences can increase the risks of injury, sexually transmitted infections (STIs), maternal and child health problems (including teen pregnancy, pregnancy complications, and fetal death), involvement in sex trafficking, and a wide range of chronic diseases and leading causes of death such as cancer, diabetes, heart disease, and suicide.

Trauma as a Risk Factor for Depression

ACEs and associated social determinants of health, such as living in under-resourced or racially segregated neighborhoods, frequently moving, and experiencing food insecurity, can cause toxic stress (extended or prolonged stress). Toxic stress from ACEs can negatively affect children's brain development, immune systems, and stress-response systems. These changes can affect children's attention, decision-making, and learning.

Children growing up with toxic stress may have difficulty forming healthy and stable relationships. They may also have unstable work histories as adults and struggle with finances, jobs, and depression throughout life. These effects can also be passed on to their own children. Some children may face further exposure to toxic stress from historical and ongoing traumas due to systemic racism or the impacts of poverty resulting from limited educational and economic opportunities. Figure 23.1 shows the mechanism by which ACEs influence health and well-being throughout the life span.

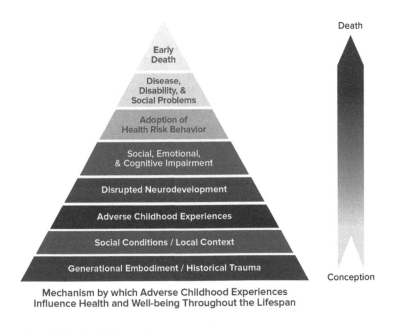

Figure 23.1. The ACE Pyramid

Centers for Disease Control and Prevention (CDC)

HOW CAN YOU PREVENT ADVERSE CHILDHOOD EXPERIENCES?

Adverse childhood experiences are preventable. To prevent ACEs, you must understand and address the factors that put people at risk of or protect them from violence.

Creating and sustaining safe, stable, and nurturing relationships and environments for all children and families can prevent ACEs and help all children reach their full potential. Table 23.1 lists the various strategies and approaches that can help in preventing ACEs.

Raising awareness of ACEs can help do the following:

- Change how people think about the causes of ACEs and who could help prevent them.
- Shift the focus from individual responsibility to community solutions.

Table 23.1. Preventing Adverse Childhood Experiences

Strategy	Approach
Strengthen economic supports to families	• Strengthening household financial security • Family-friendly work policies
Promote social norms that protect against violence and adversity	• Public education campaigns • Legislative approaches to reduce corporal punishment • Bystander approaches • Men and boys as allies in the prevention
Ensure a strong start for children	• Early childhood home visitation • High-quality childcare • Preschool enrichment with family engagement
Teach skills	• Social-emotional learning • Safe dating and healthy relationship skill programs • Parenting skills and family relationship approaches
Connect youth to caring adults and activities	• Mentoring programs • After-school programs
Intervene to lessen immediate and long-term harms	• Enhanced primary care • Victim-centered services • Treatment to lessen the harms of ACEs • Treatment to prevent problem behavior and future involvement in violence • Family-centered treatment for substance use disorders (SUDs)

Trauma as a Risk Factor for Depression

- Reduce stigma around seeking help with parenting challenges or substance misuse, depression, or suicidal thoughts.
- Promote safe, stable, and nurturing relationships and environments where children live, learn, and play.[2]

---

[2] "Fast Facts: Preventing Adverse Childhood Experiences," Centers for Disease Control and Prevention (CDC), April 6, 2022. Available online. URL: www.cdc.gov/violenceprevention/aces/fastfact.html. Accessed March 3, 2023.

Chapter 24 | The Link between Depression and Other Mental Disorders

Chapter Contents
Section 24.1—Anxiety Disorders among Women
 and Children 193
Section 24.2—Eating Disorders, Anxiety, and
 Depression 198

Section 24.1 | Anxiety Disorders among Women and Children

WHAT IS ANXIETY?
Anxiety is a feeling of worry, nervousness, or fear about an event or situation. It is a normal reaction to stress. It helps you stay alert for a challenging situation at work, study harder for an exam, or remain focused on an important speech. In general, it helps you cope.

But anxiety can be disabling if it interferes with daily life, such as making you dread nonthreatening day-to-day activities such as riding the bus or talking to a coworker. Anxiety can also be a sudden attack of terror when there is no threat.

WHAT ARE ANXIETY DISORDERS?
Anxiety disorders happen when excessive anxiety interferes with your everyday activities, such as going to work or school or spending time with friends or family. Anxiety disorders are serious mental illnesses. They are the most common mental disorders in the United States. Anxiety disorders are more than twice as common in women as in men.

WHO GETS ANXIETY DISORDERS?
Anxiety disorders affect about 40 million American adults every year. Anxiety disorders also affect children and teens. About 8 percent of teens aged 13–18 have an anxiety disorder, with symptoms starting around the age of six.

Women are more than twice as likely as men to get an anxiety disorder in their lifetime. Also, some types of anxiety disorders affect some women more than others:
- Generalized anxiety disorder (GAD) affects more American Indian/Alaskan Native women than women of other races and ethnicities. It also affects more White women and Hispanic women than Asian or African American women.
- Social phobia and panic disorder affect more White women than women of other races and ethnicities.

WHAT CAUSES ANXIETY DISORDERS?
Researchers think anxiety disorders are caused by a combination of factors, which may include the following:
- hormonal changes during the menstrual cycle
- genetics
- traumatic events

Experiencing abuse, an attack, or sexual assault can lead to serious health problems, including anxiety, posttraumatic stress disorder, and depression.

WHAT ARE THE SIGNS AND SYMPTOMS OF AN ANXIETY DISORDER?
Women with anxiety disorders experience a combination of anxious thoughts or beliefs, physical symptoms, and changes in behavior, including avoiding everyday activities they used to do. Each anxiety disorder has different symptoms. They all involve fear and dread about things that may happen now or in the future.

Physical symptoms may include the following:
- weakness
- shortness of breath
- rapid heart rate
- nausea
- upset stomach
- hot flashes
- dizziness

Physical symptoms of anxiety disorders often happen along with other mental or physical illnesses. This can cover your anxiety symptoms or make them worse.

WHAT ARE THE MAJOR TYPES OF ANXIETY DISORDERS?
The major types of anxiety disorder are as follows:
- **GAD.** People with GAD worry excessively about ordinary, day-to-day issues, such as health, money, work, and family. With GAD, the mind often jumps

The Link between Depression and Other Mental Disorders

to the worst-case scenario, even when there is little or no reason to worry. Women with GAD may be anxious about just getting through the day. They may have muscle tension and other stress-related physical symptoms, such as trouble sleeping or upset stomach. At times, worrying keeps people with GAD from doing everyday tasks. Women with GAD have a higher risk of depression and other anxiety disorders than men with GAD. They also are more likely to have a family history of depression.

- **Panic disorder.** These disorders are twice as common in women as in men. People with panic disorder have sudden attacks of terror when there is no actual danger. Panic attacks may cause a sense of unreality, a fear of impending doom, or a fear of losing control. A fear of one's own unexplained physical symptoms is also a sign of panic disorder. People having panic attacks sometimes believe they are having heart attacks, losing their minds, or dying.
- **Social phobia.** Also called "social anxiety disorder," social phobia is diagnosed when people become very anxious and self-conscious in everyday social situations. People with social phobia have a strong fear of being watched and judged by others. They may get embarrassed easily and often have panic attack symptoms.
- **Specific phobia.** A specific phobia is an intense fear of something that poses little or no actual danger. Specific phobias could be fears of closed-in spaces, heights, water, objects, animals, or specific situations. People with specific phobias often find that facing, or even thinking about facing, the feared object or situation brings on a panic attack or severe anxiety.

HOW ARE ANXIETY DISORDERS DIAGNOSED?

Your doctor or nurse will ask you questions about your symptoms and your medical history. Your doctor may also do a physical exam or other tests to rule out other health problems that could be causing your symptoms.

Anxiety disorders are diagnosed when fear and dread of non-threatening situations, events, places, or objects become excessive and are uncontrollable. Anxiety disorders are also diagnosed if the anxiety has lasted for at least six months, and it interferes with social, work, family, or other aspects of daily life.

HOW ARE ANXIETY DISORDERS TREATED?

Treatment for anxiety disorders depends on the type of anxiety disorder you have and your personal history of health problems, violence, or abuse.

Often, treatment may include the following:
- counseling (called "psychotherapy")
- medicine
- a combination of counseling and medicine

HOW DOES COUNSELING HELP TREAT ANXIETY DISORDERS?

Your doctor may refer you for a type of counseling for anxiety disorders called "cognitive-behavioral therapy" (CBT). You can talk to a trained mental health professional about what caused your anxiety disorder and how to deal with the symptoms.

For example, you can talk to a psychiatrist, psychologist, social worker, or counselor. CBT can help you change the thinking patterns around your fears. It may help you change the way you react to situations that may create anxiety. You may also learn ways to reduce feelings of anxiety and improve specific behaviors caused by chronic anxiety. These strategies may include relaxation therapy and problem-solving.

WHAT TYPES OF MEDICINE TREAT ANXIETY DISORDERS?

Several types of medicine treat anxiety disorders. These include the following:
- **Antianxiety (benzodiazepines).** These medicines are usually prescribed for short periods of time because

The Link between Depression and Other Mental Disorders

they are addictive. Stopping this medicine too quickly can cause withdrawal symptoms.
- **Beta-blockers.** These medicines can help prevent the physical symptoms of an anxiety disorder, such as trembling or sweating.
- **Selective serotonin reuptake inhibitors (SSRIs).** These change the level of serotonin in the brain. They increase the amount of serotonin available to help brain cells communicate with each other. Common side effects can include insomnia or sedation, stomach problems, and a lack of sexual desire.
- **Tricyclics.** These types of medicines work like SSRIs. But, sometimes, they cause more side effects than SSRIs. They may cause dizziness, drowsiness, dry mouth, constipation, or weight gain.
- **Monoamine oxidase inhibitors (MAOIs).** People who take MAOIs must avoid certain foods and drinks (such as Parmesan or cheddar cheese and red wine) that contain an amino acid called "tyramine." Taking an MAOI and eating these foods can cause blood pressure levels to spike dangerously. Women who take MAOIs must also avoid certain medicines, such as some types of birth control pills, pain relievers, and cold and allergy medicines. Talk to your doctor about any medicine you take.

All medicines have risks. You should talk to your doctor about the benefits and risks of all medicines.[1]

---

[1] Office on Women's Health (OWH), "Anxiety Disorders," U.S. Department of Health and Human Services (HHS), February 17, 2021. Available online. URL: www.womenshealth.gov/mental-health/mental-health-conditions/anxiety-disorders. Accessed March 10, 2023.

Section 24.2 | Eating Disorders, Anxiety, and Depression

Psychological conditions such as depression and anxiety have been found to co-occur frequently in individuals suffering from eating disorders.

DEPRESSION

Depression is a mood disorder that comprises acute feelings of distress, helplessness, anxiety, and/or guilt. It is one of the most common mental health problems, and it can seriously affect the overall well-being and productivity of the individual. Symptoms may include:
- increased frustration
- insomnia
- reckless behavior
- loss of interest in activities that were previously enjoyed
- irritability
- feelings of insignificance or self-hatred
- tendency to abuse alcohol or drugs
- frequent feelings of fatigue or pain
- low energy level
- fluctuations in eating habits and body weight
- social withdrawal
- poor concentration
- delusions
- suicidal thoughts

Depression can be caused by a number of factors, including hormonal imbalance, traumatic experiences, previous history of substance abuse, and side effects of certain medications. It can either co-occur with or lead to the development of other mental illnesses, such as anxiety, phobias, panic disorders, and eating disorders.

It is not clear whether eating disorders take root in an individual due to existing depression or whether eating disorders cause depression. Since no two eating disorders are the same and each is a complex condition on its own, both arguments are considered valid

The Link between Depression and Other Mental Disorders

in different cases. For instance, feelings of worthlessness and moodiness are often identified as a sign of an eating disorder, which, on the other hand, may also be symptoms of depression. Likewise, a depressed person can indulge in emotional eating, which can subsequently lead to an eating disorder.

ANXIETY

It is quite normal for people to feel anxious in stressful situations, but when an individual experiences an extreme and unreasonable level of anxiety, it is characterized as a disorder. Anxiety disorder is generally identified as a combination of psychological states, such as nervousness, fear, worry, and mistrust, that extends over a long period of time and considerably affects daily activities. Anxiety may be caused by a combination of environmental, social, psychological, genetic, and physiological factors. Some examples include:

- hormonal imbalance
- substance abuse or withdrawal from an illicit drug
- history of mental illness in the family
- traumatic episodes
- current physical ailment

Types of anxiety disorders include generalized anxiety disorder (GAD), obsessive-compulsive disorder (OCD), phobias, social anxiety disorder, panic disorder, and posttraumatic stress disorder (PTSD). Each of them has its own unique symptoms, which are further categorized as physical, behavioral, emotional, and cognitive. These symptoms include sweating, irregular heartbeat, difficulty in breathing, headache, irregular sleeping patterns, nervous habits, irritability, restlessness, obsessive and unwanted thoughts, and irrational fear.

Like depression, an anxiety disorder can co-occur with eating disorders. And, similarly, an individual suffering from an anxiety disorder can develop an eating disorder to cope with anxiety.

In most cases, anxiety precedes the onset of an eating disorder, such as when an individual briefly soothes symptoms of anxiety by trying to gain a sense of control over other aspects of life, such as food, exercise, and weight. This, in the long run, can lead to the development of eating disorders.

Due to the complex nature of eating disorders in conjunction with depression or anxiety, there is a need for an intense treatment plan that analyzes the factors underlying these conditions. Since a number of similar factors can lead to the development of each of these illnesses, successful treatment requires an inclusive strategy that addresses the root cause of all the conditions and helps the individual learn to manage the co-occurring disorder separately and not associate it with food. In addition to medication and nutritional support, the treatment plan may also include various forms of therapy, such as group therapy, cognitive-behavioral therapy (CBT), and music and art therapy.

References

"Eating Disorders and Other Health Problems," Eating Disorders Victoria, June 19, 2015. Available online. URL: www.eatingdisorders.org.au/eating-disorders-a-z/eating-disorders-and-other-health-conditions/. Accessed April 25, 2023.

Ekern, Jacquelyn. "Dual Diagnosis & Co-Occurring Disorders," Eating Disorder Hope, April 25, 2012. Available online. URL: www.eatingdisorderhope.com/treatment-for-eating-disorders/co-occurring-dual-diagnosis. Accessed April 25, 2023.

Chapter 25 | Depression, Substance Use, and Addiction

Chapter Contents
Section 25.1—Substance Use and Co-occurring
  Mental Disorders 203
Section 25.2—Can Smoking Cause Depression? 208
Section 25.3—Could Drinking Be Fueling
  Your Depression? 210

Section 25.1 | Substance Use and Co-occurring Mental Disorders

A substance use disorder (SUD) is a mental disorder that affects a person's brain and behavior, leading to a person's inability to control their use of substances such as legal or illegal drugs, alcohol, or medications. Symptoms can range from moderate to severe, with addiction being the most severe form of SUDs.

Individuals who experience an SUD during their lives may also experience a co-occurring mental disorder and vice versa. Co-occurring disorders can include anxiety disorders, depression, attention deficit hyperactivity disorder (ADHD), bipolar disorder, personality disorders, and schizophrenia, among others.

While SUDs and other mental disorders commonly co-occur, that does not mean that one caused the other. Research suggests three possibilities that could explain why SUDs and other mental disorders may occur together:

- **Common risk factors can contribute to both SUDs and other mental disorders**. Both SUDs and other mental disorders can run in families, suggesting that certain genes may be a risk factor. Environmental factors, such as stress or trauma, can cause genetic changes that are passed down through generations and may contribute to the development of a mental disorder or an SUD.
- **Mental disorders can contribute to substance use and SUDs**. Studies found that people with a mental disorder, such as anxiety, depression, or posttraumatic stress disorder (PTSD), may use drugs or alcohol as a form of self-medication. However, although some drugs may temporarily help with some symptoms of mental disorders, they may make the symptoms worse over time. Additionally, brain changes in people with mental disorders may enhance the rewarding effects of substances, making it more likely they will continue to use the substance.
- **Substance use and SUDs can contribute to the development of other mental disorders**. Substance use

may trigger changes in the brain structure and function that make a person more likely to develop a mental disorder.

DIAGNOSIS AND TREATMENT

Generally, it is better to treat the SUD and the co-occurring mental disorders together rather than separately. Thus, people seeking help for an SUD and other mental disorders need to be evaluated by a health-care provider for each disorder. Because it can be challenging to make an accurate diagnosis due to overlapping symptoms, the provider should use comprehensive assessment tools to reduce the chance of a missed diagnosis and provide targeted treatment.

It is also essential that treatment, which may include behavioral therapies and medications, be tailored to an individual's specific combination of disorders and symptoms, the person's age, the misused substance, and the specific mental disorder(s). Talk to your health-care provider to determine what treatment may be best for you and give the treatment time to work.

Behavioral Therapies

Research has found several behavioral therapies that have promise for treating individuals with co-occurring substance use and mental disorders. Health-care providers may recommend behavioral therapies alone or in combination with medications.

Some examples of effective behavioral therapies for adults with SUDs and different co-occurring mental disorders include the following:
- **Cognitive-behavioral therapy (CBT).** This is a type of talk therapy aimed at helping people learn how to cope with difficult situations by challenging irrational thoughts and changing behaviors.
- **Dialectical behavior therapy (DBT).** It uses concepts of mindfulness and acceptance or being aware of and attentive to the current situation and emotional state. DBT also teaches skills that can help control intense emotions, reduce self-destructive behaviors (e.g., suicide attempts, thoughts, or urges; self-harm; and drug use), and improve relationships.

Depression, Substance Use, and Addiction

- **Assertive community treatment (ACT).** This is a form of community-based mental health care that emphasizes outreach to the community and an individualized treatment approach.
- **Therapeutic communities (TCs).** These are a common form of long-term residential treatment that focuses on helping people develop new and healthier values, attitudes, and behaviors.
- **Contingency management (CM).** The principles encourage healthy behaviors by offering vouchers or rewards for desired behaviors.

BEHAVIORAL THERAPIES FOR CHILDREN AND ADOLESCENTS

Some effective behavioral treatments for children and adolescents include the following:

- **Brief strategic family therapy (BSFT).** This therapy targets family interactions thought to maintain or worsen adolescent SUDs and other co-occurring problem behaviors.
- **Multidimensional family therapy (MDFT).** This works with the whole family to simultaneously address multiple and interacting adolescent problem behaviors, such as substance use, mental disorders, school problems, delinquency, and others.
- **Multisystemic therapy (MST).** This targets key factors associated with serious antisocial behavior in children and adolescents with SUDs.

Medications

Effective medications exist for treating opioid, alcohol, and nicotine addiction and lessening the symptoms of many other mental disorders. Some medications may be useful in treating multiple disorders.[1]

---

[1] "Substance Use and Co-Occurring Mental Disorders," National Institute of Mental Health (NIMH), March 2021. Available online. URL: www.nimh.nih.gov/health/topics/substance-use-and-mental-health. Accessed March 2, 2023.

CO-OCCURRING MAJOR DEPRESSIVE EPISODE AND SUBSTANCE USE DISORDER AMONG ADOLESCENTS

Adolescents aged 12–17 who had both a past year major depressive episode (MDE) and a past year SUD (i.e., illicit drug use disorder, alcohol use disorder (AUD), or both) were classified as having co-occurring MDE and SUD. The order of the onset of an SUD relative to the onset of an MDE among adolescents cannot be established based on the National Survey on Drug Use and Health (NSDUH) data (e.g., whether the onset of an SUD preceded the onset of an MDE, or vice versa). As noted previously, the 2020 NSDUH marked the first year in which SUDs were evaluated based on *Diagnostic and Statistical Manual of Mental Disorders, Fifth Edition* (*DSM-5*) criteria as opposed to *DSM-IV* criteria.

Among adolescents aged 12–17 in 2020, 20.9 percent (5.1 million people) had either an SUD or an MDE in the past year; 14.4 percent (3.5 million people) had an MDE but not an SUD; 3.7 percent (900,000 people) had an SUD but not an MDE; and 2.7 percent (644,000 people) had both an MDE and an SUD in the past year (see Figure 25.1 and Table 25.1).

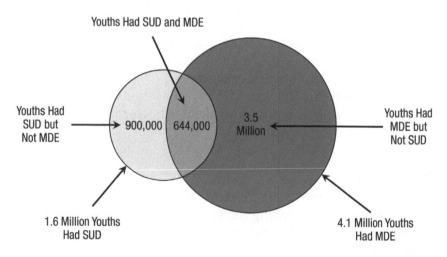

Figure 25.1. Past Year Substance Use Disorder (SUD) and Major Depressive Episode (MDE) among Youths Aged 12–17, 2020

Substance Abuse and Mental Health Services Administration (SAMHSA)

Depression, Substance Use, and Addiction

Table 25.1. Substance Use Disorder (SUD) and Major Depressive Episode (MDE) in the Past Year: Among Adolescents Aged 12 to 17; 2020

SUD or MDE Status	Number in Thousands[1]		Percentage[2]	
SUD or MDE	5,072	(218)	20.9	(0.89)
SUD but not MDE	900	(96)	3.7	(0.4)
MDE but not SUD	3,488	(186)	14.4	(0.77)
Co-occurring SUD and MDE	644	(79)	2.7	(0.33)
Co-occurring SUD and MDE with severe impairment[3]	447	(60)	1.8	(0.25)

Note: Respondents with unknown past year MDE data were excluded.

Note: SUD estimates in 2020 are based on criteria from the Diagnostic and Statistical Manual of Mental Disorders, Fifth Edition. SUD and related estimates are not comparable between 2020 and prior years of NSDUH because prior years' estimates were based on criteria from the Diagnostic and Statistical Manual of Mental Disorders (DSM), Fourth Edition. The 2020 estimates reflect additional methodological changes for the 2020 NSDUH. Due to these changes, estimates are shown for 2020 only. See the 2020 NSDUH: Methodological Summary and Definitions for details on these changes.

[1] Estimates shown are numbers in thousands with standard errors included in parentheses.
[2] Estimates shown are percentages with standard errors included in parentheses.
[3] Impairment is based on the Sheehan Disability Scale role domains, which measure the impact of a disorder on an adolescent's life. Impairment is defined as the highest severity level of role impairment across four domains: (1) chores at home, (2) school or work, (3) close relationships with family, and (4) social life. Ratings ≥ 7 on a 0 to 10 scale were considered severe impairment. Respondents with unknown impairment data were excluded.

Source: Substance Abuse and Mental Health Services Administration (SAMHSA), Center for Behavioral Health Statistics and Quality (CBHSQ), National Survey on Drug Use and Health (NSDUH), Quarters 1 and 4, 2020

SUBSTANCE USE AMONG ADOLESCENTS WITH A MAJOR DEPRESSIVE EPISODE

Adolescents aged 12–17 who had a past year MDE were more likely to use some substances in the past year or past month than their counterparts who did not have an MDE in the past year. In 2020, adolescents with a past year MDE were more likely than adolescents without a past year MDE to be past year illicit drug users (28.6%versus 10.7%) or past year marijuana users (22.0% versus 7.9%). Adolescents with a past year MDE also were more likely than those without a past year MDE to be past month binge alcohol users (6.2% versus 3.8%). Adolescents with a past year MDE were also more likely than those without a past year MDE to use tobacco

Depression Sourcebook, Sixth Edition

products or vape nicotine in the past month (12.9% versus 5.1%). Figure 25.2 shows this substance usage pattern among youth with past year MDE and youth without a past year MDE.[2]

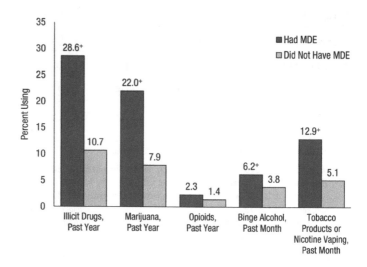

Figure 25.2. Substance Use among Youths Aged 12–17, by Past Year Major Depressive Episode (MDE), 2020

Substance Abuse and Mental Health Services Administration (SAMHSA)

Section 25.2 | Can Smoking Cause Depression?

A larger proportion of people diagnosed with mental disorders report cigarette smoking compared with people without mental disorders. Among U.S. adults in 2019, the percentage who reported past month cigarette smoking was 1.8 times higher for those with any past year mental illness than that for those without any past year mental illness (28.2% versus 15.8%). Smoking rates are

---

[2] "Key Substance Use and Mental Health Indicators in the United States: Results from the 2020 National Survey on Drug Use and Health," Substance Abuse and Mental Health Services Administration (SAMHSA), October 2021. Available online. URL: www.samhsa.gov/data/sites/default/files/reports/rpt35325/NSDUHFFRPDFWHTMLFiles2020/2020NSDUHFFR1PDFW102121.pdf. Accessed March 29, 2023.

Depression, Substance Use, and Addiction

particularly high among people with serious mental illness (those who demonstrate greater functional impairment). While estimates vary, as many as 70–85 percent of people with schizophrenia and as many as 50–70 percent of people with bipolar disorder smoke.

Rates of smoking among people with mental illness were the highest for young adults, those with low levels of education, and those living below the poverty level. Smoking is believed to be more prevalent among people with depression and schizophrenia because nicotine may temporarily lessen the symptoms of these illnesses, such as poor concentration, low mood, and stress. But it is important to note that smoking cessation has been linked with improved mental health—including reduced depression, anxiety, and stress and enhanced mood and quality of life.

Additionally, people who smoke with a mental health disorder tend to smoke more cigarettes than those in the general population. The average number of cigarettes smoked during the past month was higher among those with a mental illness than that among those without one—331 versus 310 cigarettes. High cigarette consumption is a particular problem for people with serious mental illness.[3]

Smokers are more likely to have depression than nonsmokers. Nobody knows for sure why this is. People who have depression might smoke to feel better. Or smokers might get depression more easily because they smoke. No matter what the cause, there are treatments that work for both depression and smoking.

MOOD CHANGES

Mood changes are common after quitting smoking. Some people feel increased sadness. You might be irritable, be restless, or feel down or blue. Changes in mood from quitting smoking may be part of withdrawal. Withdrawal is your body getting used to not having nicotine. Mood changes from nicotine withdrawal usually get better in a week or two. If mood changes do not get better in a couple of weeks, you should talk to your doctor. Something else, such as depression, could be the reason.

---

[3] "Do People with Mental Illness and Substance Use Disorders Use Tobacco More Often?" National Institute on Drug Abuse (NIDA), May 2022. Available online. URL: https://nida.nih.gov/publications/research-reports/tobacco-nicotine-e-cigarettes/do-people-mental-illness-substance-use-disorders-use-tobacco-more-often. Accessed March 29, 2023.

Smoking may seem to help you with depression. You might feel better at the moment. But there are many problems with using cigarettes to cope with depression. There are other things you can try to lift your mood:

- **Exercise.** Being physically active can help. Start small and build up over time. This can be hard to do when you are depressed. But your efforts will pay off.
- **Structure your day.** Make a plan to stay busy. Get out of the house if you can.
- **Be with other people.** Many people who are depressed are cut off from other people. Being in touch or talking with others every day can help your mood.
- **Reward yourself.** Do things you enjoy. Even small things add up and help you feel better.
- **Get support.** Be sure to get support. If you are feeling down after quitting smoking, talking about this with friends and family may help. Your doctor can also help.

FIND HELP 24/7

If you need help now, call a 24-hour crisis center at 800-273-TALK (800-273-8255) or 800-SUICIDE (800-784-2433) for free, private help or dial 911.

Sometimes, people who are feeling depressed think about hurting themselves or dying. If you or someone you know is having these feelings, get help now.[4]

Section 25.3 | Could Drinking Be Fueling Your Depression?

Alcohol use disorder (AUD) is a medical condition characterized by an impaired ability to stop or control alcohol use despite adverse social, occupational, or health consequences. It encompasses the

---

[4] Smokefree.gov, "Smoking and Depression," U.S. Department of Health and Human Services (HHS), July 30, 2013. Available online. URL: https://smokefree.gov/challenges-when-quitting/mood/smoking-depression. Accessed March 2, 2023.

conditions that some people refer to as alcohol abuse, alcohol dependence, alcohol addiction, and the colloquial term, alcoholism. Considered a brain disorder, AUD can be mild, moderate, or severe. Lasting changes in the brain caused by alcohol misuse perpetuate AUD and make individuals vulnerable to relapse. The good news is that no matter how severe the problem may seem, evidence-based treatment with behavioral therapies, mutual support groups, and/or medications can help people with AUD achieve and maintain recovery. According to a national survey, 14.1 million adults aged 18 and older (5.6% of this age group) had AUD in 2019. Among youth, an estimated number of 414,000 adolescents aged 12–17 (1.7% of this age group) had AUD during this time frame.

WHAT INCREASES THE RISK OF ALCOHOL USE DISORDER?

A person's risk of developing AUD depends, in part, on how much, how often, and how quickly they consume alcohol. Alcohol misuse, which includes binge drinking and heavy alcohol use, over time increases the risk of AUD. Other factors also increase the risk of AUD:

- **Drinking at an early age.** A recent national survey found that among people aged 26 and older, those who began drinking before the age of 15 were more than five times as likely to report having AUD in the past year as those who waited until the age of 21 or later to begin drinking. The risk of females in this group is higher than that of males.
- **Genetics and family history of alcohol problems.** Genetics play a role, with heritability of approximately 60 percent; however, like other chronic health conditions, AUD risk is influenced by the interplay between a person's genes and their environment. Parents' drinking patterns may also influence the likelihood that a child will one day develop AUD.
- **Mental health conditions and a history of trauma.** A wide range of psychiatric conditions—including depression, posttraumatic stress disorder, and attention deficit hyperactivity disorder—are comorbid with AUD and are associated with an increased risk of AUD. People with a history of childhood trauma are also vulnerable to AUD.

WHAT ARE THE SYMPTOMS OF ALCOHOL USE DISORDER?

Health-care professionals use criteria from the *Diagnostic and Statistical Manual of Mental Disorders, Fifth Edition (DSM-5)* to assess whether a person has AUD and to determine the severity if the disorder is present. Severity is based on the number of criteria a person meets based on their symptoms—mild (two to three criteria), moderate (four to five criteria), or severe (six or more criteria).

A health-care provider might ask the following questions to assess a person's symptoms in the past year:

- Have you had times when you ended up drinking more, or longer, than you intended?
- Have you more than once wanted to cut down or stop drinking, or tried to, but could not?
- Have you spent a lot of time drinking? Or being sick or getting over other aftereffects?
- Have you wanted a drink so badly you could not think of anything else?
- Have you found that drinking—or being sick from drinking—often interfered with taking care of your home or family? Or caused job troubles? Or school problems?
- Have you continued to drink even though it was causing trouble with your family or friends?
- Have you given up or cut back on activities that were important or interesting to you, or gave you pleasure, in order to drink?
- Have you more than once gotten into situations while or after drinking that increased your chances of getting hurt (such as driving, swimming, using machinery, walking in a dangerous area, or having unprotected sex)?
- Have you continued to drink even though it was making you feel depressed or anxious or adding to another health problem? Or after having had a memory blackout?
- Have you had to drink much more than you once did to get the effect you want? Or found that your usual number of drinks had much less effect than before?

Depression, Substance Use, and Addiction

- Have you found that when the effects of alcohol were wearing off, you had withdrawal symptoms, such as trouble sleeping, shakiness, restlessness, nausea, sweating, a racing heart, or a seizure? Or sensed things that were not there?

Any of these symptoms may be the cause for concern. The more symptoms, the more urgent the need for change.

WHAT ARE THE TYPES OF TREATMENT FOR ALCOHOL USE DISORDER?

Several evidence-based treatment approaches are available for AUD. One size does not fit all, and a treatment approach that may work for one person may not work for another. Treatment can be outpatient and/or inpatient treatment, provided by specialty programs, therapists, and doctors.

Medications

The U.S. Food and Drug Administration (FDA) currently approves three medications to help people stop or reduce their drinking and prevent relapse: naltrexone (oral and long-acting injectable), acamprosate, and disulfiram. All these medications are nonaddictive, and they may be used alone or combined with behavioral treatments or mutual support groups.

Behavioral Treatments

Behavioral treatments, also known as "alcohol counseling" or "talk therapy," provided by licensed therapists are aimed at changing drinking behavior. Examples of behavioral treatments are brief interventions and reinforcement approaches, treatments that build motivation and teach skills for coping and preventing relapse, and mindfulness-based therapies.

Mutual Support Groups

Mutual support groups provide peer support for stopping or reducing drinking. Group meetings are available in most communities, at low or no cost, at convenient times and locations—including an increasing presence online. This means they can be especially helpful to individuals at risk for relapse to drinking. Combined with medications and behavioral treatment provided by health professionals, mutual support groups can offer a valuable added layer of support.

It is to be noted that people with severe AUD may need medical help to avoid alcohol withdrawal if they decide to stop drinking. Alcohol withdrawal is a potentially life-threatening process that can occur when someone who has been drinking heavily for a prolonged period of time suddenly stops drinking. Doctors can prescribe medications to address these symptoms, making the process safer and less distressing.

CAN PEOPLE WITH ALCOHOL USE DISORDER RECOVER?

Many people with AUD do recover, but setbacks are common among people in treatment. Seeking professional help early can prevent relapse to drinking. Behavioral therapies can help people develop skills to avoid and overcome triggers, such as stress, that might lead to drinking. Medications can also help deter drinking during times when individuals may be at a greater risk of relapse (e.g., divorce, death of a family member).[5]

MYTHS AND REALITIES OF ALCOHOL, MEDICATIONS, AND MENTAL HEALTH CONDITIONS IN OLDER ADULTS

Many people have misconceptions about mental health conditions and/or substance use disorders, especially in older adults. The lack of correct information can prevent older adults from seeking and receiving help for these issues. Learning what is reality and what is a myth can help improve the quality of life (QOL) for you or someone you care about.

- **Myth**
  Only older adults who consistently drink a lot of alcohol have an alcohol problem.

---

[5] "Understanding Alcohol Use Disorder," National Institute on Alcohol Abuse and Alcoholism (NIAAA), April 2021. Available online. URL: www.niaaa.nih.gov/publications/brochures-and-fact-sheets/understanding-alcohol-use-disorder. Accessed April 24, 2023.

Depression, Substance Use, and Addiction

Reality
The key point in determining a problem is how alcohol affects the person's health, functioning, and relationships with others. For example, in people with medical conditions such as diabetes and high blood pressure, even one drink per day can be a problem.

- **Myth**
Over-the-counter (OTC) medicines and alcohol can be used together safely.
Reality
It is never safe to drink alcohol while taking medicine. Both prescription and OTC medicines can intensify the effects of alcohol. This can be dangerous or even fatal. In addition, using medicines and alcohol together, even several hours apart, can change a drug's effects. For example, the drug might not work.

- **Myth**
If alcohol and medication misuse were a problem, the doctor would tell the older adult.
Reality
Unfortunately, many doctors and other health-care professionals do not ask questions about the use of alcohol with medications. Therefore, older adults are at risk of harmful interactions of alcohol with medications. It is important for them to let their doctor know what drugs they are taking and how they use alcohol.

- **Myth**
It Is easy to tell when an older adult has an alcohol problem.
Reality
The symptoms of alcohol misuse are sometimes mistaken for signs of aging or physical illness. Alcohol misuse can mimic or intensify the signs and symptoms of many illnesses. In addition, medical problems can mask alcohol dependence.

- **Myth**
Very few women become alcoholics.

Reality
Many women have problems with alcohol. Women may not drink publicly; they may remain private about their alcohol use. Thus, people often do not know they have problems.

- **Myth**
Treating substance misuse and abuse issues in older adults is a waste of time and effort. It is too late for them to change.
Reality
Substance misuse and abuse interventions and mental health treatments are effective with older adults. They can greatly improve QOL.
- **Myth**
Feeling sad or depressed is part of growing old. There is nothing you can do to help the older adult.
Reality
Depression is common among older adults, but it is not a normal part of aging. Believing that depression is inevitable prevents older people from seeking and getting the help they need.
- **Myth**
Older adults suffering from depression or anxiety disorders lack the inner strength to fight the debilitating feelings.
Reality
Depression and anxiety disorders have many possible causes. Lack of inner strength is not one of them. Causes of depression and anxiety include heredity, stressful events such as the death of a loved one, retirement, health problems, and reactions to medicine. Drug interactions and alcohol and drug combinations can also lead to depression and anxiety.
- **Myth**
The most common sign of depression is crying.
Reality
Denial of mental health conditions is often more common and more predictable than any other

Depression, Substance Use, and Addiction

symptom. The last person to recognize a problem is often the person with the problem. Because of the strong negative prejudice and discrimination association with mental health conditions, many older adults are afraid to seek help. Other signs of depression include being easily upset and feeling fearful, forgetful, confused, hopeless, lonely, and tired. Loss of appetite is also common.

- **Myth**
  If an older adult says that drinking is his or her last remaining pleasure, it is generally best to allow the person to continue to drink. Even if it causes him or her problems, it does not matter as long as others are not being put at risk.

  Reality
  Problem drinking seriously affects physical health and QOL. It can lead to loneliness, isolation, and depression. It can also lead to forgetfulness, and it may reduce problem-solving skills. Sometimes, others unknowingly encourage drinking if they think older people have only a limited time left and, therefore, should be allowed to enjoy themselves.[6]

---

[6] "Get Connected Linking: Older Adults with Resources on Medication, Alcohol, and Mental Health," Substance Abuse and Mental Health Services Administration (SAMHSA), 2019. Available online. URL: https://store.samhsa.gov/sites/default/files/d7/priv/sma03-3824_2.pdf. Accessed March 10, 2023.

Chapter 26 | Climate Change and Depression

The threat of climate change is a key psychological and emotional stressor. Individuals and communities are affected both by direct experience of local events attributed to climate change and by exposure to information regarding climate change and its effects. For example, public communication and media messages about climate change and its projected consequences can affect perceptions of physical and societal risks and consequently affect mental health and well-being. The interactive nature and cumulative nature of climate change effects on health, mental health, and well-being are critical factors in understanding the overall consequences of climate change on human health.

EXTREME WEATHER EVENTS
In the United States, the mental health impacts of extreme weather have mainly been studied in response to hurricanes and floods and, to a lesser extent, wildfires. Though many studies discuss the mental health impacts of specific historical events, they are demonstrative of the types of mental health issues that could arise as climate change leads to further increases in the frequency, severity, or duration of some types of extreme weather. The mental health impacts of these events, such as hurricanes, floods, and drought, can be expected to increase as more people experience the stress—and often trauma—of these disasters.

Many people exposed to climate- or weather-related natural disasters experience stress reactions and serious mental health consequences, including symptoms of posttraumatic stress disorder (PTSD), depression, and general anxiety, which often occur simultaneously. Mental health effects include grief/bereavement, increased substance use or misuse, and suicidal thoughts. All of these reactions have the potential to interfere with the individual's functioning and well-being and are especially problematic for certain groups.

Exposure to life-threatening events, such as highly destructive hurricanes (e.g., Hurricane Katrina in 2005), has been associated with acute stress, PTSD, and higher rates of depression and suicide in affected communities. These mental health consequences are of particular concern for people facing recurring disasters, posing a cumulative psychological toll. Following exposure to Hurricane Katrina, veterans with preexisting mental illness had a 6.8 times greater risk of developing any additional mental illness than those veterans without a preexisting mental illness. Following hurricanes, increased levels of PTSD have been experienced by individuals who perceive members of their community as being less supportive or helpful to one another.

Depression and general anxiety are also common consequences of extreme events (such as hurricanes and floods) that involve a loss of life, resources, or social support and social networks or events that involve extensive relocation and life disruption. For example, long-term anxiety and depression, PTSD, and increased aggression (in children) have been found to be associated with floods. First responders following a disaster also experience increased rates of anxiety and depression.

Increases in predisaster rates have been observed in interpersonal and domestic violence, including intimate partner violence, particularly toward women, in the wake of climate- or weather-related disasters. High-risk coping behaviors, such as alcohol abuse, can also increase following extreme weather events. Individuals who use alcohol to cope with stress and those with preexisting alcohol use disorders (AUDs) are most vulnerable to increased alcohol use following extreme weather events.

Persons directly affected by a climate- or weather-related disaster are at increased incidences of suicidal thoughts and behaviors. Increases in both suicidal thoughts (from 2.8% to 6.4%) and

Climate Change and Depression

actual suicidal plans (from 1.0% to 2.5%) were observed in residents 18 months after Hurricane Katrina. Following Hurricanes Katrina and Rita, a study of internally displaced women living in temporary housing found reported rates of suicide attempt and completion to be 78.6 times and 14.7 times the regional average, respectively. In the six months following 1992's Hurricane Andrew, the rate of homicide-suicides doubled to two per month in Miami-Dade County, where the hurricane hit, compared to an average of one per month during the prior five-year period that did not include hurricane activity of the same scale.

Climate- or weather-related disasters can strain the resources available to provide adequate mental (or even immediate physical) health care due to the increased number of individuals who experience severe stress and mental health reactions. Communities adversely affected by these events also have diminished interpersonal and social networks available to support mental health needs and recovery due to the destruction and disruption caused by the event.

EXTREME HEAT

The majority (80.7%) of the U.S. population lives in cities and urban areas, and urbanization is expected to increase in the future. People in cities may experience greater exposure to heat-related health effects during heat waves. The impact of extreme heat on mental health is associated with an increased incidence of disease and death, aggressive behavior, violence, and suicide and increases in hospital and emergency room admissions for those with mental health or psychiatric conditions.

Individuals with mental illness are especially vulnerable to extreme heat or heat waves. In six case-control studies involving 1,065 heat-wave-related deaths, preexisting mental illness was found to triple the risk of death due to heat wave exposure. The risk of death also increases during hot weather for patients with psychosis, dementia, and substance misuse. Hospital admissions have been shown to increase for those with mental illness as a result of extreme heat, increasing ambient temperatures, and humidity. An increased death rate has also been observed in those with mental illness among cases admitted to the emergency department with a diagnosis of heat-related pathology.

People who are isolated and have difficulty caring for themselves—often characteristics of the elderly or those with a mental illness—are also at a higher risk of heat-related incidence of disease and death. Fewer opportunities for social interaction and increased isolation put people at elevated risk for not only heat-related illness and death but also a decline in mental health and, in some cases, increases in aggression and violence. Hotter temperatures and poorer air quality limit people's outdoor activities. For many, reductions in outdoor exercise and stress-reducing activities lead to diminished physical health, increased stress, and poor mental health.

There may be a link between extreme heat (climate change related or otherwise) and increasing violence, aggressive motives, and/or aggressive behavior. The frequency of interpersonal violence and intergroup conflict may increase with more extreme precipitation and hotter temperatures. These impacts can include heightened aggression, which may result in increased interpersonal violence and violent crime, negatively impacting individual and societal mental health and well-being. Given projections of increasing temperatures, there is potential for increases in human conflict, but the causal linkages between climate change and conflict are complex, and the evidence is still emerging.

THE THREAT OF CLIMATE CHANGE AS A STRESSOR

Many people are routinely exposed to images, headlines, and risk messages about the threat of current and projected climate change. Forty percent of Americans report hearing about climate change in the media at least once a month.

Noteworthy environmental changes associated with climate change constitute a powerful environmental stressor—an ongoing and stress-inducing condition or aspect of an individual's everyday environment. Equally concerning are adverse impacts relating to people's connections to place and identity and the consequent sense of loss and disconnection.

Public risk perceptions of the phenomenon and threat of climate change are associated with stigma, dread risk (such as a heightened

Climate Change and Depression

fear of low-probability, high-consequence events), and uncertainty about the future.

Many individuals experience a range of adverse psychological responses to the hybrid risk of climate change impacts. A hybrid risk is an ongoing threat or event, which is perceived or understood as reflecting both natural and human causes and processes. These responses include heightened risk perceptions, preoccupation, general anxiety, pessimism, helplessness, eroded sense of self-control and collective control, stress, distress, sadness, loss, and guilt.

Media representations of serious environmental risks, such as climate change, are thought to elicit strong emotional responses in part dependent on how climate change information is presented. People experience the threat of climate change through frequent media coverage describing events and future risks attributed to climate change. They are also directly exposed to increasingly visible changes in local environments and seasonal patterns and in the frequency, magnitude, and intensity of extreme weather events. Exposure to climate change through the media could cause undue stress if the media coverage is scientifically inaccurate or discouraging. However, effective risk communication promotes adaptive and preventive individual or collective action.

RESILIENCE AND RECOVERY

A majority of individuals psychologically affected by a traumatic event (such as a climate-related disaster) will recover over time. A set of positive changes that can occur in a person as a result of coping with or experiencing a traumatic event is known as "post-traumatic growth." An array of intervention approaches used by mental health practitioners may also reduce the adverse consequence of traumatic events. While most people who are exposed to a traumatic event can be expected to recover over time, a significant proportion (up to 20%) of individuals directly exposed develop chronic levels of psychological dysfunction, which may not get better or be resolved. Multiple risk factors contribute to these adverse psychological effects, including disaster-related factors such as physical injury, death, or loss of a loved one; loss of resources such as possessions or property; and displacement. Life events and stressors secondary to extreme events also affect mental health, including loss of jobs and social connections, financial worries, loss of social support, and family distress or dysfunction.

Disaster-related stress reactions and accompanying psychological impacts occur in many individuals directly exposed to the event and can continue over extended time periods (up to a year or more). For example, three months after Hurricane Andrew, 38 percent of children (aged 8–12 years) living in affected areas of South Florida reported symptom levels consistent with a "probable diagnosis" of PTSD. Ten months after the disaster, this proportion declined to about 18 percent, representing a substantial decrease but still indicating a significant number of individuals with serious mental health issues resulting from the disaster event.

Emerging evidence shows that individuals who are actively involved in climate change adaptation or mitigation actions experience appreciable health and well-being benefit from such engagement. These multiple psychological and environmental benefits do not necessarily minimize distress. However, when people do have distress related to relevant media exposure or to thinking about or discussing climate change, taking action to address the issue can buffer against distress. Such engagement addresses the threat and helps manage the emotional responses as people come to terms with—and adjust their understandings and lives in the context of—climate change.[1]

---

[1] GlobalChange.gov, "Mental Health and Well-Being," U.S. Global Change Research Program (USGCRP), February 1, 2023. Available online. URL: https://health2016.globalchange.gov/low/ClimateHealth2016_08_Mental_Health_small.pdf. Accessed March 23, 2023.

Chapter 27 | Other Depression Triggers

Depression affects between 15 and 20 million Americans each year. It is a medical condition that should be taken seriously. Some forms of depression are related to malfunctions in brain circuits that transmit signal-carrying chemicals called "neurotransmitters," which help regulate mood. Although these cases may not be preventable, they often respond well to treatment.

However, studies suggest that it may be possible to prevent some depressive episodes by learning to recognize and avoid common situations that serve as depression triggers. Potential environmental triggers include stressful life events, such as divorce or job loss, as well as unexpected factors that can impact emotional well-being, such as being a caregiver or spending too much time on social media. The following list describes situations that have been shown to correlate with depression and offers tips for how to avoid or cope with them.

STRESS
Some of the main sources of stress included economic worries, job security, family responsibilities, health concerns, and discrimination or harassment. Many other people simply feel overwhelmed by daily chores, obligations, and deadlines that seem to get in the way of their enjoyment of life. To prevent stress from turning into depression, experts recommend keeping a positive attitude, recognizing your own limits, and setting and enforcing personal boundaries. When tasks seem overwhelming, breaking them down into steps may make them seem more manageable. Finally, building an

emotional support network, discussing problems and concerns, and leaning on others for help as needed are important means of coping with stress.

JOB LOSS

Losing a job can cause a serious blow to a person's sense of identity and self-esteem, especially for older and highly paid workers who are likely to have more trouble finding equivalent positions. People who are fired or laid off may feel rejected, frightened, and uncertain about the future. In addition, unemployment often causes financial difficulties, which in turn can create strain in family relationships. The combination of these factors means that job loss is a leading trigger for depression. Experts recommend that people affected by job loss build a support network consisting of friends and colleagues and take advantage of career-related courses and job search resources. It is also important to stay busy and connected, structuring free time by scheduling lunches, walks, classes, or volunteer activities. Finally, after taking time to process the emotional impact of the job loss, it may be helpful to identify its positive aspects. For instance, losing a job might offer an unexpected opportunity to make a career change, pursue a new business idea, or move to a different geographic area.

FINANCIAL PROBLEMS

Money concerns and accumulated debts are a source of stress and worry for many people, especially those who feel as if they are struggling with financial problems alone. Common emotions associated with financial stress—such as shame, fear, anxiety, uncertainty—can negatively impact self-esteem and trigger depression. Research has shown that one of the key methods of combating financial stress involves formulating a plan and taking positive action. Reviewing sources of income and expenses and establishing a budget are important first steps toward increasing financial stability. People who are not good with money can take advantage of free financial services offered by many communities or borrow books on financial management from a local library. To avoid

Other Depression Triggers

becoming overwhelmed, experts recommend focusing on areas you can control and creating a long-term plan to pay down debt and build savings. Finally, it is important to remain active and stay connected to friends and family by enjoying free activities, such as a concert in a park.

DIVORCE
Divorce creates a complicated mix of emotions for those affected by it, including anger, resentment, sadness, regret, guilt, and failure. It also causes a sudden change in social status from couple to single, which can generate feelings of loneliness, fear, and uncertainty. Finally, many divorces involve stressful conflicts over financial settlements and custody of children. Taken together, the emotional upheaval of divorce becomes a potent depression trigger. Therapy—whether individual, couples, family, or support groups—can help people navigate the complicated emotions of divorce and move forward with greater confidence. It can also help resolve conflicts, reduce bitterness, and promote effective co-parenting.

INFERTILITY
The inability to have a much-desired baby is a powerful depression trigger, especially for women who suffer multiple miscarriages or have age- or health-related fertility issues. Experts suggest that people who feel despair over infertility try to take charge of the situation by investigating alternative routes to parenthood, such as adoption. Single women whose fertility window is closing due to age or health might explore such options as preserving eggs or using a sperm donor. Even if you ultimately decide not to pursue the matter, simply researching the steps involved can make you feel less vulnerable and more empowered.

"EMPTY NEST" SYNDROME
Although a child leaving home to begin college or adult life can be a joyous event, it is also a major life change for parents who suddenly must face an empty nest. Many parents struggle with feelings

of loss and uncertainty as they adjust to a new daily routine and a different self-identity. Divorced or single parents are particularly vulnerable to loneliness and depression although it also affects married couples who built their lives around their children and suddenly find that they do not share many common interests. Experts suggest that parents plan in advance to help reduce the emotional impact of empty nest syndrome. Beginning a year or more before the child leaves home, it may be helpful to sign up for a class, join a book group, plan a vacation, or schedule regular activities with friends. Although taking time to adjust is normal, the key to avoiding depression is to remain active, discover new interests, and have things to look forward to outside of the parental role.

SERIOUS ILLNESS

Being diagnosed with a serious illness is a frightening and disorienting experience that can profoundly affect a person's sense of self and outlook for the future. While the physical symptoms can be difficult enough to deal with, the emotional impact can shake the foundations of relationships and trigger depression. One of the most important steps in coping with a serious illness diagnosis is taking a proactive role in establishing a treatment plan. Patients should seek second opinions, ask for referrals to specialists, and build an effective team that includes a patient advocate or social worker as well as doctors. Experts also recommend joining a support group to gain access to the insights and understanding of people who have dealt with the same illness or condition.

HORMONE IMBALANCE

As people age, they experience fluctuation and decline in the levels of key hormones in the bloodstream. This natural process can cause a number of unpleasant symptoms, including fatigue, weight gain, hot flashes, low libido, anxiety, and depression. While the experiences of women undergoing menopause receive the most attention, men also go through midlife hormonal changes that can affect mood, energy, and sexual performance. Experts suggest that people aged 45 and older keep a record of their symptoms and

Other Depression Triggers

discuss them with a doctor. Hormonal imbalances can often be stabilized with hormone supplementation or replacement therapy. Some people also find that vitamins, herbal remedies, and stress-management techniques such as meditation and yoga can help combat mood swings associated with hormone fluctuations. Treating underlying conditions such as thyroid disorders can also help regulate hormone levels and reduce the risk of depression.

UNHEALTHY EATING HABITS

Obesity, an unhealthy diet full of refined carbohydrates, and poor sleep habits can also trigger depression. Fortunately, these triggers are among the easiest to avoid. Experts recommend evaluating your lifestyle and making gradual, long-term changes to improve your overall health and well-being. They warn against fad diets and instead suggest a diet that emphasizes fresh fruits and vegetables, whole grains, lean proteins, healthy fats, and drinking plenty of water. Consuming foods high in saturated fat or sugar—such as chips, cookies, white bread, and soda—has been shown to increase the risk of depressive episodes, so these should be avoided. In addition, experts recommend increasing physical fitness by walking or doing other activities to help maintain a healthy weight, improve mood, and stave off depression. Exercise also helps improve sleep, which is another aspect of general health that correlates to depression. Studies have shown that people who get the recommended six to eight hours of sleep per night are less likely to experience depression than those who receive more or less than the recommended amount. Some tips for improving sleep include maintaining a consistent schedule, avoiding the use of electronics in the bedroom, creating a calm, relaxing sleep environment, and employing techniques such as reading or meditation to wind down after a busy day.

NEWS AND SOCIAL MEDIA

Smartphones and other mobile devices make it easier to keep connected and up-to-date than ever before. Yet studies have shown that excessive consumption of bad news—which outweighs coverage of good news by a 17–1 margin in the modern media—can trigger anxiety and depression. Similarly, obsessive checking of social media such as Facebook, where others tend to highlight only the best aspects of their lives, can create feelings of envy, loneliness, frustration, and guilt that can trigger or worsen depression symptoms. To reduce the impact of news and social media on mood, experts suggest spending less time online and more time socializing in real life with friends and family. Spending time talking with people who care has been shown to improve mood and increase life satisfaction.

References

Brabaw, Kasandra. "Five Strange, Surprising Depression Triggers," Prevention, October 26, 2015. Available online. URL: www.prevention.com/mind-body/surprising-depression-triggers. Accessed May 2, 2023.

Haiken, Melanie. "Ten Biggest Depression Triggers, and How to Turn Them Off," Caring.com, September 5, 2016. Available online. URL: www.caring.com/articles/10-depression-triggers. Accessed May 2, 2023.

Theobald, Mikel. "Avoiding Ten Common Depression Triggers," EverydayHealth, 2016. Available online. URL: www.everydayhealth.com/hs/major-depression-health-well-being/factors-can-trigger-depression-relapse/. Accessed May 2, 2023.

Part 5 | Depression and Chronic Illnesses

Chapter 28 | Chronic Illness and Mental Health

Chapter Contents
Section 28.1—The Intersection of Depression
 and Chronic Illness...235
Section 28.2—Chronic Pain and Depression............................239
Section 28.3—Depression and Fibromyalgia............................242

Section 28.1 | The Intersection of Depression and Chronic Illness

CHRONIC ILLNESS AND MENTAL HEALTH: RECOGNIZING AND TREATING DEPRESSION

Chronic illnesses such as cancer, heart disease, or diabetes may make you likely to have or develop a mental health condition.

It is common to feel sad or discouraged after having a heart attack, receiving a cancer diagnosis, or when trying to manage a chronic condition such as pain. You may be facing new limits on what you can do and may feel stressed or concerned about treatment outcomes and the future. It may be hard to adapt to a new reality and to cope with the changes and ongoing treatment that come with the diagnosis. Favorite activities, such as hiking or gardening, may be harder to do.

Temporary feelings of sadness are expected, but if these and other symptoms last longer than a couple of weeks, you may have depression. Depression affects your ability to carry on with daily life and to enjoy family, friends, work, and leisure. The health effects of depression go beyond mood: Depression is a serious medical illness with many symptoms, including physical ones.

Some symptoms of depression include the following:
- persistent sad, anxious, or "empty" mood
- feeling hopeless or pessimistic
- feeling irritable, easily frustrated, or restless
- feeling guilty, worthless, or helpless
- loss of interest or pleasure in hobbies and activities
- decreased energy, fatigue, or feeling "slowed down"
- difficulty concentrating, remembering, or making decisions
- difficulty sleeping, early-morning awakening, or oversleeping
- changes in appetite or weight
- aches or pains, headaches, cramps, or digestive problems without a clear physical cause that do not ease even with treatment
- suicide attempts or thoughts of death or suicide

PEOPLE WITH OTHER CHRONIC MEDICAL CONDITIONS ARE AT HIGHER RISK OF DEPRESSION

The same factors that increase the risk of depression in otherwise healthy people also raise the risk in people with other medical illnesses, particularly if those illnesses are chronic (long-lasting or persistent). These risk factors include a personal or family history of depression or family members who have died by suicide.

However, some risk factors for depression are directly related to having another illness. For example, conditions such as Parkinson disease (PD) and stroke cause changes in the brain. In some cases, these changes may have a direct role in depression. Illness-related anxiety and stress can also trigger symptoms of depression.

Depression is common among people who have chronic illnesses such as:

- Alzheimer disease (AD)
- autoimmune diseases, including systemic lupus erythematosus (SLE), rheumatoid arthritis (RA), and psoriasis
- cancer
- coronary heart disease (CHD)
- diabetes
- epilepsy
- human immunodeficiency virus (HIV)/acquired immunodeficiency syndrome (AIDS)
- hypothyroidism
- multiple sclerosis (MS)
- PD
- stroke

Some people may experience symptoms of depression after being diagnosed with a medical illness. Those symptoms may decrease as they adjust to or treat the other condition. Certain medications used to treat the illness can also trigger depression.

Research suggests that people who have depression and other medical illnesses tend to have more severe symptoms of both illnesses. They may have more difficulty adapting to their medical condition, and they may have higher medical costs than those who do not have both depression and a medical illness. Symptoms of depression may continue even as a person's physical health improves.

A collaborative care approach that includes both mental and physical health care can improve overall health. Research has shown that treating depression and chronic illness together can help people better manage both their depression and their chronic disease.

CHILDREN AND ADOLESCENTS WITH CHRONIC ILLNESSES

Children and adolescents with chronic illnesses often face more challenges than their healthy peers in navigating adolescence. Chronic illnesses can affect physical, cognitive, social, and emotional development, and they can take a toll on parents and siblings. These limitations put children and adolescents at higher risk than their healthy peers of developing a mental illness.

Children and adolescents with chronic illnesses experience many forms of stress. Parents and health-care providers should be on the lookout for signs of depression, anxiety, and adjustment disorders (a group of conditions that can occur when someone has difficulty coping with a stressful life event) in young people and their families.

PEOPLE WITH DEPRESSION ARE AT HIGHER RISK FOR OTHER MEDICAL CONDITIONS

It may come as no surprise that adults with a medical illness are likely to experience depression. The reverse is also true: People of all ages with depression are at higher risk of developing certain physical illnesses.

People with depression have an increased risk of cardiovascular disease (CVD), diabetes, stroke, pain, and AD, for example. Research also suggests that people with depression may be at higher risk for osteoporosis. The reasons are not yet clear. One factor with some of these illnesses is that many people with depression may have less access to good medical care. They may have a more challenging time caring for their health—for example, seeking care, taking prescribed medication, eating well, and exercising.

Scientists are also exploring whether physiological changes seen in depression may play a role in increasing the risk of physical illness. In people with depression, scientists have found changes in the way several different systems in the body function that could have an impact on physical health, including the following:
- increased inflammation
- changes in the control of heart rate and blood circulation
- abnormalities in stress hormones
- metabolic changes such as those seen in people at risk for diabetes

DEPRESSION IS TREATABLE EVEN WHEN ANOTHER ILLNESS IS PRESENT

Depression is a common complication of chronic illness, but it does not have to be a normal part of having a chronic illness. Effective treatment for depression is available and can help even if you have another medical illness or condition.

If you or a loved one think you have depression, it is important to tell your health-care provider and explore treatment options. You should also inform your health-care provider about all your present treatments or medications for your chronic illness or depression (including prescribed medications and dietary supplements). Sharing information can help avoid problems with multiple medicines interfering with each other. It also helps your health-care provider stay informed about your overall health and treatment issues.

Treating depression with medication, psychotherapy (also known as "talk therapy"), or a combination of the two also may help improve the physical symptoms of a chronic illness or reduce the risk of future problems. Likewise, treating chronic illness and getting symptoms under control can help improve symptoms of depression.

Depression affects each individual differently. There is no "one-size-fits-all" for treatment. It may take some trial and error to find the treatment that works best.[1]

---

[1] "Chronic Illness Related to Increased Symptoms of Depression," National Institute of Mental Health (NIH), 2021. Available online. URL: www.nimh.nih.gov/health/publications/chronic-illness-mental-health#pub3. Accessed March 3, 2023.

Section 28.2 | Chronic Pain and Depression

Chronic low back pain is one of the most common types of pain, affecting about 50 million adult Americans. Many of these people rely on strong pain medications, including opioids, to be able to move and perform everyday activities.

Chronic pain also influences emotional and mental well-being. About one in five people with chronic low back pain experiences high levels of "negative affect" or feelings of sadness, fear about their pain, and anxiety. Most people develop these mental health symptoms after they begin experiencing pain, especially if the pain is severe all the time and interferes with their daily activities. The presence of depression and anxiety not only worsens an individual's overall well-being but in turn makes it even harder to relieve pain effectively—potentially increasing the risk of opioid use and misuse.

The Helping to End Addiction Long-term[SM] Initiative, or the NIH HEAL Initiative[SM], initiated the Back Pain Consortium (BACPAC) Research Program to help reduce reliance on opioid pain medications and the associated risks for patients with chronic low back pain by seeking to identify effective alternative treatment options that can be adapted to an individual's needs. As part of this program, HEAL researchers led by Ajay D. Wasan, M.D., M.Sc., from the University of Pittsburgh, tested a combination of antidepressant medications and physical therapy in people with both chronic low back pain and mood disorders.

THE INTERACTION OF PAIN AND MOOD-RELATED DISORDERS

People experiencing chronic pain and depression or anxiety tend to experience greater pain and disability than those without these conditions. They also do not respond as well to many pain treatments—including medications, nerve blocks, physical therapy, or surgery—compared to people without depression or anxiety. As a result, they are three to four times more likely to be prescribed opioid pain medications.

Together, these factors put people with chronic pain and mood-related disorders at increased risk of opioid misuse and overdose. "In fact," says Dr. Wasan, "negative affect is one of the main risk factors for misusing prescription opioids to cope with mood-related issues."

TREATMENT APPROACHES FOR PAIN AND MOOD-RELATED DISORDERS

To improve pain treatment and help reduce reliance on opioid medications in people with both chronic low back pain and mood-related disorders, Dr. Wasan and his team investigated a combination of two approaches: treatment with antidepressant medications and a special type of physical therapy. Both treatments have previously been shown to improve outcomes for people experiencing chronic pain, but testing them together is new.

Antidepressant therapy mainly targets a person's mood, but it can also provide pain relief and increase the ability to function.

Fear-avoidance physical therapy (also called "fear-of-movement physical therapy") is based on the observation that many people with chronic low back pain are so afraid of experiencing pain; they avoid movement as much as possible. Doing so leads to underuse of affected muscles, disability, and depression—all of which can worsen pain, setting off a vicious cycle. Fear-avoidance physical therapy aims to break this cycle and focuses on getting patients active and moving. This approach has also been shown to improve both physical and mental well-being and function.

TREATING PAIN AND MOOD TOGETHER IMPROVES OUTCOMES

In previous research, Dr. Wasan's team assigned 71 patients with chronic low back pain and high negative affect to either antidepressant therapy, fear-avoidance physical therapy, a combination of both treatments, or a control condition that included education about pain management only. After four months of treatment, people who received the combination therapy appeared to do better with respect to both health conditions:

- About 75–80 percent of participants in this group showed improvements in depression and anxiety.
- About 40 percent showed improvements in both pain and function.

"You may think this outcome seems obvious, that using a combination of two or more treatments that address different aspects of a patient's pain experience is better than relying on one approach alone," says Dr. Wasan. However, he adds, it is a new approach because to date very few studies have assessed the effectiveness of treatment combinations (also called "multimodal treatments") in people with chronic pain and especially in those with coexisting mood disorders.

AN EXPANDED STUDY TO DETERMINE EFFECTIVENESS

Encouraged by these initial findings, through the BACPAC program, Dr. Wasan conducted a larger, phase 2 clinical trial to determine the effectiveness of the antidepressant/physical therapy treatment combination in a larger group of patients.

"We're trying to improve negative affect, which in itself is important to do," explains Dr. Wasan, "but we are also looking at whether treatment can improve patients' pain and physical function, and in those who are prescribed opioids, if it can reduce opioid misuse."

For this study, they are using a type of physical therapy they call enhanced fear-avoidance rehabilitation—"enhanced" because they have added a mobile app that individuals can use in between their physical therapy sessions. This app includes, for example, education about pain and helpful instructional videos.

The study recruited 300 patients with chronic low back pain and high levels of both depression and anxiety; some of these individuals may be currently taking opioid pain medications.

The participants were randomly split into three groups that receive either antidepressant therapy only, specialized physical therapy only, or both. In the first phase of the study, the patients received their assigned treatment for four months. The researchers then compared the proportion of patients in each group who showed improvements in both pain and self-reported physical function (such as their ability to walk) or who showed improvements in depression symptoms. Additionally, they determined whether treatment reduced the need for opioid medications and any potential opioid misuse.

In a second four-month phase, participants who showed a response after the first phase continued their treatment, whereas participants who received only antidepressants or specialized physical therapy and showed no improvement were randomly reassigned to the same treatment or switched to another approach.

PATIENT-CENTERED TREATMENT

Through this combination strategy, the researchers sought to increase the overall number of patients who showed a treatment response and identify factors that predict treatment outcomes.

One of the main goals of the NIH HEAL Initiative's BACPAC program is to personalize interventions for chronic low back pain based on individual characteristics and preferences. Ultimately, BACPAC research projects aim to create a predictive tool that balances the many factors that contribute to chronic low back pain (which differ among people) and suggest a personalized treatment plan based on the specifics of that individual's characteristics.

"We feel that this novel multimodal combination approach of medication and physical therapy can really cause a shift in current treatment strategies," says Dr. Wasan. "We are confident that the community practice environment is poised to adopt the strategy too."[2]

Section 28.3 | Depression and Fibromyalgia

WHAT IS FIBROMYALGIA?

Fibromyalgia is a condition that causes pain all over the body (also referred to as "widespread pain"), sleep problems, fatigue, and often emotional and mental distress. People with fibromyalgia may be more sensitive to pain than people without fibromyalgia. This is called "abnormal pain perception processing." Fibromyalgia affects

---

[2] "Chronic Pain And Depression," National Institutes of Health (NIH), December 28, 2022. Available online. URL: https://heal.nih.gov/news/stories/treating-pain-mood-chronic-back-pain. Accessed March 3, 2023.

about 4 million U.S. adults, about 2 percent of the adult population. The cause of fibromyalgia is not known, but it can be effectively treated and managed.

WHAT ARE THE SIGNS AND SYMPTOMS OF FIBROMYALGIA?
The most common symptoms of fibromyalgia are:
- pain and stiffness all over the body
- fatigue and tiredness
- depression and anxiety
- sleep problems
- problems with thinking, memory, and concentration
- headaches, including migraines

Other symptoms may include the following:
- tingling or numbness in hands and feet
- pain in the face or jaw, including disorders of the jaw known as "temporomandibular joint syndrome" (TMJ syndrome)
- digestive problems, such as abdominal pain, bloating, constipation, and even irritable bowel syndrome (IBS)

WHAT ARE THE RISK FACTORS FOR FIBROMYALGIA?
Known risk factors include the following:
- **Age**. Fibromyalgia can affect people of all ages, including children. However, most people are diagnosed during middle age, and you are more likely to have fibromyalgia as you get older.
- **Lupus or rheumatoid arthritis (RA)**. If you have lupus arthritis or RA, you are more likely to develop fibromyalgia.

Some other factors have been weakly associated with the onset of fibromyalgia, but more research is needed to see if they are real. These possible risk factors include the following:
- sex (Women are twice as likely to have fibromyalgia as men.)
- stressful or traumatic events, such as car accidents and posttraumatic stress disorder (PTSD)

- repetitive injuries, such as frequent knee bending
- illness (such as viral infections)
- family history
- obesity

WHAT ARE THE COMPLICATIONS OF FIBROMYALGIA?

Fibromyalgia can cause pain, disability, and a lower quality of life (QOL). U.S. adults with fibromyalgia may have the following complications:
- **More hospitalizations.** If you have fibromyalgia, you are twice as likely to be hospitalized as someone without fibromyalgia.
- **Lower QOL.** Women with fibromyalgia may experience a lower QOL.
- **Higher rates of major depression.** Adults with fibromyalgia are more than three times more likely to have major depression than adults without fibromyalgia. Screening and treatment for depression are extremely important.
- **Higher death rates from suicide and injuries.** Death rates from suicide and injuries are higher among fibromyalgia patients, but overall mortality among adults with fibromyalgia is similar to the general population.
- **Higher rates of other rheumatic conditions.** Fibromyalgia often co-occurs with other types of arthritis such as osteoarthritis, RA, systemic lupus erythematosus (SLE), and ankylosing spondylitis (AS).

HOW IS FIBROMYALGIA DIAGNOSED?

Doctors usually diagnose fibromyalgia using the patient's history, physical examination, x-rays, and blood work.

HOW IS FIBROMYALGIA TREATED?

Fibromyalgia can be effectively treated and managed with medication and self-management strategies.

Chronic Illness and Mental Health

Fibromyalgia should be treated by a doctor or team of healthcare professionals who specialize in the treatment of fibromyalgia and other types of arthritis, called "rheumatologists." Doctors usually treat fibromyalgia with a combination of treatments, which may include the following:
- medications, including prescription drugs and over-the-counter pain relievers
- aerobic exercise and muscle-strengthening exercise
- patient education classes, usually in primary care or community settings
- stress management techniques such as meditation, yoga, and massage
- good sleep habits to improve the quality of sleep
- cognitive-behavioral therapy (CBT) to treat underlying depression

CBT is a type of talk therapy meant to change the way people act or think.

In addition to medical treatment, people can manage their fibromyalgia with the self-management strategies described below, which are proven to reduce pain and disability, so they can pursue the activities important to them.

HOW CAN YOU IMPROVE YOUR QUALITY OF LIFE?
- **Get physically active**. Experts recommend that adults be moderately physically active for 150 minutes per week. Walk, swim, or bike 30 minutes a day for five days a week. These 30 minutes can be broken into three separate 10-minute sessions during the day. Regular physical activity can also reduce the risk of developing other chronic diseases such as heart disease and diabetes.
- **Go to recommended physical activity programs**. Those concerned about how to safely exercise can participate in physical activity programs that are proven effective for reducing pain and disability related to arthritis and improving mood and the ability to move. Classes take place at local Ys, parks, and community centers. These classes can help you feel better.

- **Join a self-management education class.** These programs help people with arthritis or other conditions—including fibromyalgia—be more confident in how to control their symptoms and how to live well and understand how the condition affects their lives.[3]

---

[3] "Fibromyalgia," Centers for Disease Control and Prevention (CDC), January 6, 2020. Available online. URL: www.cdc.gov/arthritis/basics/fibromyalgia.htm. Accessed April 6, 2023.

Chapter 29 | Arthritis–Mental Health Connection

About one in five U.S. adults with arthritis has symptoms of anxiety or depression. These symptoms are more common in adults with arthritis who are women; are younger; are identified as lesbian, gay, bisexual, and transgender (LGBT); have chronic pain or other co-occurring chronic conditions; or are disabled, unemployed, or otherwise unable to work.

Because anxiety is often perceived as normal, people do not always seek mental health services for it. Left untreated, anxiety can lead to greater problems. In fact, chronic anxiety can increase someone's risk of developing depression.

Arthritis, anxiety, and depression can each have negative effects on overall health and quality of life (QOL). Feelings of sadness or worry can interfere with a person's ability and motivation to care for themselves properly and manage daily life, let alone manage their arthritis or other health conditions. That is why it is important for people who have arthritis to take care of their mental health symptoms as well as their arthritis symptoms.

SYMPTOMS OF ANXIETY AND DEPRESSION

Some common symptoms of anxiety are:
- worry or irritability
- restlessness (unable to stay still or stop racing thoughts)
- trouble focusing
- trouble sleeping
- muscle tension, rapid heartbeat, shortness of breath, dizziness, or digestive problems without a clear physical cause or that do not ease with treatment

Some common symptoms of depression are:
- sadness, emptiness, or hopelessness
- feelings of guilt or worthlessness
- lack of interest in hobbies and activities
- fatigue, or lack of energy
- appetite and/or weight changes
- thoughts of death or suicide
- aches or pains, headaches, cramps, or digestive problems without a clear physical cause or that do not ease with treatment

It is important to seek treatment when symptoms of anxiety or depression appear. Health-care providers can treat or refer patients with arthritis experiencing these symptoms to mental health professionals and community resources. Some of these resources, such as evidence-based self-management education and physical activity programs, may even address mental health and arthritis together. Self-management education workshops teach skills to help people cope with symptoms such as pain, reduce stress, and make healthy lifestyle choices. Physical activity can lead to benefits such as reduced arthritis pain, increased mobility, and improved mood.

GUIDANCE FOR HEALTH-CARE PROVIDERS

Over 58 million U.S. adults have arthritis. About 10 million adults with arthritis report either anxiety or depression symptoms, according to a 2018 Centers for Disease Control and Prevention (CDC) analysis. These symptoms were more common among adults aged 18–44 than among older adults. One in five adults with arthritis had anxiety symptoms, compared to about one in nine adults without arthritis. Depression symptoms were more than twice as common among adults with arthritis as those without arthritis (12.1% versus 4.7%).

Not only are symptoms of anxiety and depression common among U.S. adults with arthritis, but these symptoms have also been associated with reduced response to arthritis treatment and poorer QOL. Improving mental health can even reduce pain, independent of other pain management strategies. Health-care

Arthritis–Mental Health Connection

providers can empower patients to improve their mental health and manage their arthritis in the following two ways:
- **Ask your arthritis patients about depression and anxiety.** The U.S. Preventive Services Task Force (USPSTF) recommends depression screening for all adults. The Substance Abuse and Mental Health Services Administration (SAMHSA) encourages universal screening for both anxiety and depression.
- **Offer treatment and/or referrals to services.** When treating mental health conditions in your arthritis patients, encourage strategies that address both physical and mental health. Refer patients to self-management education workshops, where they can learn proven ways to manage symptoms, reduce stress, and take medicines the right way. Also, encourage patients to be physically active on their own or by taking part in a structured, arthritis-appropriate physical activity program. Research shows that self-management education and physical activity can help improve mood, increase energy, and/or reduce symptoms of anxiety, depression, and arthritis.[1]

---

[1] "The Arthritis-Mental Health Connection," Centers for Disease Control and Prevention (CDC), October 12, 2021. Available online. URL: www.cdc.gov/arthritis/communications/features/arthritis-mental-health.htm. Accessed March 14, 2023.

Chapter 30 | Depression and Attention Deficit Hyperactivity Disorder

Attention deficit hyperactivity disorder (ADHD) is a neurological disorder that affects a person's ability to control their behavior and pay attention to tasks.

WHAT CAUSES ATTENTION DEFICIT HYPERACTIVITY DISORDER?
Attention deficit hyperactivity disorder has many causes. Among these causes are:
- familial (ADHD often runs in families.)
- abnormal brain development
- brain injuries occurring before, during, or after birth

WHY IS ATTENTION DEFICIT HYPERACTIVITY DISORDER CONSIDERED A NEUROLOGICAL CONDITION?
Brain images of children with ADHD may show differences compared to children without ADHD. For example, in some children with ADHD, certain parts of the brain are smaller or less active than the brains of children without ADHD. These changes may be linked to specific brain chemicals that are needed for tasks such as sustaining attention and regulating activity levels.

WHAT ARE SOME OF THE OTHER CONDITIONS THAT ARE COMMON IN CHILDREN WITH ATTENTION DEFICIT HYPERACTIVITY DISORDER?

Some children with ADHD may also have learning disabilities, behavioral disorders, or disorders of mood, such as depression. Problems with planning, memory, schoolwork, motor skills, social skills, control of emotions, and response to discipline are common. Sleep problems can also be more frequent.

WHAT IS THE RISK OF HAVING ATTENTION DEFICIT HYPERACTIVITY DISORDER IF OTHER FAMILY MEMBERS HAVE ATTENTION DEFICIT HYPERACTIVITY DISORDER?

Children who have ADHD usually have at least one close biological (blood) relative who also has ADHD. At least one-third of all fathers who had ADHD in their youth have children with ADHD. Research has shown that ADHD can have a genetic basis, which means that it is likely that a person diagnosed with ADHD has a close relative with similar symptoms.[1]

DEPRESSION IN CHILDREN WITH ATTENTION DEFICIT HYPERACTIVITY DISORDER

Occasionally, being sad or feeling hopeless is a part of every child's life. When children feel persistent sadness and hopelessness, it can cause problems. Children with ADHD are more likely than children without ADHD to develop childhood depression. Children may be more likely to feel hopeless and sad when they cannot control their ADHD symptoms and the symptoms interfere with doing well at school or getting along with family and friends.

Examples of behaviors often seen when children are depressed include:

- feeling sad or hopeless a lot of the time
- not wanting to do things that are fun
- having a hard time focusing
- feeling worthless or useless

---

[1] "About Attention Deficit Hyperactivity Disorder," National Human Genome Research Institute (NHGRI), November 15, 2012. Available online. URL: www.genome.gov/Genetic-Disorders/Attention-Deficit-Hyperactivity-Disorder. Accessed March 6, 2023.

Depression and Attention Deficit Hyperactivity Disorder

Children with ADHD often have a hard time focusing on things that are not very interesting to them. Depression can make it hard to focus on things that are normally fun. Changes in eating and sleeping habits can also be a sign of depression. For children with ADHD who take medication, changes in eating and sleeping can also be side effects from the medication rather than signs of depression. Talk with your health-care provider if you have concerns.

TREATMENT FOR DEPRESSION IN CHILDREN WITH ATTENTION DEFICIT HYPERACTIVITY DISORDER

The first step to treatment is to talk with a health-care provider to get an evaluation. Some signs of depression, such as having a hard time focusing, are also signs of ADHD, so it is important to get a careful evaluation to see if a child has both conditions. A mental health professional can develop a therapy plan that works best for the child and family. Early treatment is important and can include child therapy, family therapy, or a combination of both. The school can also be included in therapy programs. For very young children, involving parents in treatment is very important. Cognitive-behavioral therapy (CBT) is one form of therapy that is used to treat depression, particularly in older children. It helps the child change negative thoughts into more positive, effective ways of thinking. Consultation with a health provider can help determine if medication should also be part of the treatment.[2]

---

[2] "Other Concerns and Conditions with ADHD," Centers for Disease Control and Prevention (CDC), August 9, 2022. Available online. URL: www.cdc.gov/ncbddd/adhd/conditions.html#Anxiety. Accessed March 6, 2023.

Chapter 31 | Depression and Brain Injury

Each year in the United States, traumatic brain injury (TBI) results in approximately 2.8 million emergency department visits, hospitalizations, or deaths. TBIs account for almost 2 percent of all emergency department visits, and more than one-quarter million Americans are hospitalized each year with a TBI. Heightened public awareness of sports-related concussions and TBIs incurred in combat in Iraq and Afghanistan has contributed to a marked increase in emergency department visits over the past two decades; however, the greatest increase has been in the rate of fall-related TBIs among older adults. Potentially hundreds of thousands more individuals sustain TBI each year but are not included in the data sets used to form these estimates because they do not seek medical treatment or because they are treated in physicians' offices, urgent care clinics, or federal, military, or Veterans Affairs hospitals.

WHAT IS A TRAUMATIC BRAIN INJURY?

A TBI is an alteration in brain function, or other evidence of brain pathology, caused by an external force. External forces include the head being struck by an object, the head striking an object, and the head accelerating or decelerating without direct external trauma as occurs in shaken baby syndrome or from a blast or explosion. The requirement for TBI to be due to an external force clearly separates it from other "acquired brain injuries" that occur after birth, such as strokes, anoxia/hypoxia (when the brain is denied oxygen), or electrical shock. Furthermore, the requirement that TBI includes both an external force and alteration in brain function distinguishes a TBI from injury to the head alone, such as abrasions or contusions to the face or scalp.

The "fingerprint" of TBI is that frontal areas of the brain, including the frontal lobes, are the most likely to be injured, regardless of the point of impact to the head. Once there is enough force from a blow to the head, shaking, or a blast to cause the brain to jiggle within the cranial vault, then bony ridges on the undersurface of the skull cause damage to the frontal lobes and anterior tips of the temporal lobes. Shearing and tearing of neuronal pathways connecting to the prefrontal cortex also occur if there is sufficient force. Together, wherever else there may be damage to the brain, there is also damage in the frontal areas.

HOW COMMON IS TRAUMATIC BRAIN INJURY?

A history of having at least one TBI that caused loss of consciousness may have occurred to as many as one in five adults. And almost 1 in 20 may have had a moderate or severe TBI, a level of severity that is quite likely to have residual effects, even if not causing disability. While the prevalence of disability caused by TBI is estimated to be 1.1 percent among U.S. adults, when all long-term consequences are considered, the prevalence rate is substantially higher.

There is less known about the prevalence of TBI among children though, in Ohio state, two of every three TBIs reported by adults occurred before age 20.[1]

WHAT ARE THE LINKS BETWEEN BEHAVIORAL HEALTH AND TRAUMATIC BRAIN INJURY?

There is a well-documented association between TBI and behavioral health comorbidities, including depression, anxiety, suicide, and substance use disorders. Table 31.1 shows the prevalence of TBI in behavioral health settings and among populations of persons with significant behavioral health needs.

---

[1] "Treating Patients with Traumatic Brain Injury," Substance Abuse and Mental Health Services Administration (SAMHSA), August 15, 2021. Available online. URL: https://store.samhsa.gov/sites/default/files/pep21-05-03-001.pdf. Accessed April 26, 2023.

Depression and Brain Injury

Table 31.1. Prevalence of Lifetime TBI in Vulnerable Populations

	TBI with Loss of Consciousness (%)	Moderate or Severe TBI (%)
General population of noninstitutionalized adults	22	5
Substance use disorder treatment settings	53	17
Psychiatric inpatient unit	36	20
Prisoners	50	14
Homeless persons	47	25

An exhaustive review found that the incidence of major depressive and posttraumatic stress disorders exceeded population rates after TBI, commonly emerging in the first year though onset could be delayed with more severe injuries. A population-based study in Denmark analyzed medical and behavioral health registries data for 1.4 million citizens and found that those with a history of TBI were 65 percent more likely to subsequently be diagnosed with schizophrenia, 59 percent more likely to be diagnosed with depression, and 28 percent with bipolar disorder. When compared to persons who had fractures not involving the skull or spine, the likelihood of subsequent schizophrenia and depression remained significantly higher.

Children (aged 6–15) hospitalized in a general hospital (n = 42) with mild TBI versus (n = 35) orthopedic controls demonstrated that there was a 35.7 percent prevalence rate of mood disorders at six months post injury versus 11.4 percent of the orthopedic control. The prevalence of anxiety disorders was 21.4 percent in the mild TBI group compared to 2.8 percent in the orthopedic control.

Substance use disorders are frequent prior to TBI, and intoxication frequently leads to brain injuries. While drinking may decline immediately post injury, for many, it resumes over time. Further, recent studies have also suggested that childhood TBI may predispose individuals to adult high-risk substance use. A birth cohort in New Zealand found that by age 25, those hospitalized with their first mild TBI before age six were three times more likely to have a diagnosis of either alcohol or drug dependency. Those hospitalized with the first TBI between the ages of 16–21 were three times more likely to be diagnosed with drug dependency.

Researchers recently described how the opioid epidemic created a "perfect storm" for persons with TBI. Persons with TBI were more likely to be prescribed opioids than those without, were at greater vulnerability to developing a substance use disorder, and faced greater challenges in substance use disorder treatment.

The risk of committing suicide is two to four times greater for individuals with TBI than for the general population. Even mild brain injury increases risk. When a mental illness or substance use disorder co-occurs with TBI, the risk for attempted or completed suicide is further increased and may remain elevated for up to 15 years post injury. In suicide prevention, there is growing recognition that among persons with brain injury, a risk assessment must focus more on the opportunity and less on emotional distress.

MENTAL HEALTH DISORDERS ARE COMMON FOLLOWING MILD HEAD INJURY

A study revealed that approximately one in five individuals might experience mental health symptoms up to six months after mild traumatic brain injury (mTBI), suggesting the importance of follow-up care for these patients. Scientists also identified factors that may increase the risk of developing posttraumatic stress disorder (PTSD) and/or major depressive disorder following mild mTBI or concussion through analysis of the Transforming Research and Clinical Knowledge in Traumatic Brain Injury (TRACK-TBI; https://tracktbi.ucsf.edu/) study cohort. The study was supported by the National Institute of Neurological Disorders and Stroke (NINDS), part of the National Institutes of Health (NIH). The findings were published in *JAMA Psychiatry*.

"Mental health disorders after concussion have been studied primarily in military populations, and not much is known about these outcomes in civilians," said Patrick Bellgowan, Ph.D., NINDS

Depression and Brain Injury

program director. "These results may help guide follow-up care and suggest that doctors may need to pay particular attention to the mental state of patients many months after injury."

In the study, Murray B. Stein, M.D., M.P.H., professor at the University of California San Diego, and his colleagues investigated mental health outcomes in 1,155 people who had experienced an mTBI and were treated in the emergency department. At 3, 6, and 12 months after injury, study participants completed various questionnaires related to PTSD and major depressive disorder. For a comparison group, the researchers also surveyed individuals who had experienced orthopedic traumatic injuries, such as broken legs, but did not have head injuries.

The results showed that at three and six months following injury, people who had experienced mTBI were more likely than orthopedic trauma patients to report symptoms of PTSD and/or major depressive disorder. For example, three months after injury, 20 percent of mTBI patients reported mental health symptoms compared to 8.7 percent of orthopedic trauma patients. At six months after injury, mental health symptoms were reported by 21.2 percent of people who had experienced head injuries and 12.1 percent of orthopedic trauma patients.

Dr. Stein and his team also used the data to determine risk factors for PTSD and major depressive disorder after mTBI. The findings revealed that lower levels of education, self-identifying as African American, and having a history of mental illness increased risk. In addition, if the head injury was caused by an assault or other violent attack, it increased the risk of developing PTSD, but not major depressive disorder. However, the risk of mental health symptoms was not associated with other injury-related occurrences such as duration of loss of consciousness or posttraumatic amnesia.

"Contrary to common assumptions, mild head injuries can cause long-term effects. These findings suggest that follow-up care after a head injury, even for mild cases, is crucial, especially for patients showing risk factors for PTSD or depression," said Dr. Stein.

This study is part of the NIH-funded TRACK-TBI (https://tracktbi.ucsf.edu/) initiative, which is a large, long-term study of patients treated in the emergency department for mTBI. The goal of the study is to improve understanding of the effects of concussions by establishing a comprehensive database of clinical measures, including brain images, blood samples, and outcome data for 3,000 individuals, which may help identify biomarkers of TBI and risk factors for various outcomes and improve our ability to identify and prevent adverse outcomes of head injury. To date, more than 2,700 individuals have enrolled in TRACK-TBI.

A recent study coming out of TRACK-TBI suggested that many TBI patients were not receiving recommended follow-up care.

"TRACK-TBI is overturning many of our long-held beliefs around mTBI, particularly in what happens with patients after they leave the emergency department. We are seeing more evidence about the need to monitor these individuals for many months after their injury to help them achieve the best recovery possible," said Geoff Manley, M.D., professor at the University of California San Francisco, senior author of the current study and principal investigator of TRACK-TBI.

Future research studies will help identify mental health conditions, other than PTSD and major depressive disorder, that may arise following mTBI. In addition, more research is needed to understand the biological mechanisms that lead from mTBI to mental health problems and other adverse outcomes, such as neurological and cognitive difficulties.[2]

---

[2] News and Events, "Mental Health Disorders Common Following Mild Head Injury," National Institutes of Health (NIH), January 30, 2019. Available online. URL: www.nih.gov/news-events/news-releases/mental-health-disorders-common-following-mild-head-injury. Accessed April 26, 2023.

Chapter 32 | Depression and Cancer

Depression is a disorder with specific symptoms that can be diagnosed and treated. For every 10 patients diagnosed with cancer, about two patients become depressed. The numbers of men and women affected are about the same.

A person diagnosed with cancer faces many stressful issues. These may include the following:
- fear of death
- changes in life plans
- changes in body image and self-esteem
- changes in day-to-day living
- worry about money and legal issues

Sadness and grief are common reactions to a cancer diagnosis. A person with cancer may also have other symptoms of depression, such as:
- feelings of disbelief, denial, or despair
- trouble sleeping
- loss of appetite
- anxiety or worry about the future

Not everyone who is diagnosed with cancer reacts in the same way. Some cancer patients may not have depression or anxiety, while others may have major depression or an anxiety disorder.

Signs that you have adjusted to the cancer diagnosis and treatment include the following:
- being able to stay active in daily life
- continuing in your roles as spouse, parent, or employee

- being able to manage your feelings and emotions related to your cancer

Some cancer patients may have a higher risk of depression. There are known risk factors for depression after a cancer diagnosis. Anything that increases your chance of developing depression is called a "risk factor for depression." Factors that increase the risk of depression are not always related to the cancer.

Risk factors related to cancer that may cause depression include the following:
- learning you have cancer when you are already depressed
- having cancer pain that is not well controlled
- being physically weakened by the cancer
- having pancreatic cancer
- having advanced cancer or a poor prognosis
- feeling you are a burden to others
- taking certain medicines, such as:
  - corticosteroids
  - procarbazine
  - L-asparaginase
  - interferon alfa
  - interleukin-2
  - amphotericin B

Risk factors not related to cancer that may cause depression include the following:
- a personal history of depression or suicide attempts
- a family history of depression or suicide
- a personal history of mental problems, alcoholism, or drug abuse
- not having enough support from family or friends
- stress caused by life events other than cancer
- having other health problems, such as stroke or heart attack that may also cause depression

There are many medical conditions that can cause depression.

Depression and Cancer

Medical conditions that may cause depression include the following:
- pain that does not go away with treatment
- abnormal levels of calcium, sodium, or potassium in the blood.
- not enough vitamin B_{12} or folate in your diet
- anemia
- fever
- too much or too little thyroid hormone
- too little adrenal hormone
- side effects caused by certain medicines

Family members also have a risk of depression. Anxiety and depression may occur in family members who are caring for loved ones with cancer. Family members who talk about their feelings and solve problems together are less likely to have high levels of depression and anxiety.

TYPES OF DEPRESSION IN CANCER PATIENTS
There are different types of depression.

The type of depression depends in part on the symptoms the patient is having and how long the symptoms have lasted. Major depression is one type of depression. Treatment depends on the type of depression. Major depression has specific symptoms that last longer than two weeks.

It is normal to feel sad after learning you have cancer, but a diagnosis of major depression depends on more than being unhappy.

Symptoms of major depression include the following:
- feeling sad most of the time
- loss of pleasure and interest in activities you used to enjoy
- changes in eating and sleeping habits
- slow physical and mental responses
- feeling restless or jittery
- unexplained tiredness
- feeling worthless, hopeless, or helpless

- feeling a lot of guilt for no reason
- not being able to pay attention
- thinking the same thoughts over and over
- frequent thoughts of death or suicide

The symptoms of depression are not the same for every patient. Your health-care provider will talk with you to find out if you have symptoms of depression.

DIAGNOSIS OF DEPRESSION IN CANCER PATIENTS

Your health-care provider will want to know how you are feeling and may want to discuss the following:
- your feelings about having cancer (Talking with your doctor about this may help you see if your feelings are normal sadness or more serious.)
- your moods (You may be asked to rate your mood on a scale.)
- any symptoms you may have and how long the symptoms have lasted
- how the symptoms affect your daily life, such as your relationships, your work, and your ability to enjoy your usual activities
- other parts of your life that are causing stress
- how strong your social support system is
- all the medicines you are taking and other treatments you are receiving (Sometimes, side effects of medicines or cancer seem like symptoms of depression. This is more likely during active cancer treatment or if you have advanced cancer.)

This information will help you and your doctor find out if you are feeling normal sadness or have depression.

Checking for depression may be repeated at times when stress increases, such as if cancer gets worse or if it comes back after treatment.

Depression and Cancer

In addition to talking with you, your doctor may do the following to check for depression:
- **Physical exam and history**. An exam of the body to check general signs of health, including checking for signs of disease, such as lumps or anything else that seems unusual. A history of your health habits, past illnesses including depression, and treatments will also be taken. A physical exam can help rule out other causes of your symptoms.
- **Laboratory tests**. Medical procedures that test samples of tissue, blood, urine, or other substances in the body. These tests help diagnose disease, plan and check treatment, or monitor the disease over time. Lab tests are done to rule out a medical condition that may be causing symptoms of depression.
- **Mental status exam**. An exam is done to get a general idea of your mental state by checking the following:
  - how you look and act
  - your mood
  - your speech
  - your memory
  - how well you pay attention and understand simple concepts

TREATMENT FOR DEPRESSION IN CANCER PATIENTS

The decision to treat depression depends on how long it has lasted and how much it affects your life.

You may have depression that needs to be treated if you are not able to perform your usual activities, you have severe symptoms, or the symptoms do not go away. Treatment for depression may include talk therapy, medicines, or both.

Counseling or talk therapy helps some cancer patients with depression.

Your doctor may suggest you see a psychologist or psychiatrist for the following reasons:
- Your symptoms have been treated with medicine for two to three weeks and are not getting better.

- Your depression is getting worse.
- The antidepressants you are taking are causing unwanted side effects.
- Your depression keeps you from continuing with your cancer treatment.

Most counseling or talk therapy programs for depression are offered in both individual and small group settings. These programs include the following:
- crisis intervention
- psychotherapy
- cognitive-behavioral therapy (CBT)

More than one type of therapy program may be right for you. A therapy program can help you learn about the following:
- coping and problem-solving skills
- relaxation skills and ways to lower stress
- ways to get rid of or change negative thoughts
- giving and accepting social support
- cancer and its treatment

Talking with a clergy member may also be helpful for some people.

Antidepressants may help relieve depression and its symptoms. You may be treated with a number of medicines during your cancer care. Some anticancer medicines may not mix safely with certain antidepressants or with certain foods, herbals, or nutritional supplements. It is important to tell your health-care providers about all the medicines, herbals, and nutritional supplements you are taking, including medicines used as patches on the skin, and any other diseases, conditions, or symptoms you have. This can help prevent unwanted reactions with antidepressant medicine.

When you are taking antidepressants, it is important that you use them under the care of a doctor. Some antidepressants take from three to six weeks to work. Usually, you begin at a low dose that is slowly increased to find the right dose for you. This helps avoid side effects. Antidepressants may be taken for a year or longer.

Depression and Cancer

There are different types of antidepressants. Most antidepressants help treat depression by changing the levels of chemicals called "neurotransmitters" in the brain, while some affect cell receptors. Nerves use these chemicals to send messages to one another. Increasing the amount of these chemicals helps improve mood. The different types of antidepressants act on these chemicals in different ways and have different side effects.

Several types of antidepressants are used to treat depression:
- **Selective serotonin reuptake inhibitors (SSRIs).** These are medicines that stop serotonin (a substance that nerves use to send messages to one another) from being reabsorbed by the nerve cells that make it. This means there is more serotonin for other nerve cells to use. SSRIs include drugs such as citalopram, fluoxetine, and vilazodone.
- **Serotonin norepinephrine reuptake inhibitors (SNRIs).** These are medicines that stop the brain chemicals serotonin and norepinephrine from being reabsorbed by the nerve cells that make it. This means there is more serotonin and norepinephrine for other nerve cells to use. Some SNRIs may also help relieve neuropathy caused by chemotherapy or hot flashes caused by menopause. SNRIs include older drugs, such as tricyclic antidepressants, as well as newer drugs such as venlafaxine.
- **Norepinephrine-dopamine reuptake inhibitors (NDRIs).** These are medicines that stop the brain chemicals norepinephrine and dopamine from being reabsorbed. This means there is more norepinephrine and dopamine for other nerve cells to use. The only NDRI currently approved to treat depression is bupropion.

The following antidepressants may also be used:
- mirtazapine
- trazodone
- monoamine oxidase inhibitors (MAOIs)

Other medicines may be given along with antidepressants to treat other symptoms. Benzodiazepines may be given to decrease anxiety, and psychostimulants may be given to improve energy and concentration.

The antidepressant that is best for you depends on several factors.

Choosing the best antidepressant for you depends on the following:
- your symptoms
- side effects of the antidepressant
- your medical history
- other medicines you are taking
- how you or your family members responded to antidepressants in the past
- the form of medicine you are able to take (such as a pill or a liquid)

You may have to try different treatments to find the one that is right for you.

Your doctor will watch you closely if you need to change or stop taking your antidepressant.

You may need to change your antidepressant or stop taking it if severe adverse effects occur or your symptoms are not getting better. Check with your doctor before you stop taking an antidepressant. For some types of antidepressants, your doctor will reduce the dose slowly. This is to prevent side effects that can occur if you suddenly stop taking the medicine.

It is important for you to know what to expect when you change or stop antidepressants. Your doctor will watch you closely while lowering or stopping doses of one medicine before starting another.

DEPRESSION IN CHILDREN WITH CANCER

Some children have depression or other problems related to cancer.

Most children cope well with cancer. However, a small number of children may have:
- depression or anxiety
- trouble sleeping

Depression and Cancer

- problems getting along with family or friends
- problems following the treatment plan

These problems can affect the child's cancer treatment and enjoyment of life. They can occur at any time from diagnosis to well after treatment ends. Survivors of childhood cancer who have severe late effects from cancer treatment may be more likely to have symptoms of depression.

A mental health specialist can help children with depression.

Assessment for depression includes looking at the child's symptoms, behavior, and health history.

As in adults, children with cancer may feel depressed but do not have the medical condition of depression. Depression lasts longer and has specific symptoms. The doctor may assess a child for depression if a problem, such as not eating or sleeping well, lasts for a while. To assess for depression, the doctor will ask about the following:

- how the child is coping with illness and treatment
- past illnesses and how the child coped with the illness
- the child's sense of self-worth
- homelife with family
- the child's behavior, as seen by the parents, teachers, or others
- how the child is developing compared with other children his or her age

The doctor will talk with the child and may use a set of questions or a checklist that helps diagnose depression in children.

The symptoms of depression are not the same in every child.

A diagnosis of depression depends on the symptoms and how long they have lasted. Children who are diagnosed with depression have an unhappy mood and at least four of the following symptoms every day for two weeks or longer:

- appetite changes
- not sleeping or sleeping too much
- being unable to relax and be still (such as pacing, fidgeting, and pulling at clothing)
- frequent crying

- loss of interest or pleasure in usual activities
- lack of emotion in children younger than six years
- feeling very tired or having little energy
- feelings of worthlessness, blame, or guilt
- unable to think or pay attention and frequent daydreaming
- trouble learning in school, not getting along with others, and refusing to go to school in school-aged children
- frequent thoughts of death or suicide

Talk therapy is the main treatment for depression in children. The child may talk to the counselor alone or with a small group of other children. Talk therapy may include play therapy for younger children. Therapy will help the child cope with feelings of depression and understand their cancer and treatment.

Antidepressants may be given to children with major depression and anxiety. In some children, teenagers, and young adults, antidepressants may make depression worse or cause thoughts of suicide. The U.S. Food and Drug Administration (FDA) has warned that patients younger than the age of 25 who are taking antidepressants should be watched closely for signs that the depression is getting worse and for suicidal thinking or behavior.

SUICIDE RISK IN PATIENTS WITH CANCER

Cancer patients may feel hopeless at times and think about suicide.

Cancer patients sometimes feel hopeless. Talk with your doctor if you feel hopeless. There are ways your doctor can help you.

Feelings of hopelessness may lead to thinking about suicide. If you or someone you know is thinking about suicide, get help as soon as possible.

Certain factors may add to a cancer patient's risk of thinking about suicide.

Some of these factors include the following:
- having a personal history of depression, anxiety, or other mental health problem or suicide attempts

Depression and Cancer

- having a family member who has attempted suicide
- having a personal history of drug or alcohol abuse
- feeling hopeless or that you are a burden to others
- not having enough support from family and friends
- being unable to live a normal, independent life because of problems with activities of daily living, pain, or other symptoms
- being within the first three to five months of your cancer diagnosis
- having advanced cancer or a poor prognosis
- having cancer of the prostate, lung, head and neck, or pancreas
- not getting along well with the treatment team

An assessment is done to find the reasons for feeling hopeless or thoughts of suicide.

Talking about thoughts of hopelessness and suicide with your doctor gives you a chance to describe your feelings and fears and may help you feel more in control. Your doctor will try to find out what is causing your hopeless feelings, such as:

- symptoms that are not well controlled
- fear of having a painful death
- fear of being alone during your cancer experience

You can find out what may be done to help relieve your emotional and physical pain.

Controlling symptoms caused by cancer and cancer treatment is important to prevent suicide.

Cancer patients may feel desperate to stop any discomfort or pain they have. Keeping pain and other symptoms under control will help to:

- relieve distress
- make you feel more comfortable
- prevent thoughts of suicide

Treatment may include antidepressants. Some antidepressants take a few weeks to work. The doctor may prescribe other medicines that work quickly to relieve distress until the antidepressant begins to work. For your safety, it is important to have frequent contact with a health-care professional and avoid being alone until your symptoms are controlled. Your health-care team can help you find social support.[1]

---

[1] "Depression (PDQ®)—Patient Version," National Cancer Institute (NCI), July 9, 2019. Available online. URL: www.cancer.gov/about-cancer/coping/feelings/depression-pdq. Accessed March 3, 2023.

Chapter 33 | Depression and Diabetes

Mental health affects so many aspects of daily life such as how you think and feel, handle stress, relate to others, and make choices. Having a mental health problem could make it harder to stick to your diabetes care plan.

THE MIND–BODY CONNECTION
Thoughts, feelings, beliefs, and attitudes can affect how healthy your body is. Untreated mental health issues can make diabetes worse, and problems with diabetes can make mental health issues worse. But, fortunately, if one gets better, the other tends to get better, too.

DEPRESSION: MORE THAN JUST A BAD MOOD
Depression is a medical illness that causes feelings of sadness and often a loss of interest in activities you used to enjoy. It can get in the way of how well you function at work and home, including taking care of your diabetes. When you are not able to manage your diabetes well, your risk goes up for diabetes complications such as heart disease and nerve damage.

People with diabetes are two to three times more likely to have depression than people without diabetes. Only 25–50 percent of people with diabetes who have depression get diagnosed and treated. Treating depression with therapy or medicine or both is usually very effective. Without treatment, depression often gets worse, not better.

Symptoms of depression can be mild to severe and include the following:
- feeling sad or empty
- losing interest in favorite activities
- overeating or not wanting to eat at all
- not being able to sleep or sleeping too much
- having trouble concentrating or making decisions
- feeling very tired
- feeling hopeless, irritable, anxious, or guilty
- having aches or pains, headaches, cramps, or digestive problems
- having thoughts of suicide or death

If you think you might have depression, get in touch with your doctor right away for help getting treatment. The earlier your depression is treated, the better it is for you, your quality of life (QOL), and your diabetes.

DIABETES DISTRESS

You may sometimes feel discouraged, worried, frustrated, or tired of dealing with daily diabetes care. Maybe you have been trying hard but not seeing results. Or you have developed a health problem related to diabetes in spite of your best efforts.

Those overwhelming feelings, known as "diabetes distress," may cause you to slip into unhealthy habits, stop checking your blood sugar, and even skip the doctor's appointments. It happens to many people with diabetes, often after years of good management. In any 18-month period, 33–50 percent of people with diabetes have diabetes distress.

Diabetes distress can look like depression or anxiety, but it cannot be treated effectively with medication. Instead, these approaches have been shown to help:
- Make sure you are seeing an endocrinologist for your diabetes care. He or she is likely to have a deeper understanding of diabetes challenges than your regular doctor.

Depression and Diabetes

- Ask your doctor to refer you to a mental health counselor who specializes in chronic health conditions.
- Get some one-on-one time with a diabetes educator, so you can solve the problem together.
- Focus on one or two small diabetes management goals instead of thinking you have to work on everything all at once.
- Join a diabetes support group, so you can share your thoughts and feelings with people who have the same concerns (and learn from them too).[1]

DEPRESSION: MORE COMMON IN WORKERS WITH DIABETES

Diabetes affects more than 34 million adults in the United States. A study from the National Institute for Occupational Safety and Health (NIOSH) has found that workers with diabetes may be at increased risk for depression. Among workers with diabetes, young adults and women are most likely to experience depression. The study was published online on August 25, 2021, in the journal *Diabetes Spectrum*.

"This study illustrates that for working-age people, having diabetes puts them at an even greater risk for depression," said study author and NIOSH Epidemiologist Harpriya Kaur, Ph.D. "In addition, we found certain factors, specifically age, gender, and co-existing chronic conditions, are associated with depression among workers with diabetes."

Researchers looked at data from the 2014–2018 Behavioral Risk Factor Surveillance System (BRFSS), the world's largest telephone survey, from all 50 states as well as the District of Columbia and three U.S. territories to identify study participants. For their analysis, they included respondents who reported being employed at the time of the survey and as having diabetes—a total of 84,659 people.

Researchers found that the prevalence of depression among workers with diabetes was 30 percent higher than that among those

---

[1] "Diabetes and Mental Health," Centers for Disease Control and Prevention (CDC), November 3, 2022. Available online. URL: www.cdc.gov/diabetes/managing/mental-health.html. Accessed March 3, 2023.

without diabetes, and among survey respondents, the prevalence of depression decreased with age.

Young adult workers with diabetes, aged 18–34 years, were found to have the highest prevalence of depression—nearly 30 percent reported experiencing depression compared to just over 11 percent of workers surveyed over the age of 65. Additionally, for young adult workers with diabetes, those who had another chronic condition were almost three times as likely to report depression.

When researchers looked at the data by gender, female workers with diabetes in all age groups were more likely to self-report depression than their male counterparts.

"A strength of this study is the large population-based sample that allowed us to explore the relationship between diabetes and depression among workers by age group and other characteristics including demographics and physical health conditions," said Dr. Kaur. "Having a better understanding of which groups may be at greatest risk can help inform preventive measures such as tailored educational messages and health promotion resources in the workplace."[2]

---

[2] "Depression More Common in Workers with Diabetes," Centers for Disease Control and Prevention (CDC), August 25, 2021. Available online. URL: www.cdc.gov/niosh/updates/upd-08-25-21.html. Accessed March 3, 2023.

Chapter 34 | Depression and Heart Disease

Mental health is an important part of overall health and refers to a person's emotional, psychological, and social well-being. Mental health involves how we think, feel, act, and make choices.

Mental health disorders can be short- or long-term and can interfere with a person's mood, behavior, thinking, and ability to relate to others. Various studies have shown the impact of trauma, depression, anxiety, and stress on the body, including stress on the heart.

WHAT MENTAL HEALTH DISORDERS ARE RELATED TO HEART DISEASE?

Some of the most commonly studied mental health disorders associated with heart disease or related risk factors include the following:

- **Mood disorders.** People living with mood disorders, such as major depression or bipolar disorder, find that their mood affects both psychological and mental well-being nearly every day for most of the day.
- **Anxiety disorders.** People respond to certain objects or situations with fear, dread, or terror. Anxiety disorders include generalized anxiety, social anxiety, panic disorders, and phobias.
- **Posttraumatic stress disorder (PTSD).** People can experience PTSD after undergoing a traumatic life experience, such as war, natural disaster, or any other serious incident.

- **Chronic stress.** People are in a state of uncomfortable emotional stress—accompanied by predictable biochemical, physiological, and behavioral changes—that is constant and persists over an extended period of time.

There may be other behavioral health disorders, such as substance use disorders (SUDs), that are connected to heart disease.

WHAT IS THE CONNECTION BETWEEN MENTAL HEALTH DISORDERS AND HEART DISEASE?

A large and growing body of research shows that mental health is associated with risk factors for heart disease before a diagnosis of a mental health disorder and during treatment. These effects can arise both directly, through biological pathways, and indirectly, through risky health behaviors.

People experiencing depression, anxiety, stress, and even PTSD over a long period of time may experience certain physiologic effects on the body, such as increased cardiac reactivity (e.g., increased heart rate and blood pressure), reduced blood flow to the heart, and heightened levels of cortisol. Over time, these physiologic effects can lead to calcium buildup in the arteries, metabolic disease, and heart disease.

Evidence shows that mental health disorders—such as depression, anxiety, and PTSD—can develop after cardiac events, including heart failure, stroke, and heart attack. These disorders can be brought on after an acute heart disease event from factors including pain, fear of death or disability, and financial problems associated with the event.

Some literature notes the impact of medicines used to treat mental health disorders on cardiometabolic disease risk. The use of some antipsychotic medications has been associated with obesity, insulin resistance, diabetes, heart attacks, atrial fibrillation (AF), stroke, and death.

Mental health disorders such as anxiety and depression may increase the chance of adopting behaviors such as smoking, inactive lifestyle, or failure to take prescribed medications. This is because people experiencing a mental health disorder may have fewer healthy coping strategies for stressful situations, making it difficult for them to make healthy lifestyle choices to reduce their risk for heart disease.

WHAT GROUPS HAVE HIGHER RATES OF HEART DISEASE FROM MENTAL HEALTH DISORDERS?

Specific populations that include the following show higher rates of heart disease as a result of preexisting mental health disorders:

- **Veterans.** Studies found that veterans are at a higher risk for heart disease, mainly due to PTSD as a result of combat.
- **Women.** Studies exclusively focused on women found that PTSD and depression may have damaging effects on physical health, particularly with increased risk for morbidity and mortality related to coronary heart disease (CHD).
- **Couples with someone who has PTSD.** Comparative studies found that couples where one or both partners had PTSD experienced more severe conflict, greater anger, and increased cardiovascular reactivity to conflict discussions than couples where neither partner had PTSD. Anger and physiological stress responses to couple discord might contribute to CHD and heart disease risk within these relationships.
- **Racial and ethnic minorities.** Lastly, studies focused on racial or ethnic minority groups found that depression, stress, and anxiety due to disparities in social determinants of health, adverse childhood experiences (ACEs), and racism/discrimination could place certain subpopulations at a higher risk for hypertension, cardiovascular reactivity, heart disease, and poor heart health outcomes.

WHAT CAN BE DONE FOR PEOPLE WITH MENTAL HEALTH DISORDERS?

Addressing mental health disorders early by providing access to appropriate services and support to increase healthy behaviors (e.g., increased physical activity, improved diet quality, and reduced smoking) can reduce someone's risk of experiencing a heart disease event.

Below are some actions that health-care systems, health-care professionals, and individuals can take to promote heart disease prevention and support mental health.

Actions for Health-Care Systems
- Set up multidisciplinary teams that include both mental health and heart disease professionals.
- Employ clinical decision support or electronic health record systems to coordinate care among the multidisciplinary teams.

Actions for Health-Care Professionals
- Learn more about the link between mental health and heart disease.
- Talk to your patients about the relationship between mental health and heart disease.
- Incorporate mental health screening and treatment into care surrounding a major heart disease event and chronic disease.
- Involve individuals and their family members in communication and decision making regarding treatment following a heart disease event.
- For patients with severe mental health disorders and pre-existing heart disease or its risk factors:
- Consider prescribing or switching a patient to a psychotropic medication with lower risk for heart disease, while weighing any clinical benefits and potential for adverse events.
- Consider the potential interactions between prescribed medicines for heart disease and prescribed psychotropic medications.
- Monitor heart health outcomes and risk factors, and adjust doses of heart disease medicines if required.

Depression and Heart Disease

Actions for Individuals
- Recognize the signs and symptoms of mental health disorders and heart disease.
- Talk with your health-care professionals about potential heart conditions in relation to your mental health disorder and treatment options.
- Know that your family history and genetic factors likely play some role in your risk for heart disease.
- Know which conditions increase the risk of heart disease.
- Maintain a healthy lifestyle.[1]

---

[1] "Heart Disease and Mental Health Disorders," Centers for Disease Control and Prevention (CDC), May 6, 2020. Available online. URL: www.cdc.gov/heartdisease/mentalhealth.htm#:~:text=People%20experiencing%20depression%2C%20anxiety%2C%20stress,and%20heightened%20levels%20of%20cortisol. Accessed March 3, 2023.

Chapter 35 | Depression and Human Immunodeficiency Virus

WHAT IS HUMAN IMMUNODEFICIENCY VIRUS?

Human immunodeficiency virus (HIV) is the virus that causes acquired immunodeficiency syndrome (AIDS). HIV can be transmitted during sexual intercourse, by sharing syringes, or during pregnancy, childbirth, or breastfeeding.

HIV weakens the immune system by destroying $CD4^+$ T cells, a type of white blood cell that is important for fighting off infections. The loss of these cells means that people living with HIV are more vulnerable to other infections and diseases.

Today, effective anti-HIV medications allow people with HIV to lead long, healthy lives. When taken as prescribed, these daily medications, called "antiretroviral therapy" (ART), can suppress the amount of virus in the blood to a level so low that it is undetectable by standard tests.[1]

HOW CAN HIV AFFECT YOUR MENTAL HEALTH?

- Having HIV can be a source of major stress.
- HIV may challenge your sense of well-being or complicate existing mental health conditions.
- HIV, and some opportunistic infections, can also affect your nervous system and can lead to changes in your behavior.

---

[1] "HIV and AIDS and Mental Health," National Institute of Mental Health (NIH), November 2022. Available online. URL: www.nimh.nih.gov/health/topics/hiv-aids#part_2496. Accessed March 14, 2023.

Good mental health will help you live your life to the fullest and is essential to successfully treating HIV.[2]

WHY ARE PEOPLE WITH HIV AND AIDS AT HIGHER RISK OF MENTAL DISORDERS?

The stress associated with living with a serious illness or condition, such as HIV, can affect a person's mental health. People with HIV have a higher chance of developing mood, anxiety, and cognitive disorders. For example, depression is one of the most common mental health conditions faced by people with HIV.

It is important to remember that mental disorders are treatable. People who have a mental disorder can recover.

HIV and related infections can also affect the brain and the rest of the nervous system. This may change how a person thinks and behaves. Also, some medications used to treat HIV may have side effects that affect a person's mental health.

Situations that can contribute to mental health problems for anyone are as follows:
- having trouble getting mental health services
- experiencing a loss of social support, resulting in isolation
- experiencing a loss of employment or worries about being able to perform at work
- dealing with loss, including the loss of relationships or the death of loved ones

In addition, people with HIV may also experience situations that negatively impact their mental health, such as:
- having to tell others about an HIV diagnosis
- managing HIV medicines and medical treatment
- facing stigma and discrimination associated with HIV/AIDS

---

[2] "Stigma and Mental Health," Centers for Disease Control and Prevention (CDC), May 20, 2021. Available online. URL: www.cdc.gov/hiv/basics/livingwithhiv/mental-health.html. Accessed March 14, 2023.

Depression and Human Immunodeficiency Virus

Understanding how living with HIV can affect mental health and knowing what resources are available can make it easier for people to manage their overall health and well-being.[3]

HIV AND DEPRESSION
One of the most common mental health conditions that people with HIV face is depression.

What Are the Symptoms of Depression?
Symptoms of depression that can affect your day-to-day life include:
- persistent sadness
- anxiety
- feeling empty
- feelings of helplessness
- negativity
- loss of appetite
- disinterest in engaging with others[4]

HOW CAN PEOPLE WITH HIV IMPROVE THEIR MENTAL HEALTH?
Research shows that HIV treatment should begin as soon as possible after diagnosis to achieve the best health outcomes. Following a treatment plan, such as taking the medications prescribed by a healthcare provider, is critical for controlling and suppressing the virus.

Following the treatment plan can be difficult, but there are strategies that can help, such as following a treatment plan, creating a routine, setting an alarm, and downloading a reminder app on a smartphone.

Starting ART can affect mental health in different ways. Sometimes, ART can relieve anxiety because knowing that you are taking care of yourself can provide a sense of security. However, coping with the reality of living with a chronic illness such as HIV can be challenging. In addition, some antiretroviral medicines may

---
[3] See footnote [1].
[4] See footnote [2].

cause symptoms of depression, anxiety, and sleeplessness and may make some mental health issues worse.

For these reasons, it is important for people with HIV to talk to a health-care provider about their mental health before starting ART. These conversations should continue throughout treatment.

People with HIV should talk with their providers about any changes in their mental health, such as thinking or how they feel about themselves and life in general. People with HIV should also discuss any alcohol or substance use with their providers.

People with HIV should also tell their health-care provider about any over-the-counter or prescribed medications they may be taking, including any mental health medications, because some of these drugs may interact with antiretroviral medications.[5]

---

[5] See footnote [1].

Chapter 36 | Depression and Multiple Sclerosis

Depression is common in the general population, but depression is even more common in people with multiple sclerosis (MS). Approximately 50 percent of people with MS will experience an episode of major depression, a clinical diagnosis that requires at least two weeks with five or more depressive symptoms. Major depression is not only more common in people with MS than in the general population, but it is also more common in people with MS than in people with other chronic diseases. Although major depression is a serious condition, remember that effective treatment is available.

WHY SHOULD SOMEONE BE CONCERNED IF THEY ARE DEPRESSED?

Depression is a serious condition and, if left untreated, can lead to chronic depression. Depression is a medical disorder that can be mild, severe, or even life-threatening. Not only can it affect a person's quality of life (QOL), but it can also interfere with relationships, jobs, and a person's overall health. People with depression are at higher risk for suicide, and the suicide rate is even higher for those with both MS and major depression. Depression is not something to ignore or "just get over." It is a disorder that requires close monitoring and treatment.

HOW CAN YOU TELL IF YOU HAVE MAJOR DEPRESSION?

The two main symptoms that may indicate major depression are persistent sadness and loss of interest in usually enjoyable activities.

A person may also sleep too much or too little, eat too much or too little, feel excessively guilty, and have decreased concentration or decreased energy. Some might be irritable, be angry, have feelings of hopelessness, or have thoughts of hurting themselves or others. Often, signs and symptoms of depression, such as fatigue or difficulty with concentration, can mimic symptoms of MS. Everyone feels down or overwhelmed every once in a while, but when a person feels this way for more than two weeks or is starting to have difficulty enjoying life, it is time for a more complete evaluation by a heath-care provider.

WHAT SHOULD YOU DO IF YOU THINK YOU ARE DEPRESSED?

If you think you are depressed, talk to a health-care provider. This could be your primary care team, neurologist, or rehabilitation doctor. These providers can help with diagnosing and treating depression, or they may refer you to a behavioral health specialist such as a psychiatrist or psychologist for further assessment and treatment. If a person is having thoughts of suicide, immediate attention is required: Dial 988 for the National Suicide and Crisis Lifeline, and press 1 specifically for veterans.

HOW IS MAJOR DEPRESSION TREATED?

Treatment options for major depression may include antidepressant medication, counseling, lifestyle modifications, and support, as well as complementary and alternative medicine (CAM). Effective treatment often includes a combination of these therapies. There are many antidepressant medications, and some have the added benefit of treating pain, insomnia, or fatigue. For some people, treating their depression also reduces some of their MS symptoms such as fatigue, impaired cognition, and memory difficulties. Although each person responds to medications uniquely, overall, antidepressants are well tolerated. Other substances can interfere with the effectiveness of antidepressants, and a health-care provider should be informed about all medications and supplements you are taking, as well as alcohol and drug use before starting an antidepressant. Antidepressants can take as long as six to eight weeks to work, so do not become discouraged if results are not seen immediately.

If you have depression, talk with your MS care team. Depression can be treated successfully![1]

Coping Strategies for People with Multiple Sclerosis

MS is an unpredictable disease that is often accompanied by stress. Anxiety, depression, and other psychiatric problems are often experienced by people with MS. The rates of these problems in people with MS are higher than those in people who do not have MS. People with psychiatric problems in connection with MS tend to report lower satisfaction with life. Additionally, studies show that psychiatric problems can result in the worsening of MS disability.

While psychological and social stress is common in those with MS, some people also experience posttraumatic stress disorder (PTSD). PTSD is a disorder involving prolonged reactions in those who have undergone a scary or dangerous event. PTSD can be due to trauma from the battlefield, sexual assault, childhood abuse, or even a traumatizing medical diagnosis or procedure. A pilot study from the VA MS Center of Excellence East showed that a prior diagnosis of PTSD in those with MS may be linked with increases in the number of relapses (1.2 relapses in MS participants with PTSD in the two years of the study compared to 0.37 in MS participants without PTSD). Those with MS and PTSD were also likely to have new magnetic resonance imaging (MRI) brain lesions (60% of MS participants with PTSD had new lesions in the two years of the study compared to 16.7% of MS participants without PTSD).

It is thought that PTSD and the stress related to it may potentially lead to additional neurochemical changes, leading to further inflammation, which leads to relapses and brain lesions. On the other hand, PTSD could lead to decreased adherence to MS medications, but there was no correlation with this in the study. Given that psychiatric conditions associated with MS can lead to stress,

---

[1] "Questions and Answers about Depression," U.S. Department of Veterans Affairs (VA), November 18, 2022. Available online. URL: www.va.gov/MS/Veterans/symptoms_of_MS/Questions_and_Answers_About_Depression.asp. Accessed March 6, 2023.

which can lead to worsened outcomes, strategies should be implemented to reduce stress. Coping is a behavioral strategy that can help mitigate stress.

Art Therapy

One strategy for coping with MS-related stress is art therapy. While art as a form of therapy has been around for centuries, art therapy has become popular over the years to help people cope with chronic medical conditions. Artwork such as painting, writing, or creating music can help people with MS bring their stress and worries into the open, which can help decrease the stress. Studies have shown that art therapy in those with MS can also help increase confidence and improve emotional well-being. Art therapy can also help those who are more disabled work on improved arm control.

Mindfulness

Another coping strategy shown to be useful is mindfulness. Mindfulness is defined as focusing on the present moment while understanding and accepting one's feelings, thoughts, and sensations. Practicing mindfulness originated in Eastern philosophy as a method for relaxation. Mindfulness has been shown to also help with managing anxiety, depression, and chronic pain. Classes in mindfulness can be taken and typically last around eight weeks. They tend to relate to different types of meditation such as being aware of the number and length of breaths being taken at a time, body awareness, and yoga.

Exercise

Exercise is another excellent way to cope. Exercises such as jogging, swimming, and using a stationary bicycle have been shown to be helpful for those with and without MS. Your health-care team, including the physical and occupational therapist, can help create a personalized program for you to address your specific abilities and needs. Another type of exercise worth seeking out is yoga. Yoga involves breathing and stretches that center on the spine. Depending on one's balance, changes can be made to ensure safety.

Depression and Multiple Sclerosis

Another similar exercise to yoga is tai chi, which is more "gentle." Tai chi also involves breathing, slow movement, and relaxation.

Pets

Finally, studies have shown that having a pet helps some people cope with a health problem. Being around pets can help take your mind away from dealing with the stress with MS. It can also help with the stress of psychiatric conditions related to MS. A service pet is another option for those who need assistance with medical issues such as vision or walking. For those who do not want to own a pet, health-care programs are increasingly adopting a pet program where specially trained pets work with people.

These are just a few of the coping strategies of many that exist. Combining multiple coping skills can be ideal. Discussion of these coping strategies with your treatment team, including physicians, mental health providers, physical therapists, occupational therapists, and social workers, to optimize their effectiveness is essential.[2]

---

[2] "Coping Strategies for People with Multiple Sclerosis," U.S. Department of Veterans Affairs (VA), March 3, 2022. Available online. URL: www.va.gov/MS/Veterans/complementary_and_alternative_medicine/Coping_Strategies_for_People_with_MS.asp. Accessed March 6, 2023.

Chapter 37 | Depression and Neurological Disorders

Chapter Contents
Section 37.1—Genetic Overlap between Alzheimer Disease and Depression 295
Section 37.2—Depression, a Nonmotor Manifestation of Parkinson Disease.. 298
Section 37.3—Depression in Epilepsy 302

Chapter 3 | Psychiatric and Neurological Disorders

Section 37.1 | Genetic Overlap between Alzheimer Disease and Depression

Some cases of Alzheimer disease (AD) may be driven by the genetic risk factors that can underlie depression, according to a data-mining study supported by the National Institute on Aging (NIA) by researchers at Emory University School of Medicine. The results, published in *Biological Psychiatry*, suggest that the activity of at least seven genes may help explain why depression appears to increase the chances one may experience AD.

First, the researchers sought links between the two disorders by analyzing the data of more than 1.2 million individuals of European descent who took part in several genome-wide association studies (GWASs). These types of studies aim to find one-letter changes in DNA sequences, called "single nucleotide polymorphisms"—or "SNPs" for short—that appear often on the chromosomes of individuals who experience a particular disease.

Although several other studies have suggested that there is a relationship between depression and AD, previous attempts to search for genomic links between the two disorders have produced mixed results. But those investigations relied on a single GWAS of each disease.

In contrast, for this study, the scientists searched the combined results of several depression and Alzheimer GWASs. Generally, combining data increases the chances of detecting reliable signals. They also used advanced analysis techniques for assessing how the SNPs may influence genetic activity.

Initially, the team discovered that there is a shared genetic risk between the two disorders. In other words, they saw a correlation between the SNPs carried by people with AD and those observed in individuals who experienced depression.

The researchers then used a different analysis technique to determine whether there may be a causal link between the diseases. They found that the SNPs associated with depression also raised the chances that an individual may develop AD. However, the opposite was not observed. The SNPs associated with AD did not raise the risk that an individual would also experience depression.

Further support for these findings was obtained when the researchers reanalyzed the combined results from two other aging studies known as "ROS/MAP." They found an association between participants who had higher genetic risk scores for depression and the appearance of several dementia hallmarks, including a faster decline in the ability to remember past experiences. Those who had higher scores experienced a hastier decline in memory.

To understand which genes may be behind the association, the researchers studied the brains of individuals who participated in the ROS/MAP studies. Specifically, they looked at proteins and messenger RNA (mRNA) transcripts. When a gene is turned on, its DNA sequence is copied, or transcribed, into mRNA and then often translated into a protein. So measuring the levels of both proteins and mRNA can help a scientist gauge gene activity.

They found that changes in the activity of at least seven proteins may underlie the genomic causal link between depression and AD discovered in this study. Notably, changes in the levels of two of these proteins, called "RAB27B" and "DDAH2," were associated with every AD hallmark measured in the aging studies.

In a similar type of data-mining study published in *Nature Communications*, the researchers found that AD and other neurodegenerative disorders may share at least 13 genetic links with several psychiatric disorders.

Overall, the results of the Emory study not only strengthened the apparent links between the two disorders but also provided insights into how certain genes may play a critical role in driving the increased risk for AD associated with depression. Such genes may be important targets for developing drugs to treat both depression and dementia.[1]

---

[1] National Institute on Aging (NIA), "Genetic Risk Factors That Underlie Depression May Also Drive Alzheimer's Disease," National Institutes of Health (NIH), September 15, 2022. Available online. URL: www.nia.nih.gov/news/genetic-risk-factors-underlie-depression-may-also-drive-alzheimers-disease. Accessed April 18, 2023.

Depression and Neurological Disorders

MENTAL HEALTH DISPARITIES IN ADULTS WITH DEMENTIA

Alzheimer disease and related conditions that involve loss of mental clarity (dementia) turn daily life tasks into challenges.

African Americans and Hispanics are more likely than non-Hispanic Whites to experience dementia as they age. While depression and anxiety are often associated with dementia, African Americans and Hispanics with these mental health issues are less likely than their White counterparts to be diagnosed and treated. Researchers found that people who reported feelings of serious depression and restlessness had an increased risk of having AD and related dementias. The study also showed to what extent these serious signs of mental illness exist in African Americans and Hispanics compared with Whites.

A national survey from 2007 to 2015 included more than 31,000 Americans, aged 65 and older, who each completed five questionnaires over a two-year period. The surveys captured the participants' race/ethnicity and answers to questions regarding their feelings of depression and restlessness during the past 30 days. Health providers verified diagnoses of AD and other conditions among the survey respondents.

The study results showed that the prevalence of AD and related dementias was highest for African Americans (7.1%), followed by Hispanics (5.7%) and then Whites (4.5%). Self-reported experiences of serious depression and restlessness were also higher in the minority groups.

Serious mental distress is both a potential complication and a trigger of dementia, so it is difficult to determine whether the dementia is causing mental distress or vice versa. However, better diagnosis and management of mental illness may help protect individuals from disease progression. Because of the underdiagnosis of depression and anxiety in older racial/ethnic minorities, self-reported feelings of serious mental distress may be a better predictor of risk for dementia than diagnosis by a psychiatrist.

Racism and cultural barriers might contribute to the higher levels of serious mental distress among African Americans and Hispanics with AD and associated dementias. Identifying culturally acceptable treatments for mental illness could help close the gap between these minority groups and Whites. Also, studying the effects of social stresses across the lifespan may shed light on further ways to improve minority mental health in aging populations.[2]

Section 37.2 | Depression, a Nonmotor Manifestation of Parkinson Disease

Parkinson disease (PD) is a movement disorder of the nervous system that gets worse over time. As nerve cells (neurons) in parts of the brain weaken, are damaged, or die, people may begin to notice problems with movement, tremors, stiffness in the limbs or the trunk of the body, or impaired balance. As symptoms progress, people may have difficulty walking, talking, or completing other simple tasks. Not everyone with one or more of these symptoms has PD, as the symptoms appear in other diseases as well.

There is no cure for PD, but research is ongoing, and medications or surgery can often provide substantial improvement in motor symptoms.

The four primary symptoms of PD are as follows:
- **Tremor.** Shaking or tremors often begins in a hand although sometimes a foot or the jaw is affected first. The tremor associated with PD has a characteristic rhythmic back-and-forth motion that may involve the thumb and forefinger and appear as a "pill-rolling." It is most obvious when the hand is at rest or when a person is under stress. This tremor usually disappears during sleep or improves with a purposeful, intended movement.
- **Rigidity.** Muscle stiffness, or resistance to movement, affects most people with PD. The muscles remain

---

[2] "Study Sheds Light on Mental Health Disparities in Adults with Dementia," National Institute on Minority Health and Health Disparities (NIMHD), January 14, 2022. Available online. URL: www.nimhd.nih.gov/news-events/research-spotlights/dementia.html. Accessed April 18, 2023.

Depression and Neurological Disorders

constantly tense and contracted so that the person aches or feels stiff. The rigidity becomes obvious when another person tries to move the individual's arm, which will move only in short, jerky movements known as "cogwheel rigidity."
- **Bradykinesia.** This is a slowing down of spontaneous and automatic movement that can be particularly frustrating because it may make simple tasks difficult. Activities once performed quickly and easily—such as washing or dressing—may take much longer. There is often a decrease in facial expressions (also known as "masked face").
- **Postural instability.** Impaired balance and changes in posture can increase the risk of falls.

PD does not affect everyone the same way. The rate of progression and the particular symptoms differ among individuals. PD symptoms typically begin on one side of the body. However, the disease eventually affects both sides although symptoms are often less severe on one side than on the other.

People with PD often develop a so-called parkinsonian gait that includes a tendency to lean forward, taking small quick steps as if hurrying (called "festination"), and reduced swinging in one or both arms. They may have trouble initiating movement (start hesitation), and they may stop suddenly as they walk (freezing).

The following are a few other problems that may accompany PD:
- **Depression.** Some people lose their motivation and become dependent on family members.
- **Emotional changes.** Some people with PD become fearful and insecure, while others may become irritable or uncharacteristically pessimistic.
- **Difficulty with swallowing and chewing.** Problems with swallowing and chewing may occur in the later stages of the disease. Food and saliva may collect in the mouth and back of the throat, which can result in choking or drooling. Getting adequate nutrition may be difficult.

- **Speech changes.** About half of all individuals with PD have speech difficulties that may be characterized as speaking too softly or in a monotone. Some may hesitate before speaking, slur, or speak too fast.
- **Urinary problems or constipation.** Bladder and bowel problems can occur due to the improper functioning of the autonomic nervous system, which is responsible for regulating smooth muscle activity.
- **Skin problems.** The skin on the face may become oily, particularly on the forehead and at the sides of the nose. The scalp may become oily, too, resulting in dandruff. In other cases, the skin can become very dry.
- **Sleep problems.** Common sleep problems with PD include difficulty staying asleep at night, restless sleep, nightmares and emotional dreams, and drowsiness or sudden sleep onset during the day. Another common problem is "REM behavior disorder," in which people act out their dreams, potentially resulting in injury to themselves or their bed partners. The medications used to treat PD may contribute to some sleep issues. Many of these problems respond to specific therapies.
- **Dementia or other cognitive problems.** Some people with PD develop memory problems and slow thinking. Cognitive problems become more severe in the late stages of PD, and some people are diagnosed with Parkinson disease dementia (PDD). Memory, social judgment, language, reasoning, or other mental skills may be affected.
- **Orthostatic hypotension.** It is a sudden drop in blood pressure when a person stands up from a lying down or seated position. This may cause dizziness, lightheadedness, and, in extreme cases, loss of balance or fainting. Studies have suggested that in PD, this problem results from a loss of nerve endings in the sympathetic nervous system, which controls heart rate, blood pressure, and other automatic functions in the body. The medications used to treat PD may also contribute.

Depression and Neurological Disorders

- **Muscle cramps and dystonia.** The rigidity and lack of normal movement associated with PD often cause muscle cramps, especially in the legs and toes. PD can also be associated with dystonia—sustained muscle contractions that cause forced or twisted positions. Dystonia in PD is often caused by fluctuations in the body's level of dopamine (a chemical in the brain that helps nerve cells communicate and is involved with movement).
- **Pain.** Muscles and joints may ache because of the rigidity and abnormal postures often associated with the disease.
- **Fatigue and loss of energy.** Many people with PD often have fatigue, especially late in the day. Fatigue may be associated with depression or sleep disorders, but it may also result from muscle stress or from overdoing activity when the person feels well. Fatigue may also result from akinesia, which is trouble initiating or carrying out movement.
- **Sexual dysfunction.** Because of its effects on nerve signals from the brain, PD may cause sexual dysfunction. PD-related depression, or the use of certain medications, may also cause decreased sex drive and other problems.
- **Hallucinations, delusions, and other psychotic symptoms.** These symptoms can be caused by the drugs prescribed for PD.[3]

MANAGING DEPRESSION IN PARKINSON DISEASE

Depression is the most common emotional problem found in persons with PD. It causes immense personal suffering and is associated with increased disability and burden to caregivers. Despite the adverse consequences of depression in PD, there are virtually no studies to guide clinical treatment. Several studies are currently examining the effectiveness of antidepressant medication

---

[3] "Parkinson's Disease," National Institute of Neurological Disorders and Stroke (NINDS), March 8, 2023. Available online. URL: www.ninds.nih.gov/health-information/disorders/parkinsons-disease. Accessed April 18, 2023.

for depression in PD. However, there have been no studies to examine the effectiveness of nonmedication approaches, such as cognitive-behavioral therapy (CBT), despite the success of these techniques in other populations. CBT teaches people with PD to become more aware of their thoughts and feelings and to change thinking patterns and behaviors that may be related to symptoms of depression.[4]

Section 37.3 | Depression in Epilepsy

For many of the 3.4 million people with epilepsy in the United States, the neurological disorder is just one of the health challenges they face daily.

As many as 30 percent of adults living with epilepsy also suffer from serious mental health conditions, such as severe depression, schizophrenia, or bipolar disorder. Research indicates that mental health conditions can bring on or exacerbate epilepsy, and vice versa, often complicating medical treatment and making epilepsy worse.

Epilepsy and mental illness are both stigmatizing conditions. Trying to manage treatment, the doctor's appointments, and daily activities, while also struggling with the stigma surrounding two complex conditions, can be difficult. Added to this are the challenges of unemployment, poverty, and social isolation commonly experienced by people with epilepsy and people with mental illness. Epilepsy health and social service providers determined there was a need for community-based programs to help adults with epilepsy and co-occurring mental health conditions manage their disorders.[5]

---

[4] "Coping with Depression in Parkinson's Disease," National Institute of Neurological Disorders and Stroke (NINDS), July 25, 2022. Available online. URL: www.ninds.nih.gov/health-information/clinical-trials/coping-depression-parkinsons-disease. Accessed April 18, 2023.

[5] "TIME: Targeted Self-Management for Epilepsy and Mental Illness," Centers for Disease Control and Prevention (CDC), December 6, 2021. Available online. URL: www.cdc.gov/epilepsy/communications/success-stories/time.htm. Accessed April 18, 2023.

Depression and Neurological Disorders

WHAT IS THE RISK IF YOU HAVE EPILEPSY?
- Twenty-five to fifty-five percent of epilepsy patients have depression.
- The suicide rate is higher for people with epilepsy.
- Those with depression have a worse quality of life (QOL).
- Treating depression in people with epilepsy has poor outcomes due to:
  - the focus on seizures
  - fear of medication interactions (antidepressants and anticonvulsants)
  - poor understanding of how the diseases are linked

WHY ARE EPILEPSY PATIENTS LIKELY TO BECOME DEPRESSED?
- psychological stress caused by life with epilepsy
- medication side effects
- the cause of epilepsy (traumatic brain injury (TBI), stroke, etc.) that may cause depression
- epilepsy itself

CAN DEPRESSION BE TREATED?
Depression in patients with epilepsy can be treated in the following ways:
- medications
- therapy
- electroconvulsive therapy (ECT)
- instilling hope

The vagus nerve stimulator was initially developed as a treatment for epilepsy but is now approved by the U.S. Food and Drug Administration (FDA) for depression, and its effectiveness is controversial, and the mechanism is poorly understood.[6]

---

[6] "Epilepsy and Depression," Centers for Disease Control and Prevention (CDC), August 28, 2012. Available online. URL: www.epilepsy.va.gov/Library/EpilepsyDepression.pdf. Accessed April 18, 2023.

TARGETED SELF-MANAGEMENT FOR EPILEPSY AND MENTAL ILLNESS

The Case Western Reserve University (CWRU) developed Targeted Self-Management for Epilepsy and Mental Illness (TIME). TIME is a psychosocial treatment program that blends education, goal setting, and behavioral modeling in a group format. The research suggests that this approach is highly effective in empowering patients to take ownership of their care to significantly reduce their depressive symptoms.

The curriculum-based, in-person intervention consists of 12 weekly sessions of 60–90 minutes. Each session is co-facilitated by a nurse and a peer educator, which is a person with epilepsy who serves as a guide to support intervention participants. "The nurse represents knowledge or serves as the content expert, while the peer educator represents someone with personal experience," said Dr. Martha Sajatovic, a professor of psychiatry and neurology at CWRU and principal investigator of TIME. "The peer educator is TIME's secret sauce."

The peer educator plays a key role, and not because he or she is the model of perfection, said Dr. Sajatovic. "Our premise has always been that we learn a lot more from our mistakes than our successes," she said. "So, we wanted the peer educator to be someone who has the courage to share their experiences—how they struggled with behavior change and what they learned. To say, 'I tried this, it didn't work for me, and this is how I adjusted.'"

A veteran researcher and clinician, Dr. Sajatovic has studied self-management of chronic health conditions for almost two decades. She and colleagues modeled the curriculum for TIME on a previous program targeting people with serious mental illness who also had diabetes. "In both cases, you're dealing with two significant disorders," she said. To adapt that curriculum to people with mental illness and epilepsy, she and colleagues solicited input from a stakeholder advisory group, which included a social services agency in Cleveland called the "Epilepsy Association," the major provider of epilepsy-specific community-based services in Northeast Ohio.

"We had a series of meetings with patients in treatment for epilepsy, family members, health professionals, and other community

Depression and Neurological Disorders

advocates," said Dr. Sajatovic. Over a series of months, this group adapted the program for patients with epilepsy and tested it in a randomized control trial.

The Epilepsy Association also helped with participant recruitment. "The best way to do recruitment is through community engagement," said Kari Colón-Zimmermann, a research coordinator at CWRU and a co-author on TIME. "We shook every tree," she said, recalling that they recruited one of their first peer educators when this individual was going through a challenging time that included staying at a homeless shelter. This individual later went on to become very empowered, helping himself and many others. "Once the groups got going, they became our best advertisement."

However, there was the issue of access to the program itself. "We started in-person, in the middle of a bad winter," said Dr. Sajatovic. "Pretty soon we discovered that people with epilepsy without transportation were having a hard time coming in. So, we started using the speaker phone. If people couldn't come in, they could call in—and they almost always do," said Dr. Sajatovic. As members of a group that meets regularly, they feel accountable to one another. "We've had people call in from buses stuck in traffic, and their cars as they're heading out of town—even from their hospital beds."

The study compared TIME with regular treatment over a 16-week time period in 44 adults with epilepsy and comorbid mental illness. Notably, about 70 percent of the participating adults were unemployed, and most had an income of less than $25,000 a year. The study team was successful in reaching a diverse group of study participants: 57 percent were African American; most participants had generalized seizures.

TRIAL RESULTS

The trial found a robust reduction in depressive symptoms, assessed by the Montgomery Asberg Depression Rating Scale (MADRS). Average participation in TIME group sessions was 90 percent. Of the 19 individuals assigned to TIME who completed the study, only one did not attend a single session, while six attended all but one session and eight attended all sessions. About 92 percent reported that TIME addressed issues important to their situation.

Having demonstrated that TIME can empower patients to improve their QOL without using medicines, Dr. Sajatovic and colleagues at Case Western Reserve partnered with the Epilepsy Association and the Alcohol, Drug Addiction and Mental Health Services Board of Cuyahoga County, Ohio, on Community-TIME (C-TIME), an initiative to assess using TIME in a community setting. Despite a sample size of just 30 individuals, the study again found a significant reduction in depressive symptoms, as well as a patient satisfaction rate of over 90 percent. This study demonstrated that C-TIME could be successfully used in the community. Dr. Sajatovic and her team have presented their research to national groups (e.g., American Epilepsy Society, National Association of County Behavioral Health and Disability Directors) and continue to seek more partners to adopt the intervention.[7]

---

[7] See footnote [1].

Chapter 38 | Depression and Stroke

A stroke, sometimes called a "brain attack," occurs when something blocks the blood supply to part of the brain or when a blood vessel in the brain bursts.

In either case, parts of the brain become damaged or die. A stroke can cause lasting brain damage, long-term disability, or even death.

WHAT HAPPENS IN THE BRAIN DURING A STROKE?

The brain controls our movements, stores our memories, and is the source of our thoughts, emotions, and language. The brain also controls many functions of the body, such as breathing and digestion.

To work properly, your brain needs oxygen. Your arteries deliver oxygen-rich blood to all parts of your brain. If something happens to block the flow of blood, brain cells start to die within minutes because they cannot get oxygen. This causes a stroke.

QUICK TREATMENT IS CRITICAL FOR STROKE

A stroke is a serious medical condition that requires emergency care. Act fast. Call 911 right away if you or someone you are with shows any signs of a stroke.

Time lost is brain lost. Every minute counts.

WHAT ARE THE TYPES OF STROKE?

There are two types of stroke:
- ischemic stroke
- hemorrhagic stroke

A transient ischemic attack (TIA) is sometimes called a "ministroke." It is different from the major types of stroke because blood flow to the brain is blocked for only a short time—usually no more than five minutes.

Ischemic Stroke

Most strokes are ischemic strokes. An ischemic stroke occurs when blood clots or other particles block the blood vessels to the brain.

Fatty deposits called "plaque" can also cause blockages by building up in the blood vessels.

Hemorrhagic Stroke

A hemorrhagic stroke happens when an artery in the brain leaks blood or ruptures (breaks open). The leaked blood puts too much pressure on brain cells, which damages them.

High blood pressure and aneurysms—balloon-like bulges in an artery that can stretch and burst—are examples of conditions that can cause a hemorrhagic stroke.

Transient Ischemic Attack ("ministroke")

TIAs are sometimes known as "warning strokes." It is important to know the following:
- A TIA is a warning sign of a future stroke.
- A TIA is a medical emergency, just like a major stroke.
- Strokes and TIAs require emergency care. Call 911 right away if you feel signs of a stroke or see symptoms in someone around you.
- There is no way to know in the beginning whether symptoms are from a TIA or from a major type of stroke.
- Like ischemic strokes, blood clots often cause TIAs.
- More than a third of people who have a TIA and do not get treatment have a major stroke within one year. As many as 10–15 percent of people will have a major stroke within three months of a TIA.

Depression and Stroke

Recognizing and treating TIAs can lower the risk of a major stroke. If you have a TIA, your health-care team can find the cause and take steps to prevent a major stroke.[1]

CARING FOR SOMEONE WITH EMOTIONAL AND BEHAVIORAL NEEDS
Depression after Stroke

After a stroke, your loved one may have many negative feelings. Your loved one may think that things will never get better. This is not true—help is available!

Almost half of all stroke survivors have depression. Depression is a normal response to the losses that occur from a stroke.

What Are the Signs and Symptoms of Depression in People with Stroke?

Here is a list of the signs and symptoms of depression in people with stroke. Five or more of these signs or symptoms that last more than two weeks are warning signals for depression.

- sadness or an "empty" mood
- feeling guilty, worthless, or helpless
- problems concentrating, remembering, or making decisions
- appetite and/or weight changes
- feeling hopeless
- lack of energy or feeling tired and "slowed down"
- problems with sleep, such as trouble getting to sleep, staying asleep, or sleeping too much
- feeling restless or irritable
- loss of interest or pleasure in hobbies and activities, including sex, that were once enjoyed

---

[1] "About Stroke," Centers for Disease Control and Prevention (CDC), November 2, 2022. Available online. URL: www.cdc.gov/stroke/about.htm. Accessed March 6, 2023.

Depression Sourcebook, Sixth Edition

What Do You Need to Know?
- Depression is real. People need help when they have depression.
- Physical and emotional changes are common after a stroke. Accept your loved one's changes.
- Expect improvements over time. Things often get better.

Why Is It Important to Get Help?
Treatment of depression will help stroke survivors recover faster. It will make your job as a caregiver easier. For instance, treating depression helps with the following:
- thinking skills and memory
- physical recovery and rehabilitation
- language and speech
- emotions and motivation

What Treatments Should You Discuss with Your Health-Care Team?
Get help from your health-care team quickly. The stroke survivor and family members may explain away the person's depression. Make sure that the stroke survivor receives treatment.
- Medicines, such as antidepressants, improve symptoms.
- Psychotherapy (talk therapy) is used along with medicines. Talk therapy gives your loved one a safe place to talk about feelings.
- Support groups provide help from other stroke survivors and caregivers. They know what you and your loved one are going through. There are support groups for stroke survivors and caregivers like you.

HELPFUL TIPS
- Know the warning signals of depression. Watch for the signs and symptoms of depression.
- Get help quickly.
- Be patient with your loved one. After a stroke, it will take time for your loved one to understand the changes.

Depression and Stroke

- Help your loved one exercise and take part in fun activities.
- Encourage friends and your family to visit and talk with your loved one.
- Have a good attitude. Focus on how much your stroke survivor can do. Smile and relax about things you cannot change.

REMEMBER
- Depression is real and should be treated.
- You are the key person to watch for the warning signals of depression.
- Get help quickly if you think your loved one has depression.[2]

---

[2] "RESCUE Fact Sheet—Depression after Stroke," U.S. Department of Veterans Affairs (VA), January 5, 2011. Available online. URL: www.cidrr8.research.va.gov/rescue/emotional-needs/depression.cfm#signs. Accessed March 6, 2023.

Part 6 | Diagnosis and Treatment of Depression

Chapter 39 | Recognizing Signs of Depression in You and Your Loved Ones

DEPRESSION: CONVERSATION STARTERS

Depression can be hard to talk about. But, if a friend or loved one is depressed, having a conversation about getting help can make a big difference. Use these tips to start talking.

SHOW YOU CARE

- "How are you feeling? I am here to listen to you and support you."
- "I am concerned about you. I think you may need to talk to someone about depression. I want you to get the help you need to feel better."
- "Let me tell you all the things I love about you."
- "I would really like to spend more time with you. Let us take a walk, grab something to eat, or go to a movie."

OFFER HOPE

- "You are not alone. Many people suffer from depression—it is nothing to be ashamed of."
- "Depression can be treated. Getting help is the best thing you can do."
- "Most people get better with treatment—even people who have severe depression."

- "There are different ways to treat depression, including therapy and medicine."
- "Getting more physical activity might also help you feel better."

OFFER TO HELP
- "Let me help you figure out what is going on. You can start by making an appointment with your doctor—or I can help you find someone else to talk to, such as a counselor, therapist, or social worker."
- "I can give you a ride to your therapy appointment or remind you to take your medicine."
- "You can call or text me at any time if you need support—or if you just want to talk."[1]

LIVING WELL WITH MAJOR DEPRESSIVE DISORDER
These healthy lifestyle habits, along with professional treatment, can help you manage the symptoms of major depression:
- **Focus on self-care.** Control stress with activities such as meditation or tai chi. Eat healthy, exercise, and get enough sleep. Most adults need seven to nine hours of sleep per night. Avoid using alcohol and recreational drugs, which can worsen symptoms and make depression harder to treat.
- **Set small, achievable goals.** Set realistic goals to build confidence and motivation. A goal at the beginning of treatment may be to make your bed, have lunch with a friend, or take a walk. Build up to bigger goals as you feel better.
- **Know the warning signs.** Recognize your depression triggers and talk to your doctor and/or mental health professional if you notice unusual changes in how you

---

[1] Office of Disease Prevention and Health Promotion (ODPHP), "Depression: Conversation Starters," U.S. Department of Health and Human Services (HHS), March 14, 2023. Available online. URL: https://health.gov/myhealthfinder/healthy-living/mental-health-and-relationships/depression-conversation-starters. Accessed March 14, 2023.

Recognizing Signs of Depression in You and Your Loved Ones

feel, think, or act. If needed, your doctor can safely adjust your medication. Write down how you feel day-to-day (moods, feelings, reactions) to spot patterns and understand your depression triggers.
- **Educate family and friends about major depression.** They can help you notice warning signs that your depression may be returning.
- **Seek support.** Whether you find encouragement from family members or a support group, maintaining relationships with others is important, especially in times of crisis or rough spells.
- **Stick to your treatment plan.** Even if you feel better, do not stop going to therapy or taking your medication. Abruptly stopping medication can cause withdrawal symptoms and a return of depression. Work with a doctor to adjust your doses or medication, if needed, to continue a treatment plan.[2]

---

[2] "Living Well with Major Depressive Disorder," Substance Abuse and Mental Health Services Administration (SAMHSA), September 27, 2022. Available online. URL: www.samhsa.gov/serious-mental-illness/major-depression#tips-for-living-well. Accessed March 14, 2023.

Chapter 40 | **Finding and Choosing a Therapist**

Therapists have different professional backgrounds and specialties.

The approach a therapist uses depends on the disorder being treated and the training and experience of that therapist. Therapists may combine and adapt elements of different approaches.

Once you have identified one or more possible therapists, a preliminary conversation can help you understand how treatment will proceed and decide if you feel comfortable with the therapist. Rapport and trust are essential. Discussions in therapy are deeply personal, and it is important that you feel comfortable with the therapist and have confidence in their expertise. These preliminary conversations may happen in person, by phone, or virtually. Consider trying to get answers to the following questions:
- What are the credentials and experience of the therapist? Do they have a specialty?
- What approach will the therapist take to help you? Do they practice a particular type of therapy? What is the rationale for the therapy and its evidence base?
- Does the therapist have experience in diagnosing and treating the age group (e.g., a child) and the specific condition for which treatment is being sought? If the patient is a child, how will parents or caregivers be involved in treatment?
- What are the goals of therapy? Does the therapist recommend a specific time frame or number of sessions? How will progress be assessed, and what happens if you (or the therapist) feel you are not starting to improve?

- Are medications an option? Is this therapist able to prescribe medications?
- Are meetings confidential? How is confidentiality assured? Are there limits to confidentiality?

FINDING A THERAPIST

Many types of professionals offer psychotherapy. Examples include psychiatrists, psychologists, social workers, counselors, and psychiatric nurses.

Your health insurance provider may have a list of mental health professionals participating in your plan. When talking with a prospective therapist, ask about treatment fees, whether the therapist participates in insurance plans, and whether there is a sliding scale for fees according to income.[1]

FIND A HEALTH-CARE PROVIDER OR TREATMENT

Treatment for mental illnesses usually consists of therapy, medication, or a combination of the two. Treatment can be given in person or through a phone or computer (telemental health). It can sometimes be difficult to know where to start when looking for mental health care, but there are many ways to find a provider who will meet your needs.

- **Primary care provider.** Your primary care practitioner can be an important resource, providing initial mental health screenings and referrals to mental health specialists. If you have an appointment with your primary care provider, consider bringing up your mental health concerns and asking for help.
- **Federal resources.** Some federal agencies offer resources for identifying health-care providers and help in finding low-cost health services. These include the following:
    - **The Substance Abuse and Mental Health Services Administration (SAMHSA).** For general

---

[1] "Psychotherapies," National Institute of Mental Health (NIMH), January 2023. Available online. URL: www.nimh.nih.gov/health/topics/psychotherapies. Accessed March 6, 2023.

information on mental health and to locate treatment services in your area, call the SAMHSA's National Helpline at 800-662-HELP (800-662-4357). The SAMHSA also has a Behavioral Health Treatment Services Locator on its website that can be searched by location.
- **The Health Resources and Services Administration (HRSA).** The HRSA works to improve access to health care. The HRSA website has information on finding affordable health care, including health centers that offer care on a sliding fee scale.
- **The Centers for Medicare and Medicaid Services (CMS).** This has information on its website about benefits and eligibility for mental health programs and how to enroll.
- **The National Library of Medicine (NLM) MedlinePlus.** The NLM's website has directories and lists of organizations that can help in identifying a health practitioner.
- **National agencies and advocacy and professional organizations.** Advocacy and professional organizations can be a good source of information when looking for a mental health professional. They often have information on finding a mental health professional on their website, and some have practitioner locators on their websites.
- **State and county agencies.** The website of your state or county government may have information about health services in your area. You may be able to find this information by visiting their websites and searching for the health services department.
- **Insurance companies.** If you have health insurance, a representative of your insurance company will know which local providers are covered by your insurance plan. The websites of many health insurance companies have searchable databases that allow you to find a participating practitioner in your area.

- **University, college, or medical schools.** Your local college, university, or medical school may offer treatment options. To find these, try searching on the website of local university health centers for their psychiatry, psychology, counseling, or social work departments.
- **Help for service members and their families.** Current and former service members may face different mental health issues than the general public. For resources for both service members and veterans, please visit:
  - MentalHealth.gov (www.mentalhealth.gov/get-help/veterans)
  - U.S. Department of Veteran Affairs (VA; www.mentalhealth.va.gov/get-help/index.asp)

DECIDING IF A PROVIDER IS RIGHT FOR YOU

Once you find a potential provider, it can be helpful to prepare a list of questions to help you decide if they are a good fit for you. Examples of questions you might want to ask a potential provider include the following:
- What experience do you have treating someone with my issue?
- How do you usually treat someone with my issue?
- How long do you expect treatment to last?
- Do you accept my insurance?
- What are your fees?

Treatment works best when you have a good relationship with your mental health professional. If you are not comfortable or are feeling like the treatment is not helping, talk with your provider or consider finding a different provider or another type of treatment.

Children and adolescents who do not have a mental health professional should consider speaking with a health-care provider or another trusted adult.

Do not stop the current treatment without talking to your health-care provider.[2]

---

[2] "Help for Mental Illnesses," National Institute of Mental Health (NIMH), November 2022. Available online. URL: www.nimh.nih.gov/health/find-help. Accessed March 6, 2023.

Chapter 41 | Diagnosing Depression

WHAT IS DEPRESSION SCREENING?
Depression screening is also called a "depression test." It is a standard set of questions that you answer to help your health-care provider find out whether you have depression.

Because depression is a common mental health problem, depression screening is often done as part of a routine health checkup. Medical experts recommend that depression screening should be done for everyone starting at the age of 12. Screening can help find depression early. And treating depression early may make recovery faster. Most people with depression will get better.

WHAT IS DEPRESSION SCREENING USED FOR?
Depression screening is used to:
- help diagnose depression
- understand how severe depression may be
- help figure out what type of depression you have

WHY DO YOU NEED DEPRESSION SCREENING?
Depression screening is often part of a routine checkup. You may also need depression screening if you show signs of depression, which may include the following:
- loss of interest or pleasure in activities you used to enjoy
- feeling sad or anxious
- feelings of guilt, worthlessness, or helplessness
- trouble sleeping (insomnia) or sleeping too much
- fatigue and lack of energy

- trouble concentrating, remembering details, or making decisions
- changes in your weight
- thoughts of hurting yourself or suicide

If you are thinking about suicide or hurting yourself, get help right away:
- Call 911 or go to your local emergency room.
- Contact a suicide hotline. In the United States, you can reach the National Suicide and Crisis Lifeline at any time:
  - Call or text 988.
  - Chat online with Lifeline Chat.
  - TTY users can use their preferred relay service or dial 711 and then 988.
- Veterans can contact the Veterans Crisis Line:
  - Call 988 and then press 1.
  - Text 838255.
  - Chat online.
- Call your mental health provider or other provider.
- Reach out to a loved one or close friend.

WHAT HAPPENS DURING DEPRESSION SCREENING?

During depression screening, you will answer a standard set of questions. Your provider may ask the questions, or you may fill out a questionnaire form to discuss with your provider later.

In general, the questions ask you about the following:
- changes you have noticed in your:
  - mood
  - sleep habits
  - appetite or weight
  - energy levels
  - ability to focus your attention
  - stress levels
- medicines you take
- alcohol and drug use
- your personal and family history of depression and other mental health conditions

Diagnosing Depression

You may also have a physical exam. There is no lab test that can diagnose depression. But your provider may order blood tests to find out if another health condition, such as anemia or thyroid disease, may be causing depression.

During a blood test, a health-care professional will take a blood sample from a vein in your arm, using a small needle. After the needle is inserted, a small amount of blood will be collected into a test tube or vial. You may feel a little sting when the needle goes in or out. This usually takes less than five minutes.

If you are being tested by a mental health provider, he or she may ask you more detailed questions about your feelings and behaviors. You may also be asked to fill out a questionnaire about these issues.

WILL YOU NEED TO DO ANYTHING TO PREPARE FOR DEPRESSION SCREENING?

You usually do not need any special preparations for a depression test or a blood test.

ARE THERE ANY RISKS IN DEPRESSION SCREENING?

There is no risk in answering questions or having a physical exam.

There is very little risk in having a blood test. You may have slight pain or bruising at the spot where the needle was put in, but most symptoms go away quickly.

WHAT DO THE RESULTS MEAN?

If you are diagnosed with depression, your provider will discuss your treatment options. Starting treatment as soon as possible may improve your chance of recovery. Treatment for depression may take time to work, but it can help reduce symptoms and shorten how long depression lasts.

Your provider may suggest that you see a mental health provider for your care. A mental health provider is a health-care professional who specializes in diagnosing and treating mental health problems. If you are already seeing a mental health provider, a depression test may help guide your treatment.

IS THERE ANYTHING ELSE YOU NEED TO KNOW ABOUT DEPRESSION SCREENING?

There are many types of mental health providers who treat depression. Your primary health-care provider can help you find the right support.

These are some of the professionals who have training to diagnose and treat depression:

- Psychiatrists are medical doctors who specialize in mental health. They can prescribe medicine.
- Psychologists generally have doctoral degrees, but they do not have medical degrees. They cannot prescribe medicine unless they have a special license. Some psychologists work with providers who can prescribe medicine. Psychologists may use one-on-one counseling and/or group therapy sessions.
- Psychiatric or mental health nurses are nurses with special training in mental health problems. Nurses who may have a master's or doctoral degree in psychiatric-mental health nursing include advanced practice registered nurses (APRNs), certified nurse practitioners (CNPs), and clinical nurse specialists (CNSs). In some states, certain nurses can prescribe medicines.
- Licensed clinical social workers have at least a master's degree in social work with special training in mental health. They cannot prescribe medicine, but they may work with providers who can prescribe medicine. Providers who are licensed clinical social workers usually have LCSW or LICSW after their names.
- Licensed professional counselors (LPCs) may also be called "clinicians" or "therapists." States have different names for these licenses, such as a licensed marriage and family therapist (LMFT). These professionals usually have a master's degree in a field related to mental health. They cannot prescribe medicine but may work with providers who can prescribe.[1]

---

[1] MedlinePlus, "Depression Screening," National Institutes of Health (NIH), December 15, 2022. Available online. URL: https://medlineplus.gov/lab-tests/depression-screening/. Accessed March 6, 2023.

Chapter 42 | Psychotherapy for Depression

Chapter Contents
Section 42.1—Elements of Psychotherapy.................................329
Section 42.2—Cognitive-Behavioral Therapy............................333
Section 42.3—Interpersonal Therapy..335
Section 42.4—Acceptance and Commitment Therapy..............337

Section 42.1 | Elements of Psychotherapy

Lots of teens have some kind of emotional problem. In fact, almost half of U.S. teens will have a mental health problem before they turn 18. The good news is that therapy can really help.

Sometimes, people are embarrassed or afraid to see a therapist. But getting help from a therapist because you are feeling sad or anxious is really not different from seeing a doctor because you broke a bone. In fact, you can feel proud for being brave enough to do what you need to do to get your life back on track.

WHAT IS THERAPY?

Therapy is when you talk about your problems with someone who is a professional counselor, such as a psychiatrist, psychologist, or social worker. Therapy is sometimes called "psychotherapy." That is because it helps with your psychology—the mental and emotional parts of your life.

If you are going through a rough time, talking to a caring therapist can be a great relief. A therapist can help you cope with sadness, worry, and other strong or scary feelings. Here are some other ways therapy can help:
- It can teach you specific skills for handling difficult situations, such as problems with your family or school.
- It can help you find healthy ways to deal with stress or anger.
- It can teach you how to build healthy relationships.
- It can help you figure out how to think about things in more positive ways.
- It can help you figure out how to boost your self-confidence.
- It can help you decide where you want to go in life and how to deal with any obstacles that may come up along the way.

Therapy may feel great right away, or it might feel strange at first. It can take a little time getting used to talking with someone new about your problems. But therapists are trained to listen well, and they want to help.

As time goes on, you should feel comfortable with your therapist. If you do not feel comfortable, or if you think you are not getting better, tell your parent or guardian. Another therapist or type of therapy might work better.

Therapists protect people's privacy. They can share what you say only in very special cases, such as if they think you are in danger. If you are concerned, though, ask about the privacy policy. It is important to feel like you can tell the truth in therapy. It works best if you are honest about any problems you are facing, including problems with drugs or alcohol or any behaviors that can hurt your body or mind.

Just because you start to see a therapist does not mean that you will see one forever. You should be able to learn skills that let you handle your problems on your own. Sometimes, a few sessions are all you need to learn skills and feel better.

WHY DO TEENS GO FOR THERAPY?

Many young people develop mental health conditions, such as depression, eating disorders, or anxiety disorders. If you have a mental health problem, remember there are treatments that work, and you can feel better. Also, some teens go to therapy to get help through a tough time, such as their parents getting divorced or having too much stress at school.

If you feel out of control, or you feel like a mental health problem keeps you from enjoying life, get help. Reach out to a parent or guardian or another trusted adult.

WHAT ARE SOME KINDS OF THERAPY?

There are different kinds of therapy to help you feel better. The best treatment depends on the type of problem that you are facing.

You may have one-on-one talk therapy. This is when you talk to a therapist alone. Or you may join group therapy, where you work with a therapist and other people who are having similar issues. You may also do art therapy, where you paint or draw.

Psychotherapy for Depression

One kind of talk therapy that tends to work well for depression, anxiety, and several other problems is cognitive-behavioral therapy (CBT). This type of therapy teaches you how to think and act in healthier ways.

Sometimes, your therapist will suggest that you take medicine in addition to therapy, which can often be a helpful combination.

WHAT ABOUT ONLINE SUPPORT GROUPS?

There are lots of support groups available on the Internet, including ones to help you handle your feelings. Chat rooms and other online options may help you feel less alone. But if you are having trouble coping, it is important to work with a therapist or other mental health professional.

Remember to be careful about getting information online. Some people use the Internet to promote unhealthy behaviors, such as cutting and dangerous eating habits.

WHAT SHOULD YOU DO TO GET STARTED WITH THERAPY?

If you need help finding a therapist, you can start by talking to your doctor, school nurse, or school counselor. If your family has insurance, the insurance company can tell you which therapists are covered under your plan. You and your parent or guardian can also look online for mental health treatment.

If you need help paying for therapy, you can ask a parent or guardian if they have health insurance that might help pay for therapy. If your family does not have insurance, they can find out about getting it through healthcare.gov. You may also be able to get free or low-cost therapy at a mental health clinic, hospital, university, or other places.[1]

VARIOUS COMPONENTS OF PSYCHOTHERAPY

A variety of different kinds of psychotherapies and interventions have been shown to be effective for specific disorders.

---

[1] girlshealth.gov, "Going to Therapy," Office on Women's Health (OWH), January 7, 2015. Available online. URL: www.girlshealth.gov/feelings/therapy/index.html. Accessed April 26, 2023.

Psychotherapists may use one primary approach or incorporate different elements depending on their training, the condition being treated, and the needs of the person receiving treatment.

Here are examples of the different elements that psychotherapies can include:

- helping a person become aware of automatic ways of thinking that are inaccurate or harmful (e.g., having a low opinion of their abilities) and then finding ways to question those thoughts, understanding how the thoughts affect their emotions and behavior, and changing self-defeating patterns, in an approach known as "CBT"
- identifying ways to cope with stress and developing specific problem-solving strategies
- examining a person's interactions with others and teaching social and communication skills
- applying mindfulness and relaxation techniques, such as meditation and breathing exercises
- using exposure therapy (a type of CBT) for people with anxiety disorders, in which a person spends brief periods in a supportive environment learning to tolerate the distress caused by certain items, ideas, or imagined scenes until, over time, the fear associated with those things dissipates
- tracking emotions and behaviors to raise awareness of their impact on each other
- using supportive counseling to help a person explore troubling issues and receive emotional support
- creating a safety plan to help a person who has thoughts of self-harm or suicide recognize warning signs and use coping strategies, such as contacting friends, family, or emergency personnel

Note that there are many different types of psychotherapy. Therapies are often variations of an established approach, such as CBT. There is no formal approval process for psychotherapies like there is for medications by the U.S. Food and Drug Administration (FDA).

Psychotherapy for Depression

However, for many therapies, research involving large numbers of patients has provided evidence that the treatment is effective. These evidence-based therapies have been shown to reduce symptoms of depression, anxiety, and other mental disorders.[2]

Section 42.2 | Cognitive-Behavioral Therapy

Cognitive-behavioral therapy for depression (CBT-D) is an effective treatment for depression. It is a highly recommended treatment for many individuals with depression.

CBT-D is a short-term psychotherapy (or "talk therapy") for treating symptoms of depression which may include:
- feeling sad, depressed, or hopeless
- lack of interest or pleasure in activities
- feeling worthless or having excessive guilt
- being irritable or agitated
- difficulty making decisions or concentrating
- loss of energy or fatigue
- increase or decrease in appetite or sleep

The overall goal of CBT-D is to improve the symptoms of depression by helping you develop balanced and helpful thoughts about yourself, others, and the future and by helping you spend more time engaging in pleasurable or productive activities. CBT-D helps achieve personal goals and solve problems by learning and practicing new skills. CBT-D can help improve the quality of your life and overall level of functioning.

CBT-D is one of the most studied and effective therapies developed for depression. It is based on decades of research and has been shown to be very effective with veterans, specifically. Over 75 percent of people treated for depression show noticeable improvement following CBT-D. This treatment is at least as effective as

---

[2] "Psychotherapies," National Institute of Mental Health (NIMH), January 2023. Available online. URL: www.nimh.nih.gov/health/topics/psychotherapies. Accessed March 22, 2023.

medications though both CBT and medications can be helpful in the treatment of depression for some people. Many veterans with a history of depression continue to enjoy treatment benefits long after completing CBT-D.

In CBT-D, you will work with your therapist to set specific treatment goals that will help you learn new ways of thinking about situations and coping with problems that come up in the future, even after therapy has ended. These skills will relieve your depression and help you move forward in your life.

After you and your therapist have discussed your treatment goals, your therapist may be able to estimate the amount of time that will be required to attain those goals. CBT typically requires 12–16 sessions to lead to significant improvement. Sessions last about 50–60 minutes when delivered individually and 90 minutes when delivered in a group. You will meet with your therapist regularly until the treatment goals have been reached.

If you decide to participate in CBT, you will be asked to do the following:

- Attend sessions regularly.
- Work together with your therapist to set therapy goals.
- Address the most important issues during each session.
- Practice the new CBT skills in your life outside of the session.

It will be important for you to use the information that you learn during the therapy sessions and apply them to your everyday life to help you feel better.[3]

---

[3] "Cognitive Behavioral Therapy for Depression," U.S. Department of Veterans Affairs (VA), December 11, 2015. Available online. URL: www.mentalhealth.va.gov/docs/cbt_brochure.pdf. Accessed March 22, 2023.

Section 42.3 | Interpersonal Therapy

Some people experience depression because of problematic relationships. Interpersonal therapy (IPT) has been found to be most helpful for people who need to improve their communication, conflict resolution, and/or problem-solving skills. The goal of IPT is to help you solve relationship problems, such as problems with your family, friends, and coworkers.

During IPT, your therapist will:
- help improve your communication and problem-solving skills
- help you learn better ways of responding to situations that tend to result in feelings of depression
- help you learn new and better ways of relating to others

Research has shown that IPT is an effective treatment for adults with mild-to-moderate major depression. This therapy typically lasts for 16–20 sessions and should be conducted by a trained mental health provider.

TIPS FOR GETTING THE MOST OUT OF YOUR COUNSELING SESSION
- Keep all of your appointments with your counselor.
- Be honest and open about how you feel and what issues are concerning you.
- Ask whatever questions come to mind.
- Work cooperatively with your counselor and complete any "homework" assignments (these will be simple and clear) that you may be asked to do between sessions.

If your depression does not noticeably improve after 6–12 weeks, your counselor may modify your treatment or add antidepressant medication. If not, ask your counselor about whether a treatment change is right for you.[4]

---

[4] "Depression: What You Need to Know," U.S. Department of Veterans Affairs (VA), September 13, 2010. Available online. URL: www.healthquality.va.gov/guidelines/MH/mdd/MDDTool4DepressionBookletFINALHiRes.pdf. Accessed March 22, 2023.

INTERPERSONAL PSYCHOTHERAPY FOR DEPRESSED ADOLESCENTS

Interpersonal psychotherapy for depressed adolescents (IPT-A) is designed to treat adolescents with depressive disorders. It is an adaptation of interpersonal psychotherapy (IPT) for depressed adults.

In IPT-A, therapists focus on the reciprocal relationship between mood and relationships. Therapists also focus on the impact of depressive symptoms. IPT-A aims to help adolescents identify their feelings and understand how interpersonal and environmental factors impact their mood, strengthen communication and problem-solving skills, improve interpersonal skills and relationships, and manage or decrease depressive symptoms. IPT-A is an individual treatment; however, therapists might also meet with parents or guardians for one to three sessions as needed.

IPT-A is time-limited and includes three phases. During the initial phase, the therapist provides psychoeducation to the adolescent and parents about depression and explains IPT-A treatment goals. The therapist and adolescent also discuss the adolescent's most important relationships to identify strengths and problems in their communication and problem-solving skills. The therapist and adolescent also co-develop a "treatment contract" that clearly states an area of focus, goals, and expectations for treatment. During the middle phase, the therapist and adolescent explore the area of focus in greater depth. The therapist teaches the adolescent communication skills and problem-solving strategies to help them better navigate interpersonal situations. During the termination phase, the therapist and adolescent review skills learned, progress made, and feelings around ending treatment. The therapist, adolescent, and parents determine whether additional treatment is needed and how the parent can support the adolescent's continued use of new skills.

IPT-A is rated as a promising practice because at least one study achieved a rating of moderate or high on study design and execution and demonstrated a favorable effect on a target outcome.[5]

---

[5] Administration for Children and Families (ACF), "Interpersonal Psychotherapy for Depressed Adolescents," U.S. Department of Health and Human Services (HHS), February 2021. Available online. URL: https://preventionservices.acf.hhs.gov/programs/260/show. Accessed April 25, 2023.

Section 42.4 | Acceptance and Commitment Therapy

Acceptance and commitment therapy (ACT) is a transdiagnostic form of behavior therapy that incorporates mindfulness, acceptance, and behavior-change strategies to help individuals achieve behavioral goals in accordance with their personal values. It also has relevance to patients who are struggling with suicidal ideation and anxiety. Not only there is preliminary evidence that ACT is associated with reduced suicidal ideation and symptoms related to suicidal behavior, but this approach also focuses on the identification of personally held values—sources of vitality and meaning—that may engender reasons for living and future-oriented thinking.[6]

WHAT IS ACCEPTANCE AND COMMITMENT THERAPY?

Acceptance and commitment therapy aims to help you accept all of your thoughts and feelings, whether positive or negative. By accepting both happy and painful feelings, you learn not to avoid or be controlled by them. ACT also helps you identify your values, so you can live a more meaningful life, even when you have unpleasant experiences.

HOW DOES ACCEPTANCE AND COMMITMENT THERAPY WORK?

Acceptance and commitment therapy focuses on living well, not just feeling good or being happy all the time. Dr. Walser, Ph.D., a psychologist and Associate Director for Education, National Center for PTSD, Dissemination and Training Division, at the Veterans Affairs Palo Alto Health Care System says that this is because human beings are not good at turning off just one emotion. If you try to shut down painful feelings, you will also shut down joyful feelings. The goal of ACT is to help you live with all feelings, so you can experience joy, love, and any other values you have.

---

[6] Mental Illness Research, Education and Clinical Centers (MIRECC), "Acceptance and Commitment Therapy Strategies Guide for Anxiety and Trauma-Related Problems in Living," U.S. Department of Veterans Affairs (VA), November 7, 2022. Available online. URL: www.mirecc.va.gov/visn16/docs/act-strategies-guide.pdf. Accessed April 27, 2023.

In weekly ACT sessions, you can learn to change your relationship with your thoughts and feelings. You will practice exercises, such as imagining your thoughts floating away like leaves on a stream. You may also answer questions such as, "Am I willing to feel my pain, if it means I get to have love or other things in life that are important to me?"

WHY SHOULD YOU TRY ACCEPTANCE AND COMMITMENT THERAPY?

Research shows that ACT works to help many different problems. ACT has effectively treated obsessive-compulsive disorder (OCD), depression, anxiety, and chronic pain.

HOW CAN YOU TRY ACCEPTANCE AND COMMITMENT THERAPY?

You can ask your mental health provider if there are ACT-trained therapists at your local U.S. Department of Veterans Affairs (VA) facility.[7]

ACCEPTANCE AND COMMITMENT THERAPY COACH

Acceptance and commitment therapy aims to help you live with unpleasant thoughts, feelings, and impulses without avoiding them or being controlled by them. In ACT, you are encouraged to commit to actions so that you can live your life by your values, even in the face of these unpleasant experiences. The ACT Coach app was developed for veterans, service members, and other people who are in ACT with a therapist. It offers exercises, tools, information, and tracking logs, so you can practice what you are learning in your daily life.

Features
- information about what ACT is and how it works
- six critical mindfulness practice exercises including mindful breathing, mindful walking, mindful eating,

---

[7] "What Is Acceptance and Commitment Therapy (ACT)?" U.S. Department of Veterans Affairs (VA), October 18, 2022. Available online. URL: https://news.va.gov/109987/ptsd-bytes-19-acceptance-and-commitment-therapy/. Accessed March 22, 2023.

Psychotherapy for Depression

observing thoughts, observing sensations, and observing emotions
- interactive tools to facilitate value-based living, including assistance identifying values, developing a list of personal actions to support those values, and tips and reminders to help patients stay motivated to work toward living those values
- tools to track your mindfulness practice and coping strategies[8]

---

[8] "ACT Coach," U.S. Department of Veterans Affairs (VA), May 26, 2014. Available online. URL: https://mobile.va.gov/app/act-coach. Accessed March 22, 2023.

Chapter 43 | Mental Health Medications

Medications can play a role in treating mental disorders and conditions and are often used in combination with other treatment approaches such as psychotherapies and brain stimulation therapies. It is important for people to work with a health-care provider or mental health professional to develop a treatment plan that meets their needs and medical situation.

Information about medications is updated frequently. Check the U.S. Food and Drug Administration (FDA) Medication Guides (www.accessdata.fda.gov/scripts/cder/daf/index.cfm?event=medguide.page) web page for the latest warnings, patient medication guides, and newly approved medications.

ANTIDEPRESSANTS

Antidepressants are medications used to treat depression. In some cases, health-care providers may prescribe antidepressants to treat other health conditions such as anxiety, pain, and insomnia.

Commonly prescribed types of antidepressants include selective serotonin reuptake inhibitors (SSRIs), serotonin norepinephrine reuptake inhibitors (SNRIs), and norepinephrine-dopamine reuptake inhibitors (NDRIs).

These medications are commonly prescribed because they improve symptoms related to a broad group of depressive and anxiety disorders and are associated with fewer side effects than older types of antidepressants. Although older antidepressant medications, such as tricyclics and monoamine oxidase inhibitors

(MAOIs), are associated with more side effects, they may be the best option for some people.

Antidepressant medications take time to work—usually four to eight weeks—and symptoms such as problems with sleep, appetite, energy, or concentration sometimes improve before mood lifts. It is important for people to follow their health-care provider's directions and take the medication for the recommended amount of time before deciding whether it works.

Common side effects of SSRIs and other antidepressants may include upset stomach, headache, or sexual dysfunction. The side effects are generally mild and tend to improve over time. People who are sensitive to the side effects of these medications sometimes benefit from starting with a low dose, increasing the daily dose very slowly, and adjusting when they take the medication (e.g., at bedtime or with food).

Esketamine is a newer FDA-approved medication for treatment-resistant depression, which may be diagnosed when a person's symptoms have not improved after trying at least two antidepressant therapies. Esketamine is delivered as a nasal spray in a health-care provider's office, a clinic, or a hospital. It often acts rapidly—typically within a couple of hours—to relieve depression symptoms. People usually continue to take an oral antidepressant to maintain the improvement in symptoms.

Combining antidepressants with medications or supplements that also act on the serotonin system, such as "triptan" medications (often used to treat migraine headaches) and St. John's Wort (a dietary supplement), can cause a rare but life-threatening illness called "serotonin syndrome." Symptoms of serotonin syndrome include agitation, muscle twitches, hallucinations (seeing or hearing things others do not see or hear), high temperature, and unusual blood pressure changes. For most people, the risk of such extreme reactions is low. It is important for health-care providers to consider all possible interactions and use extra care in prescribing and monitoring medication combinations that carry above-average risk.

It must be noted that in some cases, children, teenagers, and young adults under 25 may experience an increase in suicidal thoughts or behavior when taking antidepressants, especially in

Mental Health Medications

the first few weeks after starting the medication or when the dose is changed. People of all ages taking antidepressants should be watched closely, especially during the first few weeks of treatment.

ANTIANXIETY MEDICATIONS

Antianxiety medications help reduce symptoms of anxiety, such as panic attacks and extreme fear and worry.

Many medications commonly used to treat depression—including SSRIs and SNRIs—may also be used to treat anxiety. In the case of panic disorder or social anxiety disorder, health-care providers typically start with SSRIs or other antidepressants as the first treatment because they have fewer side effects than other medications.

Another common type of antianxiety medication are benzodiazepines. These medications are sometimes used to treat generalized anxiety disorder.

Short half-life (or short-acting) benzodiazepines are used to treat the short-term symptoms of anxiety. Health-care providers may also prescribe beta-blockers off-label to treat short-term symptoms. People with phobias—an overwhelming and unreasonable fear of an object or situation, such as public speaking—often experience intense physical symptoms. Beta-blockers can help manage these symptoms, such as rapid heart rate, sweating, and tremors.

As short-term treatments, benzodiazepines and beta-blockers can be used as needed to reduce severe anxiety. Taking benzodiazepines over long periods may lead to drug tolerance or even dependence. To avoid these problems, health-care providers usually prescribe benzodiazepines for short periods and taper them slowly to reduce the likelihood that a person will experience withdrawal symptoms or renewed anxiety symptoms. Beta-blockers generally are not recommended for people with asthma or diabetes because they may worsen symptoms related to both conditions.

Buspirone is a different type of medication that is sometimes used to treat anxiety over longer periods. In contrast to benzodiazepines, buspirone must be taken every day for three to four weeks to reach its full effect and is not effective for treating anxiety on an "as-needed" basis.

STIMULANTS

Health-care providers may prescribe stimulant medications when treating attention deficit hyperactivity disorder (ADHD) and narcolepsy. Stimulants increase alertness, attention, and energy. They can also elevate blood pressure, heart rate, and breathing.

Prescription stimulants typically improve alertness and focus for most people, regardless of diagnosis. These medications can markedly improve daily functioning for people with significant focus problems, such as people with ADHD. Although motor hyperactivity associated with ADHD in children usually goes away by the time they reach adolescence, people with ADHD may continue to experience inattention and difficulty with focus into adulthood. As such, stimulant medications can be helpful for adults with ADHD, as well as for children and adolescents with ADHD.

Stimulant medications are safe when taken under a health-care provider's supervision and used as directed. Some children taking them may report feeling slightly different or "funny." Most side effects of stimulant medications are minor and disappear at lower doses.

Some parents worry that stimulant medications may lead to misuse or dependence, but evidence shows this is unlikely when the medications are used as prescribed. Other challenges with stimulant treatment, such as sleep disturbance and slowed growth, can generally be safely managed in collaboration with the prescribing health-care provider while continuing treatment.

ANTIPSYCHOTICS

Antipsychotic medications are typically used to treat psychosis, a condition that involves some loss of contact with reality. People experiencing a psychotic episode often experience delusions (false beliefs) or hallucinations (hearing or seeing things others do not see or hear). Psychosis can be related to drug use or a mental disorder such as schizophrenia, bipolar disorder, or severe depression (also known as "psychotic depression").

Health-care providers may also prescribe antipsychotic medications in combination with other medications to relieve symptoms associated with delirium, dementia, or other mental health

Mental Health Medications

conditions. Antipsychotic treatment for older adults necessitates additional care and consideration. The FDA requires that all antipsychotic medication labels include a black box warning stating that antipsychotics are associated with increased rates of stroke and death in older adults with dementia.

Older, first-generation antipsychotic medications are sometimes called "typical" antipsychotics or "neuroleptics." Long-term use of typical antipsychotic medications may lead to a condition involving uncontrollable muscle movements called "tardive dyskinesia" (TD). TD can range from mild to severe. People who think they might have TD should check with their health-care provider before stopping their medication.

Newer, second-generation medications are sometimes called "atypical antipsychotics." Several atypical antipsychotics may be used to treat a broader range of symptoms compared with older medications. For example, these medications are sometimes used to treat bipolar depression or depression that has not responded to antidepressant medication alone. Health-care providers may ask people taking atypical antipsychotic medications to participate in regular monitoring to check their weight, glucose levels, and lipid levels.

Some symptoms, such as feeling agitated and having hallucinations, typically go away within days of starting antipsychotic medication. Other symptoms, such as delusions, usually go away within a few weeks of starting antipsychotic medication. However, people may not experience the full effects of antipsychotic medication for up to six weeks.

If a person's symptoms do not improve with usual antipsychotic medications, they may be prescribed an atypical antipsychotic called "clozapine." People who take clozapine must have regular blood tests to check for a potentially dangerous side effect that occurs in 1–2 percent of people.

MOOD STABILIZERS

Mood stabilizers are typically used to treat bipolar disorder and mood changes associated with other mental disorders. In some cases, health-care providers may prescribe mood stabilizers to augment the effect of other medications used to treat depression. Lithium, an effective mood stabilizer, is approved for the treatment of mania and maintenance treatment of bipolar disorder. Some studies indicate that lithium may reduce the risk of suicide among people taking it for long-term maintenance. Health-care providers generally ask people who are taking lithium to participate in regular monitoring to check lithium levels and kidney and thyroid function.

Mood stabilizers are sometimes used to treat depression (usually with an antidepressant), schizoaffective disorder, disorders of impulse control, and certain mental illnesses in children. For people with bipolar depression, health-care providers typically prescribe a mood stabilizer and an antidepressant to reduce the risk of switching to mania or rapid cycling.

Some anticonvulsant medications may also be used as mood stabilizers as they may work better than lithium for some people, such as people with "mixed" symptoms of mania and depression or those with rapid-cycling bipolar disorder. Health-care providers generally ask people taking anticonvulsants to participate in regular monitoring to check medication levels and assess side effects and potential interactions with other common medications.

SPECIAL GROUPS: CHILDREN, OLDER ADULTS, AND PREGNANT WOMEN

All types of people take mental health medications, but some groups have special needs and considerations.

Children and Adolescents

Many medications used to treat mental disorders are safe and effective for children and adolescents. However, it is important to know that children may experience different reactions and side effects compared with adults, and some medications have FDA warnings about potential side effects for younger people.

In some cases, a health-care provider may prescribe an FDA-approved medication on an "off-label" basis to treat a child's symptoms even though the medication is not approved for the child's specific mental disorder or for use by people under a certain age.

Mental Health Medications

Although there has been less research on mental disorders in children than in adults, there is some evidence that medications can be helpful for children. It is important to monitor children and adolescents who take medications on an "off-label" basis.

A child's health-care provider may suggest trying nonmedication treatments, such as psychotherapies, first and may add medication later, if necessary. In other cases, the health-care provider may suggest nonmedication treatment in combination with medication.

Older Adults

People over 65 should take extra care with medications, especially if they are taking many different medications. Older adults have a higher risk of experiencing drug interactions and are often more sensitive to medications. Even healthy older adults react to medications differently compared with younger people because older adults' bodies often process and eliminate medications more slowly.

Before starting a medication, older adults and their family members should talk with a health-care provider about any effects the medication may have on physical and mental functioning. The health-care provider can also discuss strategies to make it easier to follow the treatment plan, helping to ensure that older adults take the correct medication dose at the correct time.

Women Who Are Pregnant or Who May Become Pregnant

Researchers are continuing to investigate the use of mental health medications during pregnancy. The risks associated with taking medication during pregnancy depend on the type of medication and the stage of pregnancy. While no medication is considered universally safe during pregnancy, untreated mental disorders can also pose risks to the pregnant person and the developing fetus.

Pregnant women and health-care providers can work together to develop a personalized treatment plan that considers individual needs and circumstances. It is important to weigh the benefits and risks associated with all available treatment options, including psychotherapies, medications, brain stimulation therapies, or a combination of these options. Health-care providers may closely monitor a person's physical and mental health throughout pregnancy and, after delivery, pay particular attention to signs of perinatal or postpartum depression.

Certain medications taken during pregnancy—including some benzodiazepines, mood stabilizers, and antipsychotic medications—have been linked with birth defects, but the risks vary widely and depend on the specific medication.

Antidepressants, especially SSRIs, are generally considered safe for use during pregnancy. Antidepressant medications can cross into the placenta and may reach the fetus, but the risk of birth defects and other problems is very low. Some studies have found an association between third-trimester SSRI exposure and certain symptoms, including breathing problems, in newborns. However, the FDA does not find sufficient evidence for a causal link and recommends that health-care providers treat depression during pregnancy according to the person's specific needs.

UNDERSTANDING YOUR MEDICATIONS

People respond to medications in different ways, and it may take several tries to find the medication that is most effective with the fewest side effects. In some cases, people find that a medication helps for a while, and then their symptoms come back. It often takes some time for a medication to be effective, so it is important to stick with the treatment plan and take medication as prescribed.

People should not stop taking a prescribed medication, even if they are feeling better, without the help of a health-care provider. A health-care provider can adjust the treatment plan and slowly and safely decrease the medication dose. It is important to give the body time to adjust to the change. Stopping a medication too soon may cause unpleasant or harmful side effects.

If you are prescribed a medication, do the following:
- Tell the health-care provider about all other medications, vitamins, and supplements you are already taking.
- Remind the health-care provider about any allergies and any problems you have had with medications in the past.

Mental Health Medications

- Make sure you understand how to take the medication before you start using it and take your medication as instructed.
- Talk to the health-care provider about possible side effects and what to expect when taking a medication.
- Do not take medications prescribed for another person or give your medication to someone else.
- Call a health-care provider right away if you have any problems with your medication or are worried that it might be doing more harm than good. The health-care provider will work with you to address any problems and determine next steps.
- Report serious side effects to the FDA MedWatch Adverse Event Reporting Program (www.nimh.nih.gov/health/topics/mental-health-medications#part_2365).[1]

---

[1] "Mental Health Medications," National Institute of Mental Health (NIMH), June 2022. Available online. URL: www.nimh.nih.gov/health/topics/mental-health-medications. Accessed March 6, 2023.

Chapter 44 | Combination Treatment

Depression is a complex mental illness that can result in significant disability, reduced quality of life, and societal burden. Pharmacological agents are one of several initial treatment modalities used for depression, and one of the most frequently utilized classes of drugs is the selective serotonin reuptake inhibitors (SSRIs). However, the rate of treatment response from baseline symptoms following first-line treatment with SSRIs is moderate, varying from 40 to 60 percent; remission rates vary from 30 to 45 percent. Up to one-third of persons on drug treatment will develop recurrent symptoms of depression while on therapy. Moreover, there is limited evidence identifying reliable predictors (demographic, clinical, or genetic characteristics) of individual response. Adequate response to SSRI interventions is not consistently operationalized, but it is generally accepted that a 50 percent decrease in symptom severity from baseline is sufficient. Remission from depression is defined as being free or nearly free of symptoms for the current episode.

Given the large proportion of patients who do not respond adequately to SSRIs as first-line therapy, the practitioner is faced with the dilemma of determining the presence of inadequacy of the response and then selecting a new course of action. The new course of action may vary and can include:
- an optimization strategy (altering the dose or duration of the SSRI)
- switching to other SSRIs
- switching to other classes of antidepressants

- combining SSRIs with other medications or nonpharmacological therapies
- switching to nonpharmacological interventions alone
- combinations of these

There is a need to examine the evidentiary base for these varying management strategies for patients who have failed to adequately respond to the SSRI used as first-line therapy for the index episode. For the purpose of this systematic review, treatment failure (TF) is a response of less than 50 percent change relative to baseline and primarily reflects the perspective of the clinician and researcher. It marks the threshold of change by which a clinician will seek to progress or modify treatment for the patient. The terms "failure to respond" or "nonresponder" are used in this same context; the unsatisfactory response is used to capture the perspective of the patient being treated for depression; an unsatisfactory response may include other aspects of concern not captured by a change score relative to baseline.

TF can encompass a number of subgroups of patients who do not adequately respond to interventions for their current episode of depression. TF is not consistently defined within the literature, but it is generally understood to reflect patients with depression who have not responded to one course of therapy. TF populations may include patients who would meet criteria for treatment resistance (more than two inadequate responses) subgroups based on the past treatment for prior episodes of depression. A portion of patients who have experienced TF will also go on to be defined as treatment-resistant if they also fail to respond to subsequent treatment strategies. Treatment resistance is variably defined but usually refers to patients who have failed at least two trials of medication that have been of adequate dose and duration. Some definitions suggest that the failures should be to medications of different classes, but this is not universally accepted.

Monitoring adherence to antidepressants is sometimes difficult, but nonadherence may account for up to 20 percent of patients classified as having treatment-resistant depression. Similarly, there is the potential for pseudo-resistance (nonresponse to inadequate treatment). All this would suggest the difficulty of defining and

Combination Treatment

capturing subjects who have had TF and related subgroups. It may also reflect heterogeneity across studies evaluating the efficacy of SSRIs within this patient population.

Previous literature reviews would suggest that some of the strategies to treat patients following inadequate response may not be based on evidence; this is partially attributable to the small number of studies that have evaluated the different strategies. Rhue et al. evaluated the evidence for switching SSRIs in studies where 50 percent of subjects had previously used an SSRI and not responded adequately. This review found eight randomized trials and 23 open studies (with and without comparator groups). Response rates after switching to a new therapy varied from 12 to 86 percent, and remission rates varied between 7 and 82 percent. Rates of dropouts due to harms varied from 9 to 39 percent. This review also identified some evidence showing that the number of failed responses to previous treatment with antidepressants was negatively associated with a positive response or outcome. Overall, this review showed that there was limited high-quality evidence describing optimal strategies to switch medications in persons with previous SSRI use. In addition, there were limited studies that recruited prospectively determined SSRI nonresponders. Papakostas et al. undertook a meta-analysis of four trials in subjects with TF who were randomized to switch to a non-SSRI versus another SSRI. The results suggest a modest and statistically significant advantage for remission rates when switching to non-SSRI rather than another SSRI. This review restricted eligible studies to those using three outcomes (Hamilton Depression Rating Scale, Montgomery-Asberg Depression Rating Scale, and Quick Inventory of Depressive Symptomology) and to those evaluating the acute phase of major depressive disorder (MDD). Williams et al. completed a systematic review of the treatment of depression in adolescents and children. Although this review did not focus on subjects who had failed to respond, the eligible studies did show that the rate at which children failed to respond to an initial trial of SSRIs varied from 31 to 64 percent. There was also some evidence that not all SSRIs were efficacious and that combined therapy (including an SSRI) is effective in this population.

A variety of treatment strategies aimed at helping individuals who have inadequate responses to first-line therapy with an SSRI have been developed and applied in patients with depression. The primary goal of this comparative effectiveness research (CER) is to examine the evidence guiding clinical treatment decisions and ultimately to aid clinicians in their care of patients in whom SSRI use as a first-line therapy for the index episode fails to bring about either complete or partial response or remission of depression.[1]

---

[1] Effective Health Care Program, "Depression Treatment after Unsatisfactory Response to SSRIs When Used as First-Line Therapy," Agency for Healthcare Research and Quality (AHRQ), December 2019. Available online. URL: https://effectivehealthcare.ahrq.gov/products/depression-treatment-ssri/research-protocol. Accessed March 15, 2023.

Chapter 45 | Brain Stimulation Therapies for Severe Depression

WHAT ARE BRAIN STIMULATION THERAPIES?
Brain stimulation therapies can play a role in treating certain mental disorders. Brain stimulation therapies involve activating or inhibiting the brain directly with electricity. The electricity can be given directly by electrodes implanted in the brain or noninvasively through electrodes placed on the scalp. The electricity can also be induced by using magnetic fields applied to the head. While these types of therapies are less frequently used than medication and psychotherapies, they hold promise for treating certain mental disorders that do not respond to other treatments.

Electroconvulsive therapy (ECT) is the best-studied brain stimulation therapy and has the longest history of use. Other stimulation therapies discussed here are newer and, in some cases, still experimental methods. These include:
- vagus nerve stimulation (VNS)
- repetitive transcranial magnetic stimulation (rTMS)
- magnetic seizure therapy (MST)
- deep brain stimulation (DBS)

A treatment plan may also include medication and psychotherapy. Choosing the right treatment plan should be based on a person's individual needs and medical situation and under a doctor's care.

ELECTROCONVULSIVE THERAPY

Electroconvulsive therapy uses an electric current to treat serious mental disorders. This type of therapy is usually considered only if a patient's illness has not improved after other treatments (such as antidepressant medication or psychotherapy) are tried or in cases where rapid response is needed (e.g., as in the case of suicide risk and catatonia).

Why Electroconvulsive Therapy Is Done

Electroconvulsive therapy is most often used to treat severe, treatment-resistant depression, but it may also be medically indicated in other mental disorders, such as bipolar disorder or schizophrenia. It may also be used in life-threatening circumstances, such as when a patient is unable to move or respond to the outside world (e.g., catatonia), is suicidal, or is malnourished as a result of severe depression.

ECT can be effective in reducing the chances of relapse when patients undergo follow-up treatments. Two major advantages of ECT over medication are that ECT begins to work quicker, often starting within the first week, and older individuals respond especially quickly.

How Electroconvulsive Therapy Works

Before ECT is administered, a person is sedated with general anesthesia and given a medication called a "muscle relaxant" to prevent movement during the procedure. An anesthesiologist monitors breathing, heart rate, and blood pressure during the entire procedure, which is conducted by a trained medical team, including physicians and nurses. During the procedure, the following things take place:
- Electrodes are placed at precise locations on the head.
- Through the electrodes, an electric current passes through the brain, causing a seizure that lasts generally less than one minute. Because the patient is under anesthesia and has taken a muscle relaxant, it is not painful and the patient cannot feel the electrical impulses.

Brain Stimulation Therapies for Severe Depression

- Five to ten minutes after the procedure ends, the patient awakens. He or she may feel groggy at first as the anesthesia wears off. But after about an hour, the patient is usually alert and can resume normal activities.

A typical course of ECT is administered about three times a week until the patient's depression improves (usually within 6–12 treatments). After that, maintenance ECT treatment is sometimes needed to reduce the chances that symptoms will return. ECT maintenance treatment varies depending on the needs of the individual and may range from one session per week to one session every few months. Frequently, a person who undergoes ECT also takes antidepressant medication or a mood-stabilizing medication.

Side Effects of Electroconvulsive Therapy

The most common side effects associated with ECT include:
- headache
- upset stomach
- muscle aches
- memory loss

Some people may experience memory problems, especially memories around the time of the treatment. Sometimes, the memory problems are more severe, but usually, they improve over the days and weeks following the end of an ECT course.

Research has found that memory problems seem to be more associated with the traditional type of ECT called "bilateral ECT," in which the electrodes are placed on both sides of the head.

In unilateral ECT, the electrodes are placed on just one side of the head—typically the right side because it is opposite to the brain's learning and memory areas. Unilateral ECT has been found to be less likely to cause memory problems and, therefore, is preferred by many doctors, patients, and families.

VAGUS NERVE STIMULATION

Vagus nerve stimulation works through a device implanted under the skin that sends electrical pulses through the left vagus nerve, half of a prominent pair of nerves that run from the brainstem through the neck and down to each side of the chest and abdomen. The vagus nerves carry messages from the brain to the body's major organs (e.g., heart, lungs, and intestines) and to areas of the brain that control mood, sleep, and other functions.

Why Vagus Nerve Stimulation Is Done

Vagus nerve stimulation was originally developed as a treatment for epilepsy. However, scientists noticed that it also had favorable effects on mood, especially depressive symptoms. Using brain scans, scientists found that the device affected areas of the brain that are involved in mood regulation. The pulses appeared to alter the levels of certain neurotransmitters (brain chemicals) associated with mood, including serotonin, norepinephrine, gamma-aminobutyric acid (GABA), and glutamate.

The U.S. Food and Drug Administration (FDA) approved VNS for use in treating treatment-resistant depression in certain circumstances:

- if the patient is 18 years of age or over
- if the illness has lasted two years or more
- if it is severe or recurrent
- if the depression has not eased after trying at least four other treatments

According to the FDA, it is not intended to be a first-line treatment, even for patients with severe depression. And, despite the FDA's approval, VNS remains an infrequently used treatment because results of early studies testing its effectiveness for major depression were mixed. But a newer study, which pooled together findings from only controlled clinical trials, found that 32 percent of depressed people responded to VSN and 14 percent had full remission of symptoms after being treated for nearly two years.

How Vagus Nerve Stimulation Works

A device called a "pulse generator," about the size of a stopwatch, is surgically implanted in the upper left side of the chest. Connected

Brain Stimulation Therapies for Severe Depression

to the pulse generator is an electrical lead wire, which is connected from the generator to the left vagus nerve.

Typically, 30-second electrical pulses are sent about every five minutes from the generator to the vagus nerve. The duration and frequency of the pulses may vary depending on how the generator is programmed. The vagus nerve, in turn, delivers those signals to the brain. The pulse generator, which operates continuously, is powered by a battery that lasts around 10 years, after which it must be replaced. Normally, people do not feel pain or any other sensations as the device operates.

The device can also be temporarily deactivated by placing a magnet over the chest where the pulse generator is implanted. A person may want to deactivate it if side effects become intolerable or before engaging in strenuous activity or exercise because it may interfere with breathing. The device reactivates when the magnet is removed.

VNS treatment is intended to reduce symptoms of depression. It may be several months before the patient notices any benefits, and not all patients will respond to VNS. It is important to remember that VNS is intended to be given along with other traditional therapies, such as medications, and patients should not expect to discontinue these other treatments, even with the device in place.

Side Effects of Vagus Nerve Stimulation

Vagus nerve stimulation is not without risk. There may be complications such as infection from the implant surgery, or the device may come loose, move around, or malfunction, which may require additional surgery to correct. Some patients have no improvement in symptoms, and some actually get worse.

Other potential side effects include:
- voice changes or hoarseness
- cough or sore throat
- neck pain
- discomfort or tingling in the area where the device is implanted
- breathing problems, especially during exercise
- difficulty swallowing

Long-term side effects are unknown.

REPETITIVE TRANSCRANIAL MAGNETIC STIMULATION

Repetitive transcranial magnetic stimulation uses a magnet to activate the brain. First developed in 1985, rTMS has been studied as a treatment for depression, psychosis, anxiety, and other disorders.

Unlike ECT, in which electrical stimulation is more generalized, rTMS can be targeted to a specific site in the brain. Scientists believe that focusing on a specific site in the brain reduces the chance for the types of side effects associated with ECT. But opinions vary as to what site is best.

Why Repetitive Transcranial Magnetic Stimulation Is Done

Repetitive transcranial magnetic stimulation was approved for use by the FDA as a treatment for major depression for patients who do not respond to at least one antidepressant medication in the current episode. It is also used in other countries as a treatment for depression in patients who have not responded to medications and who might otherwise be considered for ECT.

The evidence supporting rTMS for depression was mixed until the first large clinical trial, funded by the National Institute of Mental Health (NIMH), was published in 2010. The trial found that 14 percent achieved remission with rTMS compared to 5 percent with an inactive (sham) treatment. After the trial ended, patients could enter a second phase in which everyone, including those who previously received the sham treatment, was given rTMS. Remission rates during the second phase climbed to nearly 30 percent. A sham treatment is like a placebo, but instead of being an inactive pill, it is an inactive procedure that mimics real rTMS.

How Repetitive Transcranial Magnetic Stimulation Works

A typical rTMS session lasts 30–60 minutes and does not require anesthesia.

During the procedure, the following things happen:
- An electromagnetic coil is held against the forehead near an area of the brain that is thought to be involved in mood regulation.

Brain Stimulation Therapies for Severe Depression

- Then, short electromagnetic pulses are administered through the coil. The magnetic pulses easily pass through the skull and cause small electrical currents that stimulate nerve cells in the targeted brain region.

Because this type of pulse generally does not reach further than two inches into the brain, scientists can select which parts of the brain will be affected and which will not be affected. The magnetic field is about the same strength as that of a magnetic resonance imaging (MRI) scan. Generally, the person feels a slight knocking or tapping on the head as the pulses are administered.

Not all scientists agree on the best way to position the magnet on the patient's head or give the electromagnetic pulses. They also do not yet know if rTMS works best when given as a single treatment or combined with medication and/or psychotherapy.

Side Effects of Repetitive Transcranial Magnetic Stimulation

Sometimes, a person may have discomfort at the site on the head where the magnet is placed. The muscles of the scalp, jaw, or face may contract or tingle during the procedure. Mild headaches or brief light-headedness may result. It is also possible that the procedure could cause a seizure, although documented incidences of this are uncommon. Studies on the safety of rTMS found that most side effects, such as headaches or scalp discomfort, were mild or moderate, and no seizures occurred. Because the treatment is relatively new, however, long-term side effects are unknown.

MAGNETIC SEIZURE THERAPY
How Magnetic Seizure Therapy Works

Magnetic seizure therapy borrows certain aspects from both ECT and rTMS. Like rTMS, MST uses magnetic pulses instead of electricity to stimulate a precise target in the brain. However, unlike rTMS, MST aims to induce seizure-like ECT. So the pulses are given at a higher frequency than that used in rTMS. Therefore, like ECT, the patient must be anesthetized and given a muscle relaxant to prevent movement. The goal of MST is to retain the effectiveness of ECT while reducing its cognitive side effects.

MST is in the early stages of testing for mental disorders, but initial results are promising. A review article that examined the evidence from eight clinical studies found that MST triggered remission from major depression or bipolar disorder in 30–40 percent of individuals.

Side Effects of Magnetic Seizure Therapy

Like ECT, MST carries the risk of side effects that can be caused by anesthesia exposure and the induction of a seizure. Studies in both animals and humans have found that MST produces fewer memory side effects, shorter seizures, and shorter recovery time than ECT.

DEEP BRAIN STIMULATION

Deep brain stimulation was first developed as a treatment for Parkinson disease (PD) to reduce tremors, stiffness, walking problems, and uncontrollable movements. In DBS, a pair of electrodes is implanted in the brain and controlled by a generator that is implanted in the chest. Stimulation is continuous, and its frequency and level are customized to the individual.

DBS has been studied as a treatment for depression or obsessive-compulsive disorder (OCD). There is a Humanitarian Device Exemption (HDE) for the use of DBS to treat OCD, but its use in depression remains only on an experimental basis. A review of all 22 published studies testing DBS for depression found that only three of them were of high quality because they not only had a treatment group but also had a control group that did not receive DBS. The review found that across the studies, 40–50 percent of people receiving DBS showed greater than 50 percent improvement.

How Deep Brain Stimulation Works

Deep brain stimulation requires brain surgery. The head is shaved and then attached with screws to a sturdy frame that prevents the head from moving during the surgery. Scans of the head and brain

Brain Stimulation Therapies for Severe Depression

using MRI are taken. The surgeon uses these images as guides during the surgery. Patients are awake during the procedure to provide the surgeon with feedback, but they feel no pain because the head is numbed with a local anesthetic and the brain itself does not register pain.

Once ready for surgery, two holes are drilled into the head. From there, the surgeon threads a slender tube down into the brain to place electrodes on each side of a specific area of the brain. In the case of depression, the first area of the brain targeted by DBS is called "Area 25," or the subgenual cingulate cortex. This area has been found to be overactive in depression and other mood disorders. But later research targeted several other areas of the brain affected by depression. So DBS is now targeting several areas of the brain for treating depression. In the case of OCD, the electrodes are placed in an area of the brain (the ventral capsule/ventral striatum) believed to be associated with the disorder.

After the electrodes are implanted and the patient provides feedback about their placement, the patient is put under general anesthesia. The electrodes are then attached to wires that are run inside the body from the head down to the chest, where a pair of battery-operated generators are implanted. From here, electrical pulses are continuously delivered over the wires to the electrodes in the brain. Although it is unclear exactly how the device works to reduce depression or OCD, scientists believe that the pulses help to "reset" the area of the brain that is malfunctioning so that it works normally again.

Side Effects of Deep Brain Stimulation

Deep brain stimulation carries risks associated with any type of brain surgery. For example, the procedure may lead to:
- bleeding in the brain or stroke
- infection
- disorientation or confusion
- unwanted mood changes
- movement disorders
- light-headedness
- trouble sleeping

Because the procedure is still being studied, other side effects not yet identified may be possible. Long-term benefits and side effects are unknown.[1]

---

[1] "Brain Stimulation Therapies," National Institute of Mental Health (NIMH), June 2016. Available online. URL: www.nimh.nih.gov/health/topics/brain-stimulation-therapies/brain-stimulation-therapies. Accessed March 15, 2023.

Chapter 46 | Light Therapy for Seasonal Affective Disorder

Seasonal affective disorder (SAD) is a condition associated with feeling sad or blue during certain times of the year. It is a disorder that triggers symptoms of depression, most commonly in the fall or winter. In the fall and winter, there is less sunlight; hence, it is sometimes called "winter depression."

Psychiatrists and other mental health clinicians diagnose depression by documenting the low or sad mood, irritability, feelings of guilt or shame, problems with sleep, poor concentration or attention (memory problems), low energy or motivation, poor appetite, and thoughts of self-harm.

SAD can mimic other medical conditions, such as anemia, hypothyroidism, diabetes, and infections. Hence, a medical workup may be needed including levels of some vitamins, such as vitamin D.

You may have SAD if, in the last two years, you feel depressed during this season and normal during the rest of the year. You may also have SAD if the depression for which you are being treated gets worse in this season.

Your symptoms will get better on their own when a new season arrives, often in spring or summer. But treatment can make you feel better sooner.

LIGHT THERAPY

Light therapy, also called "phototherapy," generally works well for SAD. You need to sit in front of a box or lamp that gives out up to

10,000 lux of fluorescent light—more than 20 times brighter than most indoor light. Researchers think that light helps your brain make more serotonin, a neurotransmitter that affects your mood. You have to sit 12–18 inches in front of the light for 30 minutes or more a day, three times per week at least. The light must shine on your back or chest. You can read a book to pass the time. Do not stare at the light. You will feel better after one or two weeks.

You may also want to see a medical provider to consider taking medications to increase serotonin levels. Your doctor may also recommend talk therapy such as cognitive-behavioral therapy. You will learn behavioral skills to do pleasurable things during the winter, notice and change negative thoughts, or manage stress.

It is important to consider all types of treatment. Get more sun, stay active, get to a brighter place, and work toward sleeping the right amount of time.

Consider talking to a professional to identify ways of coping with SAD. Counselors are available to guide you during this time. Do not feel frightened to talk about your problems. They are there to help you.[1]

GET MORE SUN, STAY ACTIVE, AND GET TO A BRIGHTER PLACE

There is some evidence that light therapy may be useful as a preventive treatment for people with a history of SAD. The idea behind light therapy is to replace the diminished sunshine of the fall and winter months using daily exposure to a light box. Most typically, light boxes filter out the ultraviolet rays and require 20–60 minutes of exposure to 10,000 lux of cool white fluorescent light, an amount that is about 20 times greater than ordinary indoor lighting.[2]

---

[1] "Help for Veterans with Seasonal Affective Disorder," U.S. Department of Veterans Affairs (VA), February 6, 2018. Available online. URL: www.va.gov/HEALTH/NewsFeatures/2018/February/Help-for-Veterans-with-Seasonal-Affective-Disorder.asp. Accessed March 15, 2023.

[2] "Seasonal Affective Disorder and Complementary Health Approaches: What the Science Says," National Center for Complementary and Integrative Health (NCCIH), January 18, 2019. Available online. URL: www.nccih.nih.gov/health/providers/digest/seasonal-affective-disorder-and-complementary-health-approaches-science. Accessed March 15, 2023.

Chapter 47 | Depression and the Placebo Effect

THE POWER OF PLACEBO: HELPING THE BRAIN HEAL THE BODY
If you are feeling unwell, you may turn to medicine to find relief. But how do you know it was the drug that made you feel better? Sometimes, when you expect a treatment to work, it will. This phenomenon is called the "placebo effect." Scientists are looking for ways to harness this effect for medical treatments.

A placebo is an inactive substance or action that resembles a drug or medical treatment. But it is not meant to actually fix anything in your body. A pill that does not contain any medicine is one example.

Historically, placebos have been a key part of testing if a new treatment works. In some types of clinical trials, participants are given either an active treatment or a placebo. But they are not told which one they are getting. The treatment must do more to improve the participants' condition than the placebo. If both groups show similar improvement, it may be from the placebo effect, not the drug.

The placebo effect works by turning on the body's natural mechanisms for helping us feel better. Our brains make many substances that can lessen pain, stress, anxiety, and other unpleasant feelings.

Dr. Luana Colloca, a physician-scientist at the University of Maryland, Baltimore, calls this our "inner pharmacy." Just expecting to feel better can cause the release of these substances.

"Our mindset is so critical," Dr. Colloca says, "because our thoughts are not independent from our bodies' responses."

The placebo effect can be powerful. It can help with pain, fatigue, depression, anxiety, or nausea. But our inner pharmacy cannot treat everything. It cannot, for instance, make tumors go away, lower your cholesterol, or get rid of infections.

Researchers funded by the National Institute of Health (NIH) are trying to understand the brain pathways underlying the placebo effect. They are also looking for ways to use it to improve treatments.

Recent studies have been exploring if placebos can be used to cut down on how much medication people take. People with a chronic disease may need to take a drug for a long time. Researchers are testing if placebos can be used to replace some drug doses. These are called "dose-extending placebos." The drug effects might continue working for some time as if the patient had taken a real dose.

Dose-extending placebos may be particularly useful with opioids. Opioids are sometimes used to treat chronic pain. But they can be highly addictive and may pose risk of overdose or even death. Scientists are studying whether dose-extending placebos can reduce the chances of opioid addiction.

But, for a placebo to work, do you need to believe you are taking the real thing? Recent research suggests that may not be the case. That is because your expectations can also affect how well a treatment works.

For instance, if you are given a drug for pain, it may work better if you are told that it is a potent pain treatment. This approach can work for placebos, too—if you are truthfully told that it has been shown to help.

A drug may also be more effective if you have had a good experience with it before. Dr. Colloca's research has shown that even seeing someone else get relief from a treatment can make it more effective.

For these reasons, good communication between patients and health-care providers is an essential part of treatment. Having a provider you trust, who is supportive and has empathy, can produce better treatment results.[1]

---

[1] *NIH News in Health*, "The Powerful Placebo," National Institutes of Health (NIH), January 2023. Available online. URL: https://newsinhealth.nih.gov/2023/01/powerful-placebo. Accessed April 12, 2023.

Depression and the Placebo Effect

PLACEBO EFFECT IN DEPRESSION TREATMENT

A placebo is a substance, such as a pill or shot, that does not contain any active medicine. Scientists typically use placebos as controls in research studies. This helps them understand how much of a medicine's effect is due to the drug itself, versus how much is due to participants' expectations or other factors.

People who are given a placebo may report improvements in symptoms, sometimes even when they know they are taking something that does not contain real medicine. To better understand the neurochemical mechanisms underlying the placebo effect, a team led by Dr. Jon-Kar Zubieta, formerly at the University of Michigan School of Medicine and now at the University of Utah, examined such effects in depression treatment. The study was funded in part by the NIH's National Institute of Mental Health (NIMH). Results appeared online on September 30, 2015, in *JAMA Psychiatry*.

The scientists enrolled 35 people with major depression who were not taking any medications. In the first phase of the study, the participants were randomly assigned to receive placebo pills that were described as a potentially fast-acting antidepressant ("active" placebo group) or identical pills described as a placebo with no antidepressant effects ("inactive" placebo group). Each group took the pills for a week, and then after a few days, the groups switched.

At the end of each week of treatment, the participants completed a questionnaire about their depression symptoms. They also underwent a positron emission tomography (PET) brain scan to measure the activity of µ-opioid receptors, which are known to be involved in emotion, stress, social rewards, and depression. During the scan, the active placebo group received intravenous doses of saline with the understanding that it might activate brain systems involved in mood improvement. This was done to monitor the acute effects of an active placebo on brain function. The inactive placebo group received no infusions during the scan.

In the second phase of the study, all participants were treated for 10 weeks with antidepressants (usually selective serotonin reuptake inhibitors), and their depression symptoms were monitored. At the end of the study, each person was fully briefed on the study design and use of placebos.

The researchers found that the participants reported significant decreases in depression symptoms when they took the active placebo, compared to when they took the inactive placebo. These reductions were linked to increased μ-opioid receptor brain activity in regions of the brain associated with emotion and stress regulation. Notably, the increased μ-opioid activity induced by the active placebo was also associated with significantly better responses to the subsequent antidepressant treatment.

"These results suggest that some people are more responsive to the intention to treat their depression and may do better if psychotherapies or cognitive therapies that enhance the clinician-patient relationship are incorporated into their care as well as antidepressant medications," Dr. Zubieta says. "We need to find out how to enhance the natural resiliency that some people appear to have."[2]

---

[2] News and Events, "Placebo Effect in Depression Treatment," National Institutes of Health (NIH), October 19, 2015. Available online. URL: www.nih.gov/news-events/nih-research-matters/placebo-effect-depression-treatment. Accessed April 12, 2023.

Chapter 48 | Genetic Studies May Lead to Accurate Medication Dose

A U.S. Department of Veterans Affairs (VA) study found that pharmacogenomic testing can help providers avoid prescribing antidepressant medications that may have undesirable outcomes. Pharmacogenomics is the study of how genes affect the body's response to drugs.

The researchers also found that the patients who underwent genetic testing had more positive outcomes than patients in usual care. Over 24 weeks of treatment, the group with genetic testing had a drop in depression symptoms—with a peak effect at 12 weeks. Each patient in the study had major depressive disorder. Symptoms of that health condition include insomnia, loss of appetite, feelings of sadness and depression, and thoughts of dying by suicide.

The study results appeared in July 2022 in the *Journal of the American Medical Association (AMA)*.

Dr. David Oslin, director of VA's VISN 4 Mental Illness, Research, Education, and Clinical Center (MIRECC), led the study. He thinks the results will encourage providers to consider using pharmacogenomic testing, with patient consent, to help drive treatment decisions.

"From a VA policy perspective, I don't think that we would say the study is robust enough that we recommend testing everybody," says Dr. Oslin, who is also a psychiatrist at the Corporal Michael J. Crescenz VA Medical Center in Philadelphia. "The results were not a slam dunk, and in fact, an important outcome of the study is that only about 15–20 percent of the patients had genes that would significantly interfere with the prescribed medication. But I think the results favoring a positive effect on treatment, although small, will encourage providers to test patients and get this genetic information. Future research should explore if there are subgroups of patients who would benefit more from testing."

THE FOCUS ON METABOLIZING THE DRUG

In recent years, pharmacogenomic testing has received greater attention as a tool to personalize medication selection and is often used to treat patients with health conditions such as cancer and heart disease. Many in the medical community hope the testing can also be helpful in treating people with major depressive disorder. Research has been limited, however, on demonstrating improved clinical outcomes.

Currently, most of the pharmacogenomic testing focuses on a variant in the genes that encode hepatic CYP450 enzymes, a pathway that metabolizes drugs in the liver. Dr. Oslin and his team used a commercial battery of genes that focused on the CYP450 system. The battery tested eight genes, six of which test for variants in enzymes of the liver.

What Do Genes Have to Do with Antidepressants?

"The genes we tested don't actually relate to depression," Dr. Oslin says. "They relate to how a person metabolizes the drugs once they're in the body. Some of these genes will cause the medications to metabolize much faster than normal. Others will cause the drugs to metabolize much slower than normal, which means you'll end up with a lot of medication in your body."

The patients enrolled in the study were initiating or switching treatment with an antidepressant drug. The study included nearly 2,000 patients from 22 VA medical centers who were randomized evenly, with half receiving pharmacogenomic testing and the other half getting usual care. Dr. Oslin and his colleagues aimed to learn if genetic testing helped patients receive fewer medications

Genetic Studies May Lead to Accurate Medication Dose

with predicted drug-gene interactions and if that produced better outcomes.

A drug-gene interaction is an association between a medication and a genetic variant that may affect a patient's response to drug treatment. Having that information helps the provider select the appropriate dosage for a specific patient.

THE "CRUX" OF THE STUDY

The patients in the control group received genetic testing, but their providers did not see the results. That meant those providers made medication choices for their patients that were not supported by pharmacogenomic tests.

"That was really the crux of the study," Dr. Oslin says. "Does the pharmacogenetic test help you choose the medicine that you want to use with this particular patient?"

The study found a marked shift in prescribing away from medications with significant drug-gene interactions or moderate drug-gene interactions. Overall, 59 percent of the patients in the genetic testing group received a medication with no predicted drug-gene interaction, compared with 26 percent in the control group. The researchers defined that difference as "statistically significant and clinically meaningful."

Dr. Oslin says he went into the study thinking the research team would not see such a dramatic effect in predicted drug-gene interactions. He was "somewhat surprised" by the result. "There was essentially a major shift in avoiding medicines that had a predicted drug-gene interaction," he says.

To test their DNA, the patients used a cheek swab.

"Some companies do use a blood draw," Dr. Oslin explained. "There's no advantage or disadvantage to one versus the other. It really has to do with how the company processes the sample. Cheek swabs and blood samples are the most common sources of DNA. The sample is then used to look at several very specific genes that are known to relate to the metabolism of antidepressants and many other drugs. But in this study, we were interested only in antidepressants."

The researchers interviewed the patients about their depression outcomes. All three outcomes—depression remission, depression response, and symptom improvement—favored the group that received the genetic tests. They were all statistically significant over the course of 24 weeks, with a peak effect at 12 weeks. Depression outcomes were not statistically different between the groups at 24 weeks.

"We were not powered to look specifically at 24 weeks," Dr. Oslin explains. "That wasn't part of our primary hypothesis. Our primary hypothesis was an overall effect. And we showed an overall effect in all three of the ways that we measured outcomes. So, it's a glass half full, glass half empty kind of thing. Another way to think about the results is the group that had the pharmacogenetic test results had a faster response. That also was not something that we tested. But clearly if you look at 12 weeks in all three outcomes, the group that got the genetic test showed a better improvement in remission, response, and symptom improvement."

"It's important to realize that the test is not telling you whether the patient is going to respond to the treatment or not," he adds. "It's telling you something about how the patient metabolizes the medication. So it's not telling me that this is a good medicine for the patient. It's telling me not to prescribe this medicine, or perhaps to adjust the dosing, because the patient doesn't metabolize it well."

POSTTRAUMATIC STRESS DISORDER AFFECTED TREATMENT RESPONSE

In supplemental material, the researchers noted that the presence of posttraumatic stress disorder (PTSD) in patients had a profound negative impact on remission from depression. Basically, patients with PTSD responded poorly to antidepressants. "We know from the literature that PTSD doesn't respond well to antidepressants," Dr. Oslin says. The main psychotherapies for patients with PTSD, he points out, are cognitive processing therapy and prolonged exposure—both widely used in VA.

"One of the special ways that we did this study is as a pragmatic study in frontline clinical practices," Dr. Oslin says. "We used clinicians and their patients. The providers all had to say that the

Genetic Studies May Lead to Accurate Medication Dose

patients were being treated for depression. But they could have had comorbidities, and many of them had comorbid PTSD, which had a big influence on treatment outcomes in a negative way."

"For providers who would like to do pharmacogenomic testing in the future, the burden is low across the board," says Dr. Oslin. "There's no risk to patients in getting the test."

"The costs actually are very low because the results can be used over the patient's lifetime," Dr. Oslin says. "So you're not talking about a test that has a shelf life of only five minutes. And there's really no risk to getting the test. You're just getting the cheek swab or a blood test. Cost is low, risk is low, and the population benefits are probably low. But overall, this test likely benefits some patients substantially."[1]

---

[1] "Genetic Testing May Benefit Patients with Depression," U.S. Department of Veterans Affairs (VA), July 12, 2022. Available online. URL: www.research.va.gov/currents/0722-Genetic-testing-may-benefit-patients-with-depression.cfm. Accessed March 6, 2023.

Chapter 49 | Brain Biofeedback for Depressive Symptoms

Biofeedback is a process that uses your body's own signals such as heart rate and body temperature to bring about healthy changes. Neurofeedback (or EEG biofeedback) is a type of biofeedback that specifically uses brain wave signals to bring about healthy changes. Biofeedback can improve health issues that are caused or worsened by stress. Using a two-step process, biofeedback can help you relax and reduce your stress. Neurofeedback can improve health through shifting brain wave patterns in such a way there is a concomitant shift in cognition or mood. Clinical biofeedback involves interaction between a provider, a client, and a machine/device providing feedback from body-derived signals.

BIOFEEDBACK SAFETY AND EFFECTIVENESS

An evidence map of biofeedback was developed by the U.S. Department of Veterans Affairs (VA) Health Services Research and Development. Conditions with evidence of positive effect include migraine and tension-type headaches, secondary outcomes of headaches (medication intake, muscle tension, anxiety, and depression, etc.), stroke, urinary incontinence (related to prostatectomy), and fecal incontinence. Conditions with potential positive benefits include balance/gait training, fibromyalgia, and hypotension. Conditions with mixed or unclear benefits include sleep bruxism, chronic idiopathic constipation, knee osteoarthritis, and balance/gait training.

Also found was high-confidence evidence that biofeedback as an adjunctive treatment for pelvic floor muscle training (PFMT) can result in both immediate and long-term improvements in urinary incontinence for men after prostatectomy as compared with PFMT alone.

OCCUPATIONAL GUIDANCE

All biofeedback trainers must be licensed health-care professionals. Examples include but are not limited to psychology, nursing, occupational therapy, physical therapy, social work, and counseling. Additionally, they must be trained in the specific modality they offer. Professionals should consult with their local discipline leadership to ensure the biofeedback training they intend to practice is within their scope/core privileges or determine if a modification to a scope of practice or additional privileges are needed.[1]

---

[1] "Biofeedback," U.S. Department of Veterans Affairs (VA), July 11, 2022. Available online. URL: www.va.gov/WHOLEHEALTH/professional-resources/Biofeedback.asp. Accessed March 6, 2023.

Chapter 50 | Alternative and Complementary Therapies for Depression

Chapter Contents
Section 50.1—Use, Effectiveness, and Safety of Complementary and Alternative Therapies 381
Section 50.2—Meditation, Mindfulness, and Mental Health 389
Section 50.3—What the Science Says about Complementary Health Approaches for Depression 395

Section 50.1 | Use, Effectiveness, and Safety of Complementary and Alternative Therapies

Many patients receiving conventional, evidence-based treatment for mental or substance use disorders (SUDs) may also try various nonmainstream, or complementary, health approaches to treat their disorders or to relieve symptoms; some may do so without professional guidance. Patients may also independently turn to complementary products or practices to address co-occurring medical issues such as pain or to achieve personal health and wellness goals such as weight loss. At the same time, an increasing number of medical facilities and behavioral health programs are including complementary health approaches in their menu of services.

Complementary therapies vary in their safety, cost, and evidence of effectiveness. Patients may spend a great deal of time and money on products and services without knowing whether or how they work. In addition, patients may be unaware that some complementary therapies can have side effects or adversely interact with medications.

Some patients may not tell their behavioral health service practitioners about their use of complementary therapies; other patients may ask practitioners whether complementary health approaches are helpful. Practitioners may also be called on to explain the benefits of any complementary practices offered by their treatment programs.

WHAT ARE COMPLEMENTARY HEALTH APPROACHES?

The term "complementary health approaches" encompasses a group of diverse medical and health-care systems, practices, and products that are not generally considered to be part of conventional medicine. Also called "mainstream," "modern," or "Western" medicine, conventional medicine is practiced by doctors holding medical degrees and by allied health professionals, and its practices are evaluated scientifically for evidence of effectiveness.

Most Americans use nonmainstream practices as complements, rather than as alternatives, to conventional medicine. Generally speaking, complementary therapies have not been evaluated as extensively and rigorously as practices in conventional medicine.

Many complementary therapies have emerged out of ancient medical systems, such as Ayurvedic medicine from India, traditional Chinese medicine (which includes acupuncture), traditional African medicine, shamanism, and Native American healing practices. Other systems that offer complementary therapies, such as homeopathy and naturopathy, stem from practices that emerged in Europe beginning in the late 18th century.

HOW POPULAR ARE COMPLEMENTARY HEALTH APPROACHES FOR TREATMENT OF MENTAL OR SUBSTANCE USE DISORDERS?

A National Health Interview Survey (NHIS) study found that 45.4 percent of adults who were current moderate or heavier drinkers had used complementary health approaches in the preceding 12 months (reasons unspecified). The survey also found that in the preceding 12 months, 2.8 percent of adults had used complementary health approaches for anxiety, and 1.2 percent had used complementary health approaches for depression.

Another study of data from the National Comorbidity Survey Replication determined that 6.8 percent of participants with a mental disorder or SUD had used complementary therapy (alone or with treatment from another source) to treat the disorder in the 12 months before the survey interview. The study also found that in the same 12-month period, 31.3 percent of all mental health visits were to complementary health practitioners.

WHAT IS THE APPEAL OF COMPLEMENTARY HEALTH APPROACHES FOR BEHAVIORAL HEALTH TREATMENT?

For a variety of reasons, complementary health approaches can be especially appealing to behavioral health patients. Individuals who have not been successful with a particular conventional treatment may be curious about trying complementary therapies as adjuncts or treatment alternatives. Or such individuals may hope that augmenting conventional treatment will enhance their recovery. Some patients may have a lifestyle preference for products and healing systems they perceive as natural, want to avoid medication side effects, or appreciate the hands-on care they receive from a complementary health practitioner.

From the standpoint of the behavioral health treatment program, offering complementary therapy that is culturally relevant or popular in the community may attract prospective patients to the program's conventional treatment offerings and support retention. Some practices, such as meditation or movement-based therapies, may help patients gain self-efficacy skills. Complementary practices offered to groups may also enhance patients' socialization skills and support systems.

HOW EFFECTIVE ARE COMPLEMENTARY HEALTH APPROACHES?

Complementary health approaches have been insufficiently studied compared with conventional treatments. Many of the studies that have been conducted lack one or more features of the randomized controlled trial (RCT), which is the gold standard for evaluating biomedical or behavioral interventions. An RCT compares a treatment with a different treatment or with a placebo and randomly assigns subjects to experimental and control (comparison) groups. RCTs are often blinded (i.e., the subjects or the scientists administering the experiment, or both, do not know which treatment each subject is receiving) and, ideally, include sample sizes large enough for study results to achieve statistical significance. A well-designed RCT seeks to account for all possible variables that may influence the study results.

These features of the RCT can present challenges when assessing complementary practices. For example, some complementary practices involve multiple components (e.g., movement combined with meditation and deep breathing); teasing apart the effects of each component adds to the already considerable amount of time, funds, and labor required to conduct an RCT. Also, when studying interventions such as yoga or acupuncture, it is often not feasible to blind study participants and those administering the intervention. Yet another challenge is that complementary health practitioners typically customize the treatment to the individual. For purposes of an RCT, however, the intervention must be standardized, which can make a study's results less relevant to real-world application. The challenges of evaluating complementary health approaches through well-designed RCTs are prompting health researchers to explore alternative trial designs.

Another challenge in evaluating the efficacy of complementary health approaches is the ongoing debate over the value of the placebo effect. Evidence on a variety of complementary practices indicates that positive effects that occur may be attributable not to the treatment itself but rather to the interaction between the complementary health practitioner and the patient, the patient's beliefs and expectations about the treatment, and the setting and cultural context in which it is provided. Evidence that the placebo effect may play a potentially significant role in some complementary therapies has led some researchers to label complementary health approaches as "placebos." However, some researchers claim that the placebo effect is a powerful force that can be effectively harnessed through complementary health approaches to facilitate the body's ability to heal itself.

The task of helping patients make informed, evidence-based decisions about complementary health approaches is complicated by—as just described—the lack of convincing data, questions about the most appropriate means of evaluating these practices, and the unresolved controversy over the role of placebo in treatment. Presented below are summaries of the existing evidence on selected complementary health approaches for mental disorder or SUD, as provided by systematic reviews and meta-analyses.

Acupuncture

Acupuncture is a low-risk, low-cost therapy that, based on anecdotal evidence, can relieve physical withdrawal symptoms, help with relaxation, and suppress cravings for drugs and alcohol. A small percentage of substance abuse treatment programs—4.4 percent—offer acupuncture as an adjunct therapy.

Some systematic reviews have focused specifically on acupuncture for the treatment of disorders involving opioids, alcohol, and cocaine. These reviews did not find evidence of efficacy, and the authors have concluded that more research is needed. A 2009 review of clinical trials found some evidence for acupuncture's effectiveness with opioid withdrawal but not for treatment of other conditions such as alcohol withdrawal, nicotine relapse prevention, or cocaine dependence. A 2013 review of 48 RCTs testing acupuncture for use with patients who had alcohol, cocaine, nicotine, or opioid dependence concluded that nearly half of the clinical trials reviewed had at least one positive result (e.g., on craving), indicating that different types of acupuncture may have beneficial effects at different points in the withdrawal and recovery process.

A substantial number of studies have been done on acupuncture as a treatment for mental disorders. A review published by the Task Force on Complementary and Alternative Medicine (CAM) of the American Psychiatric Association (APA) concluded that the data do not suggest that acupuncture is effective in treating major depressive disorder.

Mindfulness Meditation

An increasing amount of research has focused on mindfulness meditation, with 477 articles published in academic journals in 2012 alone. In a systematic review of 14 randomized and 10 nonrandomized controlled trials, the authors found evidence that mindfulness-based interventions can reduce consumption of substances of abuse when compared with various controls, and they found preliminary evidence that the interventions can reduce cravings.

Movement Therapies

For the treatment of mental disorders or SUDs, exercise is theorized to provide social and psychological benefits by increasing socialization, improving emotional regulation, decreasing sensitivity to anxiety, and improving stress management. It is also postulated that because exercise triggers neurological effects similar to those produced by opioid drugs, exercise may serve as a substitute for substance use.

Exercise to promote physical, mental, emotional, or spiritual health is called "movement therapy." Some studies have investigated movement therapies in relation to specific mental disorders or SUDs. A 2013 meta-analysis of 37 RCTs found that exercise is moderately more effective than no therapy or a control intervention for reducing symptoms of depression. A 2011 meta-analysis of 10 RCTs found that yoga-based interventions have a statistically significant effect when used as an adjunct for treating severe mental illness, especially when current treatment modalities are inadequate or have adverse effects (e.g., weight gain, cardiovascular disease). A 2014 review of eight studies on yoga for the treatment of addictions reported that seven of those studies showed positive effects; the article authors concluded that the results are "encouraging but inconclusive" because of methodological limitations.

Although evidence of exercise's effect on mental disorders and SUDs is inconclusive, the benefits of routine physical exercise for overall health, wellness, and quality of life are well documented. At the least, exercise can be a helpful adjunct therapy to behavioral health treatment, and patients may benefit from participation in a movement-based complementary practice such as yoga, Pilates, or tai chi. A doctor's guidance on appropriate types of exercise or movement therapy is advised for patients who are pregnant, have a specific medical condition (e.g., multiple sclerosis, back injury, osteoporosis), or have not exercised in a long time.

Natural Products

Of the many dietary supplements marketed to consumers as having mental health benefits, two of the most popular are omega-3 supplements and S-adenosyl-L methionine (SAMe). Some omega-3 fatty acids are essential nutrients obtained from food sources such as fatty fish and certain plants such as flax. SAMe is a chemical that is naturally found in almost all tissues in the body. It also lists two examples kava and St. John's wort. Table 50.1 provides evidence of the effectiveness and caution of these products. Many herbal products are also marketed to consumers for the treatment of mental disorders. Among the many other botanicals marketed as treatments for mental health conditions are brook mint for anxiety or insomnia, chamomile for insomnia, lavender for anxiety or

Alternative and Complementary Therapies for Depression

Table 50.1. Examples of Natural Products Marketed to Consumers for the Treatment of Mental Disorders

Product	Example of Use	Evidence of Effectiveness	Cautions
Omega-3 fatty acids (found in fatty fish, flax, and other dietary sources)	Depression	May have benefits as an adjunct to standard pharmacologic therapy for depression.	May interact with anticoagulants.
SAMe (chemical found naturally in the body)	Depression	May have benefits as an adjunct to standard pharmacologic therapy for depression.	Close medical supervision is advised for patients with bipolar disorder or on tricyclic antidepressants.
Kava (*Piper methysticum*, plant)	Anxiety	May have an anxiolytic effect.	• Safety risks outweigh the benefits. • Adversely interacts with several classes of drugs, including some sedatives, benzodiazepines, and monoamine oxidase inhibitors (MAOIs). • Has been linked to severe liver damage. • Should not be taken with alcohol because of the risk of excessive sedation and harm to the liver.
St. John's wort (*Hypericum perforatum*, herb)	Depression	Some evidence exists to support use for treating mild-to-moderate depression in adults.	• Active compounds in St. John's wort interact with other medications to render them less effective and potentially cause serious side effects. Such herb–drug interactions have been documented for MAOIs and selective serotonin reuptake inhibitors (SSRIs) used to treat depression. Interactions have also been documented for medications to treat other conditions, including HIV/AIDS, Parkinson disease (PD), and cancer. St. John's wort can also interfere with the efficacy of oral contraceptives, anticonvulsants, immunosuppressants used with transplantation, anticoagulants, and other types of medications. • Products made from St. John's wort vary considerably in the quantity and quality of their active compounds, leading to variability in interactive and other side effects.

insomnia, linden for insomnia and nervous tension, passion flower for insomnia and anxiety, and valerian for anxiety.

RCTs and systematic reviews provide little evidence that homeopathic medicines are effective for any specific condition. The key ingredient can be extremely diluted, so the principle of action does not appear to be science-based. Even when the main ingredient is highly diluted, there may be other active ingredients in the mixture, including alcohol and metals, that can cause side effects and drug interactions.

Ayurvedic medicine has not been sufficiently studied in RCTs to determine its effectiveness. Ayurvedic medicines in the subset called "rasa shastra" have additional ingredients deliberately added; these additives may include metals, minerals, and gems. A study of 230 such products purchased over the Internet from India or the United States found that nearly 21 percent contained detectable levels of lead, mercury, or arsenic.[1]

EIGHT THINGS TO KNOW ABOUT DEPRESSION AND COMPLEMENTARY HEALTH APPROACHES

Many people with depression turn to complementary health approaches in addition to or in place of conventional treatment. Research suggests that some approaches may be modestly helpful in reducing depression symptoms. For other approaches, benefits are uncertain, or there are safety concerns.

Here are eight things you should know about complementary health approaches for depression:
- Depression can be a serious illness. Do not use a complementary health approach to replace conventional care or postpone seeing a health-care provider about symptoms of depression.
- Some evidence suggests acupuncture may modestly reduce depression symptoms.

---

[1] "Complementary Health Approaches: Advising Clients About Evidence and Risks," Substance Abuse and Mental Health Services Administration (SAMHSA), 2015. Available online. URL: https://store.samhsa.gov/sites/default/files/d7/priv/sma15-4921.pdf. Accessed April 27, 2023.

Alternative and Complementary Therapies for Depression

- Music therapy may provide short-term benefits for people with depression.
- Studies in adults, adolescents, and children have suggested that yoga may be helpful in reducing depressive symptoms.
- It is uncertain whether omega-3 fatty acid supplements are helpful for symptoms of depression.
- Some research on the herb St. John's wort (*Hypericum perforatum*) has suggested that it may be helpful for depression symptoms, but not all studies agree. There is an important concern about the safety of St. John's wort: It can interact in dangerous, sometimes life-threatening ways with a variety of medicines.
- Current scientific evidence does not support the use of other dietary supplements, including S-adenosyl-L-methionine (SAMe) or inositol, for depression.
- Take charge of your health—talk with your health-care providers about any complementary health approaches you use. Together, you can make shared, well-informed decisions.[2]

Section 50.2 | Meditation, Mindfulness, and Mental Health

WHAT IS MEDITATION AND MINDFULNESS?
Meditation has a history that goes back thousands of years, and many meditative techniques began in Eastern traditions. The term "meditation" refers to a variety of practices that focus on mind and body integration and are used to calm the mind and enhance overall well-being. Some types of meditation involve maintaining a mental focus on a particular sensation, such as breathing, a sound, a visual image, or a mantra, which is a repeated word or phrase.

---

[2] "8 Things to Know about Depression and Complementary Health Approaches," U.S. Department of Veterans Affairs (VA), January 12, 2022. Available online. URL: www.nccih.nih.gov/health/tips/things-to-know-about-depression-and-complementary-health-approaches. Accessed March 6, 2023.

Other forms of meditation include the practice of mindfulness, which involves maintaining attention or awareness of the present moment without making judgments.

Programs that teach meditation or mindfulness may combine the practices with other activities. For example, mindfulness-based stress reduction (MBSR) is a program that teaches mindful meditation, but it also includes discussion sessions and other strategies to help people apply what they have learned to stressful experiences. Mindfulness-based cognitive therapy integrates mindfulness practices with aspects of cognitive-behavioral therapy (CBT).

HOW POPULAR ARE MEDITATION AND MINDFULNESS?

Mindfulness programs for schools have become popular. These programs provide mindfulness training with the goal of helping students and educators manage stress and anxiety, resolve conflicts, control impulses, and improve resilience, memory, and concentration. The mindfulness practices and training methods used in these programs vary widely. Studies on the effectiveness of school-based mindfulness programs have had small sample sizes and been of varying quality.

HOW DO MEDITATION AND MINDFULNESS WORK?

Some research suggests that meditation and mindfulness practices may affect the functioning or structure of the brain. Studies have used various methods of measuring brain activity to look for measurable differences in the brains of people engaged in mindfulness-based practices. Other studies have theorized that training in meditation and mindfulness practices can change brain activity. However, the results of these studies are difficult to interpret, and the practical implications are not clear.

WHY DO PEOPLE PRACTICE MINDFULNESS MEDITATION?

In a U.S. survey, 1.9 percent of 34,525 adults reported that they had practiced mindfulness meditation in the past 12 months. Among those responders who practiced mindfulness meditation exclusively, 73 percent reported that they meditated for their general wellness and to prevent diseases, and most of them (approximately 92%) reported that they meditated to relax or reduce stress. In more than half of the responses, a desire for better sleep was a reason for practicing mindfulness meditation.

WHAT ARE THE HEALTH BENEFITS OF MEDITATION AND MINDFULNESS?

Meditation and mindfulness practices may have a variety of health benefits and may help people improve the quality of their lives. Recent studies have investigated if meditation or mindfulness helps people manage anxiety, stress, depression, pain, or symptoms related to withdrawal from nicotine, alcohol, or opioids.

Other studies have looked at the effects of meditation or mindfulness on weight control or sleep quality.

However, much of the research on these topics has been preliminary or not scientifically rigorous. Because the studies examined many different types of meditation and mindfulness practices and the effects of those practices are hard to measure, the results from the studies have been difficult to analyze and may have been interpreted too optimistically.

Stress, Anxiety, and Depression

- A 2021 analysis of 23 studies (1,815 participants) examined mindfulness-based practices used as a treatment for adults with diagnosed anxiety disorders. The studies included in the analysis compared the mindfulness-based interventions (alone or in combination with usual treatments) with other treatments such as CBT, psychoeducation, and relaxation. The analysis showed mixed results for the short-term effectiveness of the different mindfulness-based approaches. Overall, they were more effective than the usual treatments at reducing the severity of anxiety and depression symptoms, but only some types of mindfulness approaches were as effective as CBT. However, these results should be interpreted with caution because the risk of bias for all of the studies

was unclear. Also, the few studies that followed up with participants for periods longer than two months found no long-term effects of mindfulness-based practices.
- A 2019 analysis of 23 studies that included a total of 1,373 college and university students looked at the effects of yoga, mindfulness, and meditation practices on symptoms of stress, anxiety, and depression. Although the results showed that all the practices had some effect, most of the studies included in the review were of poor quality and had a high risk of bias.

High Blood Pressure

Few high-quality studies have examined the effects of meditation and mindfulness on blood pressure. According to a statement from the American Heart Association (AHA), the practice of meditation may have a possible benefit, but its specific effects on blood pressure have not been determined.
- A 2020 review of 14 studies (including more than 1,100 participants) examined the effects of mindfulness practices on the blood pressure of people who had health conditions such as hypertension, diabetes, or cancer. The analysis showed that for people with these health conditions, practicing mindfulness-based stress reduction was associated with a significant reduction in blood pressure.

Pain

Studies examining the effects of mindfulness or meditation on acute and chronic pain have produced mixed results.
- A 2020 report by the Agency for Healthcare Research and Quality (AHRQ) concluded that mindfulness-based stress reduction was associated with short-term (less than six months) improvement in low back pain but not fibromyalgia pain.
- A 2020 analysis of five studies of adults using opioids for acute or chronic pain (with a total of 514 participants) supported by the National Center for

Complementary and Integrative Health (NCCIH) found that meditation practices were strongly associated with pain reduction.
- Acute pain, such as pain from surgery, traumatic injuries, or childbirth, occurs suddenly and lasts only a short time. A 2020 analysis of 19 studies examined the effects of mindfulness-based therapies for acute pain and found no evidence of reduced pain severity. However, the same analysis found some evidence that the therapies could improve a person's tolerance for pain.
- A 2019 comparison of treatments for chronic pain did an overall analysis of 11 studies (697 participants) that evaluated CBT, which is the usual psychological intervention for chronic pain; four studies (280 participants) that evaluated mindfulness-based stress reduction; and one study (341 participants) of both therapies. The comparison found that both approaches were more effective at reducing pain intensity than no treatment, but there was no evidence of any important difference between the two approaches.
- A 2019 review found that mindfulness-based approaches did not reduce the frequency, length, or pain intensity of headaches. However, the authors of this review noted that their results are likely imprecise because only five studies (a total of 185 participants) were included in the analysis, and any conclusions made from the analysis should be considered preliminary.

Insomnia and Sleep Quality

Mindfulness meditation practices may help reduce insomnia and improve sleep quality.
- A 2019 analysis of 18 studies (1,654 total participants) found that mindfulness meditation practices improved sleep quality more than education-based treatments. However, the effects of mindfulness meditation approaches on sleep quality were no different than those of evidence-based treatments such as CBT and exercise.

Substance Use Disorder

Several clinical trials have investigated if mindfulness-based approaches such as mindfulness-based relapse prevention (MBRP) might help people recover from substance use disorders (SUDs). These approaches have been used to help people increase their awareness of the thoughts and feelings that trigger cravings and learn ways to reduce their automatic reactions to those cravings.

Cancer

Mindfulness-based approaches may improve the mental health of people with cancer.

- A 2019 analysis of 29 studies (3,274 total participants) of mindfulness-based practices showed that the use of mindfulness practices among people with cancer significantly reduced psychological distress, fatigue, sleep disturbance, pain, and symptoms of anxiety and depression. However, most of the participants were women with breast cancer, so the effects may not be similar for other populations or other types of cancer.

Attention Deficit Hyperactivity Disorder

Several studies have been done on using meditation and mindfulness practices to improve symptoms of attention deficit hyperactivity disorder (ADHD). However, the studies have not been of high quality, and the results have been mixed, so evidence that meditation or mindfulness approaches will help people manage symptoms of ADHD is not conclusive.

ARE MEDITATION AND MINDFULNESS PRACTICES SAFE?

Meditation and mindfulness practices usually are considered to have few risks. However, few studies have examined these practices for potentially harmful effects, so it is not possible to make definite statements about safety.

A 2020 review examined 83 studies (a total of 6,703 participants) and found that 55 of those studies reported negative experiences related to meditation practices. The researchers concluded that

Alternative and Complementary Therapies for Depression

about 8 percent of participants had a negative effect from practicing meditation, which is similar to the percentage reported for psychological therapies. The most commonly reported negative effects were anxiety and depression. In an analysis limited to three studies (521 participants) of mindfulness-based stress reduction programs, investigators found that the mindfulness practices were not more harmful than receiving no treatment.

TIPS TO CONSIDER
- Do not use meditation or mindfulness to replace conventional care or as a reason to postpone seeing a health-care provider about a medical problem.
- Ask about the training and experience of the instructor of the meditation or mindfulness practice you are considering.
- Take charge of your health—talk with your health-care providers about any complementary health approaches you use. Together, you can make shared, well-informed decisions.[3]

Section 50.3 | What the Science Says about Complementary Health Approaches for Depression

OMEGA-3 FATTY ACID SUPPLEMENTATION
At present, it is uncertain whether omega-3 fatty acid supplementation may be useful for depression. Some studies have shown small effects of adjunctive therapy in patients with a diagnosis of major depressive disorder (MDD) and on depressive patients without a diagnosis of MDD; however, most trials have been adjunctive studies. Controlled trials of omega-3 fatty acids as monotherapy

---

[3] "Meditation and Mindfulness: What You Need To Know," National Center for Complementary and Integrative Health (NCCIH), June 2022. Available online. URL: www.nccih.nih.gov/health/meditation-and-mindfulness-what-you-need-to-know. Accessed March 15, 2023.

are inconclusive compared to standard antidepressant medicines, and it remains unclear whether a mechanism is present to suggest that a pharmacologic or biologic antidepressant effect exists.

What Does the Research Show?

- A 2021 Cochrane review of 35 randomized controlled trials (34 studies involving a total of 1924 participants investigated the impact of omega-3 polyunsaturated fatty acid (PUFA) supplementation compared to placebo, and one study involving 40 participants investigated the impact of omega-3 PUFA supplementation compared to antidepressant treatment) evaluated the effect of omega-3 PUFAs on MDD. For the placebo comparison, omega-3 PUFA supplementation resulted in a small-to-modest benefit for depressive symptomology compared to placebo. The reviewers noted that this effect is unlikely to be clinically meaningful. The reviewers concluded that there is insufficient high-certainty evidence to determine the effects of omega-3 PUFAs as a treatment for MDD.
- A 2021 systematic review and meta-analysis of 31 trials involving 41,470 participants assessed the effects of long-chain omega-3s. They found that increasing long-chain omega-3 probably has little or no effect on the risk of depression symptoms (median dose 0.95 g/d, duration of 12 months) or anxiety symptoms (median dose 1.1 g/d, duration of six months).
- A 2020 network meta-analysis involving 910 participants with MDD in 10 trials with three adjuvant therapy strategies (high-dose omega-3 PUFAs, low-dose omega-3 PUFAs, and placebo) concluded that high-dose omega-3 PUFA supplementation might be superior to low-dose supplementation in the early therapy period for MDD. However, the reviewers noted that more head-to-head clinical trials need to be carried out to provide more direct comparisons and enhance the evidence of the efficacy of omega-3 PUFAs for this disorder.
- A 2020 meta-analysis of 18 randomized controlled trials involving a total of 4,052 pregnant women or postpartum

Alternative and Complementary Therapies for Depression

women concluded that omega-3 PUFAs had an overall significant but small beneficial effect on perinatal depression. The reviewers advised against prescribing omega-3 PUFAs for the treatment or prevention of depressive symptoms during pregnancy, given a lack of effect with low heterogeneity. In contrast, the reviewers noted that omega-3 PUFA supplementation may be a promising adjuvant treatment for postpartum depression.

Safety
- Omega-3 fatty acid supplements are generally safe and well-tolerated. When side effects do occur, they typically consist of minor gastrointestinal symptoms and a fishy aftertaste.
- There is some concern that omega-3 supplements may extend bleeding time. The risk appears to be minimal and should never be used in patients who take drugs that affect platelet function.
- It is important to discuss any potential herb–drug interactions with patients if they are considering using omega-3 fatty acids.
- It is uncertain whether people with fish or shellfish allergies can safely consume fish oil supplements, and they should not be used in such patients.

ST. JOHN'S WORT (*HYPERICUM PERFORATUM*)

Results of some studies suggest that St. John's wort (*Hypericum perforatum*) may have an effect on mild-to-moderate MDD for a limited number of patients, similar to standard antidepressants, but the evidence is far from definitive. Although some studies have demonstrated a slight efficacy over placebo, others contradict these findings.

Safety
- Drug interactions with St. John's wort (*Hypericum perforatum*) limit use and are important safety considerations.

- Combining St. John's wort (*Hypericum perforatum*) and certain antidepressants can lead to serotonin syndrome, with dangerous symptoms ranging from tremors and diarrhea to very dangerous confusion, muscle stiffness, drop in body temperature, and even death.
- Other side effects of St. John's wort (*Hypericum perforatum*) are usually minor and uncommon and may include upset stomach and sensitivity to sunlight. Also, St. John's wort may worsen feelings of anxiety in some people.
- A rare but possible side effect of taking St. John's wort (*Hypericum perforatum*) is psychosis. Those with certain mental health disorders, such as bipolar disorder, are at risk of experiencing this rare side effect. Therefore, it is important to discuss this potential side effect with patients who are considering using St. John's wort and encourage discontinuation of the herb if they experience a worsening of symptoms.
- Taking St. John's wort (*Hypericum perforatum*) increases the activity of the cytochrome P450 3A4 (CYP3A4) enzyme and reduces plasma concentrations and can weaken many prescription medicines, such as:
  - antidepressants
  - oral contraceptives
  - cyclosporine
  - digoxin
  - some HIV drugs, including indinavir
  - some chemotherapeutic agents, including irinotecan
  - warfarin and other anticoagulants

SAMe

Current scientific research does not support the use of S-adenosyl-L-methionine (SAMe) for the treatment of depression.

What Does the Research Show?

- A 2020 randomized, double-blind, placebo-controlled trial involving 90 participants evaluated the effects of the combination of SAMe 200 mg and *Lactobacillus plantarum* (*L. plantarum*) HEAL9 for the overall symptomatology of mild-to-moderate depression over a six-week period. A greater reduction in depressive symptoms for the combination of SAMe and *L. plantarum* compared to placebo was seen at treatment week six.

Safety
- Information on the long-term safety of SAMe is limited and inconclusive. However, in one study of alcohol-related liver disease in which participants took SAMe for two years, no serious side effects were reported.
- SAMe may decrease the effects of levodopa. It is also possible that SAMe might interact with drugs and dietary supplements that increase levels of serotonin, including some antidepressants, L-tryptophan, and St. John's wort, but the evidence for such interactions is very limited.
- SAMe promotes the growth of *Pneumocystis*, a fungus that can cause pneumonia in people with suppressed immune systems. It is possible that taking SAMe might increase the likelihood or severity of *Pneumocystis* infection in people who are HIV-positive and should never be used in these patients.
- Side effects of SAMe appear to be uncommon, and when they do occur, they are usually problems such as nausea or digestive upsets.

ACUPUNCTURE
There is some evidence that suggests acupuncture may provide a modest reduction in symptoms of depression, particularly when compared with no treatment or a control.

What Does the Research Show?
- A 2019 meta-analysis of seven trials compared the effectiveness of acupuncture therapy in patients with poststroke depression and found evidence to support the use of acupuncture for this condition. Subgroup analyses

also showed that acupuncture alone resulted in better outcomes than drug therapy in improving depressive symptoms.
- A 2019 systematic review and meta-analysis of 29 studies involving 2,268 participants (22 trials were conducted in China, and 7 were conducted outside of China) concluded that acupuncture might be a suitable adjunct to usual care and standard antidepressant medication. However, most of the trials included in the review and meta-analysis were at a high risk of bias.

Safety
- Relatively few complications from using acupuncture have been reported. Still, complications have resulted from the use of nonsterile needles and improper delivery of treatments.
- When not delivered properly, acupuncture can cause serious adverse effects, including skin infections, punctured organs, pneumothoraces, and injury to the central nervous system.

MUSIC THERAPY
There is some evidence that music therapy may provide short-term benefits for people with depression.

What Does the Research Show?
- A 2020 meta-analysis of 55 randomized controlled trials found that music therapy exhibited a significant reduction in depressive symptoms compared with the control group, and music medicine (i.e., music as therapy that is not managed by a music therapist and does not involve a therapeutic relationship) exhibited a stronger effect in reducing depressive symptoms. Among the specific music therapy methods, recreative music therapy, guided imagery and music, music-assisted relaxation, music and imagery, improvisational music therapy, and therapeutic music listening exhibited different effects.

Alternative and Complementary Therapies for Depression

Safety
There are no adverse effects associated with music therapy.

YOGA
There is some evidence that yoga may be helpful in reducing depressive symptoms.

What Does the Research Show?
- A 2020 systematic review of 27 studies evaluated yoga as an intervention for reducing anxiety and depression in children and adolescents. The reviewers concluded that yoga generally leads to some reductions in anxiety and depression in youth; however, the methodological quality of evidence included in the review was weak to moderate.

Safety
- Yoga is generally considered a safe form of physical activity for healthy people when performed properly under the guidance of a qualified instructor. However, as with other types of physical activity, injuries can occur. The most common injuries are sprains and strains. Serious injuries are rare.
- People with health conditions, older adults, and pregnant women may need to avoid or modify some yoga poses and practices.[4]

---

[4] "Depression and Complementary Health Approaches: What the Science Says," National Center for Complementary and Integrative Health (NCCIH), December 2021. Available online. URL: www.nccih.nih.gov/health/providers/digest/depression-and-complementary-health-approaches-science. Accessed April 10, 2023.

Chapter 51 | Treating Depression in Children and Adolescents

Mental health is an important part of overall health for children as well as adults. For many adults who have mental disorders, symptoms were present—but often not recognized or addressed—in childhood and adolescence. For a young person with symptoms of a mental disorder, the earlier treatment is started, the more effective it can be. Early treatment can help prevent more severe, lasting problems as a child grows up.

WARNING SIGNS

It can be tough to tell if troubling behavior in a child is just part of growing up or a problem that should be discussed with a health professional. But if there are behavioral signs and symptoms that last weeks or months, and if these issues interfere with the child's daily life at home and at school, or with friends, you should contact a health professional.

Young children may benefit from an evaluation and treatment if they:
- have frequent tantrums or are intensely irritable much of the time
- often talk about fears or worries
- complain about frequent stomachaches or headaches with no known medical cause
- are in constant motion and cannot sit quietly (except when they are watching videos or playing video games)

- sleep too much or too little, have frequent nightmares, or seem sleepy during the day
- are not interested in playing with other children or have difficulty making friends
- struggle academically or have experienced a recent decline in grades
- repeat actions or check things many times out of fear that something bad may happen

Older children and adolescents may benefit from an evaluation if they:
- have lost interest in things that they used to enjoy
- have low energy
- sleep too much or too little or seem sleepy throughout the day
- are spending more and more time alone and avoid social activities with friends or family
- diet or exercise excessively or fear gaining weight
- engage in self-harm behaviors (such as cutting or burning their skin)
- smoke, drink alcohol, or use drugs
- engage in risky or destructive behavior alone or with friends
- have thoughts of suicide
- have periods of highly elevated energy and activity and require much less sleep than usual
- say that they think someone is trying to control their mind or that they hear things that other people cannot hear

Mental illnesses can be treated. If you are a child or teen, talk to your parents, school counselor, or health-care provider. If you are a parent and need help starting a conversation with your child or teen about mental health, find resources for families from the Substance Abuse and Mental Health Services Administration (www.samhsa.gov/families). If you are unsure where to go for help, ask your pediatrician or family doctor or visit the Help for Mental Illnesses

Treating Depression in Children and Adolescents

web page of the National Institute of Mental Health (NIMH; www.nimh.nih.gov/health/find-help).

It may be helpful for children and teens to save several emergency numbers on their cell phones. The ability to get immediate help for themselves or for a friend can make a difference.
- the phone number for a trusted friend or relative
- the nonemergency number for the local police department
- the Crisis Text Line: 741741
- the Suicide & Crisis Lifeline: 988[1]

TREATMENT OPTIONS

The mental health professional will review the evaluation results to help determine if a child's behavior is related to changes or stresses at home or school or if it is the result of a disorder for which they would recommend treatment. Treatment recommendations may include the following:
- **Psychotherapy ("talk therapy")**. There are many different approaches to psychotherapy, including structured psychotherapies directed at specific conditions. Effective psychotherapy for children always includes the following:
  - parent involvement in the treatment
  - teaching the child skills to practice at home or school (between-session "homework assignments")
  - measures of progress (such as rating scales and improvements on "homework assignments") that are tracked over time
- **Medications**. As with adults, the type of medicines used for children depends on the diagnosis and may include antidepressants, stimulants, mood stabilizers, or other medications. For general information on specific classes of medications, visit the NIMH's mental

---

[1] "Child and Adolescent Mental Health," National Institute of Mental Health (NIMH), May 2021. Available online. URL: www.nimh.nih.gov/health/topics/child-and-adolescent-mental-health. Accessed March 8, 2023.

health medications web page (www.nimh.nih.gov/health/topics/mental-health-medications). Medications are often used in combination with psychotherapy. If multiple health-care providers or specialists are involved, treatment information should be shared and coordinated to achieve the best results.
- **Family counseling.** Including family members in treatment can help them understand how a child's challenges may affect relationships with parents and siblings.
- **Support for parents.** Individual or group sessions for parents that include training and the opportunity to talk with other parents can provide new strategies for supporting a child and managing difficult behavior in a positive way. The therapist can also coach parents on how to communicate and work with schools on accommodations.

WORKING WITH THE SCHOOL

Children who have behavioral or emotional challenges that interfere with success in school may benefit from plans or accommodations provided under laws that prevent discrimination against children with disabilities. Your child's health-care providers can help you communicate with the school.

A first step may be to ask the school whether accommodations such as an individualized education program may be appropriate for your child. Accommodations might include measures such as providing a child with a tape recorder for taking notes, allowing more time for tests, or adjusting seating in the classroom to reduce distraction. There are many sources of information on what schools can and, in some cases, must provide for children who would benefit from accommodations and how parents can request evaluation and services for their child. The U.S. Department of Education has detailed information on laws that establish mechanisms for providing children with accommodations tailored to their individual needs and aimed at helping them succeed in school. The department has also a website on the Individuals with Disabilities Education Act (IDEA), and its Office for Civil Rights (OCR) has information on other federal laws that prohibit discrimination based on disability in public programs, such as schools.[2]

---

[2] "Children and Mental Health: Is This Just a Stage?" National Institute of Mental Health (NIMH), 2021. Available online. URL: www.nimh.nih.gov/health/publications/children-and-mental-health#part_6394. Accessed March 8, 2023.

Chapter 52 | Treatment-Resistant and Relapsed Depression

In March 2019, the U.S. Food and Drug Administration (FDA) approved an equally remarkable new medication—esketamine—which targets treatment-resistant depression (TRD). TRD is a form of depression that does not get better even after the patient has tried at least two antidepressant therapies. Delivered intranasally in a doctor's office, clinic, or hospital, esketamine acts rapidly—within a couple of hours—to relieve depression symptoms in approximately half of the patients with TRD. Like brexanolone, esketamine also grew out of a long line of research sponsored by the National Institute of Mental Health (NIMH).

GLUTAMATE: A TARGET BEYOND MONOAMINES IN THE TREATMENT OF DEPRESSION

The possibility that ketamine might be an effective antidepressant started as an educated guess born of frustration. Through the second half of the 20th century, the science of psychopharmacology—the use of drugs to combat the devastating symptoms of mental illnesses—had led to a transformation of psychiatry. Effective, cheap, and fast, antidepressant medications became the main weapon in the fight against depression. Each decade or so, a new class of drug was developed, maintaining efficacy with fewer side effects and easier to prescribe and take.

By the 1990s, this rapid pace of incremental improvement slowed dramatically. It turns out that all of the known antidepressants targeted similar mechanisms—increasing the activity of a class of neurotransmitters called "monoamines," including serotonin, norepinephrine, and dopamine. Despite many attempts, scientists were unable to improve significantly on the monoaminergic antidepressants, leaving many people suffering from TRD.

Many pharmacologists began to believe that to make significant improvements, new drugs would need to target mechanisms beyond the monoamines. Glutamate is the major excitatory neurotransmitter in the brain, responsible for activating neurons to turn on the key circuits that drive all forms of behavior. Drs. John Krystal, M.D., Ph.D., and Dennis Charney, M.D., at Yale University, had been studying the effects of altering glutamate neurotransmission in healthy subjects and patients with schizophrenia, testing the hypothesis that changes in glutamate function might underlay psychosis. They noticed that a particular glutamate receptor blocker, ketamine, had profound psychological effects on people, inducing psychotic-like symptoms. They were aware of preclinical studies, particularly those of Phil Skolnick, Ph.D., D.Sc., and his colleagues suggesting that antagonists of one of the glutamate receptors, the NMDA receptor, had antidepressant-like properties. They also knew that glutamate has important roles in mood and in the regulation of monoamines. They wondered, might glutamate play a role in depression? Could ketamine be used to treat depression? In a small group of patients with depression, the scientists at Yale found that low doses of ketamine—lower than those that cause psychosis-like symptoms—dramatically reduced depressive symptoms. Remarkably, while monoaminergic antidepressants take weeks to work, the effects of ketamine on depression occurred within hours.

FROM KETAMINE TO ESKETAMINE: PROVING AND IMPROVING

After their initial report was published, Dr. Charney joined the NIMH as an investigator and recruited Husseini Manji, M.D., and Carlos Zarate, M.D., to build a mood disorders research program in the NIMH's Intramural Research Program (IRP).

Treatment-Resistant and Relapsed Depression

Together, Drs. Charney, Manji, and Zarate planned the first study with ketamine in TRD. In 2006, for the first time, Dr. Zarate and colleagues found that ketamine produced rapid, robust, and relatively sustained antidepressant effects in patients with TRD (in this study, patients had failed more than six antidepressants). Since then, among the key findings carried out at the NIMH by Dr. Zarate are the findings that ketamine has strong, rapid effects on TRD and bipolar depression, as well as in reducing suicidal thoughts. Furthermore, the NIMH and the NIMH-funded researchers have conducted a number of studies to better understand the mechanisms by which ketamine may produce these rapid therapeutic effects.

Several additional studies confirmed that ketamine was useful in TRD, where it provides relief from depression in about half of the patients. Other studies showed that the effects of ketamine last for several days to a few weeks and that multiple doses can provide continued relief in those who respond.

While these studies convincingly demonstrated ketamine's potential benefits, significant obstacles to its widespread use remained. Most significantly, the intravenous route of administration meant considerable expense and inconvenience to those who might benefit from ketamine. While some physicians began to study intranasal ketamine, Dr. Manji, who had left the IRP to work at Janssen Pharmaceuticals, decided to take a different tack. Like many organic molecules, ketamine consists of two different chemicals that differ only in their three-dimensional structure: so-called S-ketamine and R-ketamine. Janssen's scientists, working under Dr. Manji, reasoned that S-ketamine was the active ingredient and that if they made a pure form of S-ketamine, they could deliver more of the drug to the nasal passages. They manufactured the drug, calling it esketamine. Subsequent clinical trials demonstrated that esketamine, delivered intranasally, had robust antidepressant effects in patients with TRD. Esketamine was granted FDA approval in March 2019.

BUILDING ON SUCCESS: WHAT IS NEXT IN KETAMINE RESEARCH?

The job is not done for TRD. Ketamine and esketamine work, but both have significant drawbacks. Many patients experience uncomfortable dissociative symptoms, hypertension, or other side effects for a few hours after administration. Because of these symptoms, as well as the potential for abuse, both need to be administered in a doctor's office. These are not medications you can pick up at the pharmacy and take on your own. Dr. Zarate and others are hard at work at finding safer alternatives to ketamine by examining the mechanisms by which it works.[1]

---

[1] "New Hope for Treatment-Resistant Depression: Guessing Right on Ketamine," National Institute of Mental Health (NIMH), August 13, 2019. Available online. URL: www.nimh.nih.gov/about/director/messages/2019/new-hope-for-treatment-resistant-depression-guessing-right-on-ketamine. Accessed March 22, 2023.

Chapter 53 | **Paying for Mental Health Care**

Mental health conditions, such as depression and anxiety, can happen to anyone anytime. Talk to your doctor or health-care provider about depression or anxiety symptoms.

MEDICARE HELPS COVER MENTAL HEALTH SERVICES

Medicare Part A (Hospital Insurance) helps pay for mental health services if you are an inpatient in a general hospital or psychiatric hospital that only cares for people with mental health conditions. Part A covers semiprivate rooms, meals, general nursing, drugs (including methadone to treat an opioid use disorder), and other related services and supplies. If you are in a psychiatric hospital (instead of a general hospital), Part A only pays for up to 190 days of inpatient psychiatric hospital services during your lifetime.

Medicare Part B (Medical Insurance) helps cover mental health services you generally get outside a hospital and services a hospital provides in its outpatient department.

Part B helps pay for these services if your doctor accepts Medicare:
- one depression screening each year
- individual and group psychotherapy
- family counseling if the main purpose is to help with your treatment
- testing to see if you are getting the services you need and if your current treatment is helping you
- psychiatric evaluation
- medication management

- certain prescription drugs that are not usually "self-administered," like some injections
- diagnostic tests
- partial hospitalization

Part B covers opioid use disorder treatment services that opioid treatment programs provide. The services include:
- medication (such as methadone, buprenorphine, naltrexone, and naloxone)
- counseling
- drug testing
- individual and group therapy
- intake activities
- periodic assessments

Part B also covers one alcohol misuse screening each year for adults with Medicare (including pregnant individuals) who use alcohol but do not meet the medical criteria for alcohol dependency. If you have a substance use disorder or a co-occurring mental health disorder, you can get telehealth services from home.

Medicare drug coverage (Part D) helps cover drugs you may need to treat a mental health condition. Medicare drug plans are required to cover nearly all antidepressants and antipsychotics.

WHAT DO YOU PAY?

For inpatient mental health services, you pay:
- a one-time hospital deductible for each benefit period
- days 1–60: no coinsurance amount for each benefit period
- days 61–90: a coinsurance amount per day of each benefit period
- days 91 and beyond: a coinsurance amount for each "lifetime reserve day" after day 90 of each benefit period (up to 60 days over your lifetime)

Part B covers certain doctors' services, outpatient care, medical supplies, and preventive services. This includes mental health

Paying for Mental Health Care

services that doctors and other health-care professionals provide if you are admitted as a hospital inpatient. You pay 20 percent of the Medicare-approved amount for these mental health services while you are a hospital inpatient.

For prescription drugs, the amount you pay depends on if you have a Medicare drug plan and which one you have. If you have limited income and resources and meet certain conditions, you may qualify for Extra Help from Medicare to help pay the costs of Medicare drug coverage.[1]

---

[1] "Medicare & Your Mental Health Benefits," Centers for Medicare & Medicaid Services (CMS), September 2022. Available online. URL: www.medicare.gov/publications/11358-medicare-and-your-mental-health-benefits-getting-started.pdf. Accessed May 15, 2023.

Part 7 | Strategies for Managing Depression

Chapter 54 | **Understanding Mental Illness Stigma**

ATTITUDES TOWARD MENTAL ILLNESS STIGMA

People's beliefs and attitudes toward mental illness set the stage for how they interact with, provide opportunities for, and help support a person with mental illness. People's beliefs and attitudes toward mental illness also frame how they experience and express their own emotional problems and psychological distress and whether they disclose these symptoms and seek care. About one in four U.S. adults (26.2%) aged 18 and older, in any given year, has a mental disorder (e.g., mood disorder, anxiety disorder, impulse control disorder, or substance use disorder), meaning that mental disorders are common and can affect anyone. Many adults with common chronic conditions, such as arthritis, cancer, diabetes, heart disease, and epilepsy, experience concurrent depression and anxiety—further complicating self-management of these disorders and adversely affecting the quality of life.

Attitudes and beliefs about mental illness are shaped by personal knowledge about mental illness, knowing and interacting with someone living with mental illness, cultural stereotypes about mental illness, media stories, and familiarity with institutional practices and past restrictions. When such attitudes and beliefs are expressed positively, they can result in supportive and inclusive behaviors (e.g., willingness to date a person with a mental illness or to hire a person with a mental illness). When such attitudes and beliefs are expressed negatively, they may result in avoidance, exclusion from daily activities, and, in the worst case, exploitation and discrimination.

Stigma has been described as a cluster of negative attitudes and beliefs that motivate the general public to fear, reject, avoid, and discriminate against people with mental illnesses. When stigma leads to social exclusion or discrimination ("experienced" stigma), it results in unequal access to resources that all people need to function well: educational opportunities, employment, a supportive community (including friends and family), and access to quality health care. These types of disparities in education, employment, and access to care can have cumulative long-term negative consequences.

For example, a young adult with untreated mental illness who is unable to graduate from high school is less likely to find a good-paying job that can support his or her basic needs, including access to health care. These disadvantages can cause a person to experience more negative outcomes. Being unemployed, living at or below the poverty line, being socially isolated, and living with other social disadvantages can further deflate self-esteem, compounding mental illness symptoms, and add to the burden of stigma. Sometimes, stigma is simply felt in the absence of being discriminated against and results from internalizing perceived negative attitudes associated with a characteristic (e.g., age), a disorder (e.g., human immunodeficiency virus (HIV)/acquired immunodeficiency syndrome (AIDS)), a behavior (e.g., smoking), or other factors (e.g., place of birth).

Whether stigma is experienced as social exclusion or discrimination or felt as a pervasive and underlying sense of being different from others, it can be debilitating for people and poses a challenge to public health prevention efforts. Different opinions exist regarding the implications of different labels associated with describing mental illness (e.g., brain disease) and felt or experienced stigma. However, the prevailing view of health-related stigma is that it refers to perceived, enacted, or anticipated avoidance or social exclusion and not to an individual blemish or mark. Different methods exist for measuring health-related stigma, and challenges and limitations associated with distinguishing between felt versus experienced stigma in attitudinal research have been described.

WHAT ARE THE CONSEQUENCES OF NEGATIVE ATTITUDES TOWARD MENTAL ILLNESS?

Only about 20 percent of adults with a diagnosable mental disorder or with a self-reported mental health condition saw a mental health provider in the previous year. The embarrassment associated with accessing mental health services is one of the many barriers that cause people to hide their symptoms and prevent them from getting the necessary treatment for their mental illness symptoms. Stigma poses a barrier to public health primary prevention efforts designed to minimize the onset of mental illness, as well as with secondary prevention efforts aimed at promoting early treatment to prevent the worsening of symptoms over time.

Stigma can also interfere with the self-management of mental disorders (tertiary prevention). Untreated symptoms can have grave consequences for people living with mental illness and negatively impact families affected by these disorders. For example, most people with serious and persistent mental illness (mental disorders that interfere with some area of social functioning) are unemployed and live below the poverty line, and many face major barriers to obtaining decent, affordable housing. These individuals may need a number of additional social supports (e.g., job training, peer support networks) to live successfully in the community, but such support may not be available. Other individuals with depression and anxiety might avoid disclosing their symptoms and instead adopt unhealthy behaviors to help them cope with their distress (e.g., smoking, excessive alcohol use, binge eating). These behaviors can increase their risk of developing chronic diseases, worsening their overall health over time. Studies have found an increased risk of death at younger ages for people with mental illness.

Attitudes toward mental illness can also influence how policymakers allocate public resources to mental health services, pose challenges for staff retention in mental health settings, result in poorer quality of medical care administered to people with mental illness, and create fundraising challenges for organizations who serve people with mental illness and their families. State-level factors such as unemployment levels and access to mental health services and the presence or absence of other state resources may affect public attitudes and merit study.

WHY IS IT IMPORTANT TO TRACK ATTITUDES TOWARD MENTAL ILLNESS?

People's attitudes and beliefs predict their behavior. People's beliefs and attitudes about mental illness might predict whether they disclose their symptoms and seek treatment and support. Knowledge and beliefs that can aid in the recognition, management, or prevention of mental health disorders are defined as mental health literacy. Tracking attitudes toward mental illness can serve as an indicator of the public's mental health literacy. In a study of U.S. adults, only about one-fourth agreed that people are caring and sympathetic to people with mental illness. When asked about how much it would be worth to avoid mental illness compared to general medical illnesses, the public was less willing to pay to avoid mental health treatment than they were to pay to avoid physical health treatment. These studies provide important snapshots of attitudes toward mental illness across the country; however, studies that examine attitudes in-depth, such as distinguishing between attitudes relative to perceived or experienced stigma; studies that link attitudes to actual behavior; or studies that track attitudes toward mental illness at the state level do not occur routinely. These limited, cross-sectional studies tell us little about how attitudes shift in relation to historical events (e.g., media oversensationalization of the rare violence associated with a person with mental illness), how attitudes shift over time in the same people, and how these attitudes differ within a state relative to characteristics of the state, such as the average unemployment rate or per capita expenditures on state mental health agencies.[1]

---

[1] "Attitudes toward Mental Illness: Results from the Behavioral Risk Factor Surveillance System," Centers for Disease Control and Prevention (CDC), 2012. Available online. URL: www.cdc.gov/hrqol/Mental_Health_Reports/pdf/BRFSS_Full%20Report.pdf. Accessed March 10, 2023.

Chapter 55 | Well-Being Concepts

Chapter Contents

Section 55.1—Well-Being and Satisfaction with Life 425
Section 55.2—Self-Management Support: Beyond
        the Medical Model 427

Section 55.1 | Well-Being and Satisfaction with Life

Well-being is a positive outcome that is meaningful for people and many sectors of society because it helps people perceive that their lives are going well. Good living conditions (e.g., housing, employment) are fundamental to well-being. Tracking these conditions is important for public policy. However, many indicators that measure living conditions fail to measure what people think and feel about their lives, such as the quality of their relationships, their positive emotions, and resilience; the realization of their potential; or their overall satisfaction with life that is their "well-being." Well-being generally includes global judgments of life satisfaction and feelings ranging from depression to joy.

HOW IS WELL-BEING DEFINED?

Well-being includes the presence of positive emotions and moods (e.g., contentment, happiness), the absence of negative emotions (e.g., depression, anxiety), and satisfaction with life, fulfillment, and positive functioning. In simple terms, well-being can be described as judging life positively and feeling good. For public health purposes, physical well-being (e.g., feeling very healthy and full of energy) is also viewed as critical to overall well-being.

Different aspects of well-being are:
- physical well-being
- economic well-being
- social well-being
- development and activity
- emotional well-being
- psychological well-being
- life satisfaction
- domain-specific satisfaction
- engaging in activities and work

HOW DOES WELL-BEING RELATE TO HEALTH PROMOTION?

Health is more than the absence of disease; it is a resource that allows people to realize their aspirations, satisfy their needs, and cope with the environment in order to live a long, productive, and fruitful life. In this sense, health enables social, economic, and personal development fundamental to well-being. Health promotion is the process of enabling people to increase control over and improve their health.

Environmental and social resources for health can include the following:
- peace
- economic security
- stable ecosystem
- safe housing

Individual resources for health can include the following:
- physical activity
- healthful diet
- social ties
- resiliency
- positive emotions
- autonomy

Health promotion activities aimed at strengthening such individual, environmental, and social resources may ultimately improve well-being.

WHY IS WELL-BEING USEFUL FOR PUBLIC HEALTH?
Well-being integrates mental health (mind) and physical health (body), resulting in holistic approaches to disease prevention and health promotion. Well-being is a valid population outcome measure beyond morbidity, mortality, and economic status that tells how people perceive their life is going from their own perspective. Well-being is an outcome that is meaningful to the public. Advances in psychology, neuroscience, and measurement theory suggest that well-being can be measured with some degree of accuracy. Results from studies find that well-being is associated with the following:
- self-perceived health
- longevity

Well-Being Concepts

- healthy behaviors
- mental and physical illness
- social connectedness
- productivity
- factors in the physical and social environment

Well-being is associated with numerous health, job, family, and economically related benefits. For example, higher levels of well-being are associated with decreased risk of disease, illness, and injury; better immune functioning; speedier recovery; and increased longevity. Individuals with high levels of well-being are more productive at work and are more likely to contribute to their communities.[1]

Section 55.2 | Self-Management Support: Beyond the Medical Model

Self-management support is the help given to people with chronic conditions that enables them to manage their health on a day-to-day basis. Self-management support can help and inspire people to learn more about their conditions and to take an active role in their health care.

Self-management support goes beyond simply supplying patients with information. It includes a commitment to patient-centered care, providing clear and useful information to patients, helping patients set goals and make plans to live a healthier life, creating a team of clinicians and administrative staff with clearly understood roles and responsibilities, and using office systems to support follow-up and tracking of patients.

Self-management support includes the following:
- providing compassionate, patient-centered care
- involving the whole care team in planning, carrying out, and following up on patient visits

---

[1] "Well-Being Concepts," Centers for Disease Control and Prevention (CDC), October 31, 2018. Available online. URL: www.cdc.gov/hrqol/wellbeing.htm. Accessed March 14, 2023.

- planning patient visits that focus on prevention and care management rather than critical or acute care
- involving the patient in goal setting
- providing customized education and skills training, using materials appropriate for different cultures and health literacy levels
- making referrals to community-based resources, such as programs that help patients quit smoking or follow an exercise plan
- following up with patients through email, phone, text messaging, or mailings to support them in taking good care of themselves

WHY IS SELF-MANAGEMENT SUPPORT IMPORTANT?

Managing chronic illness and changing behavior are challenging and take time for everyone involved—providers, patients, and caregivers. Yet it is often patients themselves who are called on to manage the broad range of factors that contribute to their health. Common sense suggests—and health-care experts agree—that people with chronic care needs should receive support to help them manage their health as effectively as possible. Using self-management support in primary care can have a positive effect on the care and health outcomes of people with chronic conditions, as well as provider and patient satisfaction.

Helping patients make good choices and maintain healthy behaviors requires a collaborative relationship between the primary care clinical team and patients and their families. Learning how to incorporate self-management support into practice can support patients in building the skills and confidence they need to lead healthier lives.

HOW CAN SELF-MANAGEMENT SUPPORT BE PUT INTO ACTION?

Incorporating self-management support into the daily routine of clinical practice can be challenging, but there are many helpful programs and resources available, including the following specific strategies.

Well-Being Concepts

- **Defining and sharing the roles and responsibilities of the practice care team.** To provide effective self-management support, a team of clinicians and administrative staff need to coordinate closely with each other to provide care before, during, and after the patient visit. Successful teams are made up of clinical and administrative staff whose roles are planned in advance. Some roles and responsibilities include the following:
  - gathering clinical data before a visit
  - setting agendas for the visit
  - helping patients set health goals
  - developing action plans for achieving goals
  - tracking health outcomes
  - referring patients to community programs
- **Using tools and techniques to improve self-management support.** Self-management support includes a variety of techniques and tools that help patients choose and maintain healthy behaviors. Primary care staff can ease into a self-management support program by learning how to use tools such as action plans, goal-setting worksheets, and problem-solving techniques to support and motivate patients.
- **Learning new skills, such as motivational interviewing and reflective listening.** The best use of self-management support is the collaborative interaction between the clinician and the patient. Motivating, listening, and coaching are important self-management support skills that can make the clinician–patient interaction stronger and in which all members of the care team can become knowledgeable. Through ongoing training and practice, supporting patients and their families in self-care will become part of day-to-day care.
- **Selecting understandable, actionable educational materials and using them effectively.** Many print and audiovisual educational materials do not communicate

effectively. Handing out even well-designed materials is not likely to promote patient self-management. Primary care staff can start by choosing materials that diverse patients can understand and act on and then reviewing the material with the patient and confirming understanding.[2]

SELF-MANAGEMENT INTERVENTIONS

It can often take a few weeks before you feel an improvement from counseling or medications. In the meantime, there are a number of things you can do to help yourself.

The following are the activities that can help you in managing depression:

- **Engage in fun physical activities and exercise**. Regular exercise can improve your mood. Even taking a short walk every day may help you feel a little better.
- **Make time for activities you enjoy**. Even though you may not feel as motivated or happy as you used to, commit to scheduling a fun activity (such as a favorite hobby) at least a few times a week.
- **Spend time with people who can support you**. It is easy to avoid contact with people when you are feeling down. But it is during these times that you actually need the support of friends and family. Try explaining to them what you are feeling. If you do not feel comfortable talking about it, that is all right. Just asking them to be with you, maybe during an activity, is a good first step. It is suggested to meet a friend for coffee or to play cards, take a walk with a neighbor, or work in the garden with your spouse.
- **Practice relaxation**. For many people, the changes that come with depression can be stressful. Since physical relaxation can lead to mental relaxation,

---

[2] U.S. Department of Health and Human Services (HHS), "Self-Management Support," Agency for Healthcare Research and Quality (AHRQ), November 27, 2013. Available online. URL: www.ahrq.gov/ncepcr/tools/self-mgmt/self.html. Accessed April 25, 2023.

Well-Being Concepts

try deep breathing, taking a hot shower, or just finding a quiet, comfortable, and peaceful place. Say comforting things to yourself, such as, "It is going to get better."

- **Pace yourself**. Set simple goals and take small steps. It is easy to feel overwhelmed by problems and decisions, and it can be hard to deal with them when you are feeling sad, have little energy, or are not thinking as clearly as usual. Some problems and decisions can be delayed, but others cannot. Try breaking down a large problem into smaller ones and then taking one small step at a time to solve it. Give yourself credit for each step you take.
- **Avoid making major life decisions while feeling depressed**. Major decisions might include changing jobs, making a financial investment, moving, divorcing, or making a major purchase. If you feel you must make a major decision about your life, ask your care provider or someone you trust to help you.
- **Eat nutritious, balanced meals**. Many people find that when they eat more nutritious, balanced meals, they feel better not only physically but also emotionally and mentally. To learn about choosing healthy foods, talk with a nutritionist. Avoid using alcohol and drugs of abuse. Alcohol is a depressant and can add to feeling down and alone. It can also interfere with the help you may receive from antidepressant medication.
- **Develop healthy sleep habits**. Sleep problems are common for those with depression. Getting enough sleep can help you feel better and more energetic.
- **Follow your care provider's instructions about your treatment and communicate openly**. It is very important to take your medicine as prescribed each day and to keep your appointments with your provider, even when you begin to feel better. Ask your provider if you have any questions or concerns about your treatment. Tell your provider about your feelings,

activities, sleep and eating patterns, unusual symptoms, or physical problems.
- **Tell someone if you are thinking about death or hurting yourself.** Thoughts of death may accompany depression. Always discuss this symptom with your care provider. If you are thinking about hurting yourself, tell your provider or a trusted friend, your spouse, or a relative who can get you immediate emergency professional help.
- **Remain hopeful—depression is treatable.** With treatment, most people with depression can begin to feel better, but it may take some time. Remember that negative thinking (blaming yourself, feeling hopeless, expecting failure, and other similar thoughts) is part of depression. As the depression lifts, negative thinking will also lift.

You do not have to do all of these things right away! Start slowly and take small steps on your way to feeling better. Work with your provider(s) to select the activities that fit your own situation, lifestyle, and needs.[3]

---

[3] "Depression: What You Need to Know," U.S. Department of Veterans Affairs (VA), September 13, 2010. Available online. URL: www.healthquality.va.gov/guidelines/MH/mdd/MDDTool4DepressionBookletFINALHiRes.pdf. Accessed March 14, 2023.

Chapter 56 | Relationship between Psychological Resilience and Mental Health

Chapter Contents
Section 56.1—Understanding Individual Resilience 435
Section 56.2—Building Resilience in Children and
          Youth Dealing with Trauma 440

Section 56.1 | Understanding Individual Resilience

Everyone goes through tough times in life. But many things can help you survive—and even thrive—during stressful periods. There is no one-size-fits-all approach. Learning healthy ways to cope and how to draw from resources in your community can help you build resilience.

"Resilience is the extent to which we can bounce back from adverse events, cope with stress, or succeed in the face of adversity," says Dr. Cindy Bergeman, a psychology professor at the University of Notre Dame.

You are not born with resilience. "It's not something you either have or don't have," says Dr. Alexandra Burt, a child development expert at Michigan State University.

"Resilience is a process in which many factors—including family, community, and cultural practices—interact. It boosts wellness and protects you from risks to your well-being. For many people, these risks are compounded by hardship and discrimination," adds Dr. Lisa Wexler, who studies suicide prevention at the University of Michigan.

Researchers are studying what helps people become more resilient. Creating healthy habits and taking care of yourself can help. And so can family, friends, and your connection to community and culture.

FINDING YOUR STRENGTHS

Stress can cause wear and tear on the body and brain. Chronic stress has been linked to an increased risk of many health conditions. These include heart disease, high blood pressure (HBP), depression, and anxiety.

Many stressful situations cannot easily be changed by one person. And some—such as parenting or a challenging job—can be things you want to do, even if they are taxing.

But resilience is not just about eliminating stress. It is also about tapping into your strengths. Researchers call these protective factors. "They can buffer stress or directly promote well-being—and sometimes even do both," Dr. Wexler says.

Your strengths include those of your neighborhood and community. Different cultures have developed different ways to help people cope. The ceremonies, teachings, and cultural practices that are meaningful to you can help, Dr. Wexler says.

Other protective factors involve nurturing your body. "Being able to manage your stress is key to what underlies resilience. And a healthy body is going to deal with stress much better," says Dr. Bergeman.

Other tools are emotional, like expressing your feelings rather than bottling them up, she explains. Looking at problems from different angles can help, too.

"Can you see a difficulty in a more positive way?" Dr. Bergeman asks. "For example, you can look at a stressful situation as a growth opportunity instead of thinking of it as a threat. Ask yourself: What can I learn from this situation?"

Meeting your own needs also makes a difference. "We're often so busy trying to take care of other people that we don't do good self-care. I encourage people to do something that they enjoy every single day. Many people feel guilty about that. But it really helps us replenish our emotional reserves, just like a meal fills our physical reserves," says Dr. Bergeman.

In times of stress, self-care can be the opposite of selfishness. Adults who take time for themselves can better help nurture resilience in children, says Dr. Burt. "One of the best things any parent can do for their child is to be well and healthy themselves. That makes it a lot easier for you to provide the support your child needs."

TAPPING INTO RESOURCES

Another part of resilience is about using the resources available to you. More and more, researchers are understanding that resilience does not happen in a vacuum.

"The presence of resilience in a person is related to the supports around them," Dr. Burt says. For example, she and her team found that growing up in a very impoverished neighborhood can change

Relationship between Psychological Resilience and Mental Health

the way a child's brain develops. But, when adults in the community work together to support and monitor neighborhood children, it helps protect the children's brains despite their circumstances. "A child can be resilient because they have these resilience-promoting things around them," Dr. Burt explains.

Supportive adults do not have to be a parent or relative, Dr. Burt says, though they often are. Some kids do not have supportive families.

"That supportive person can also be a teacher, or someone else who's important to them. Just one person who they really feel has their back," she says.

Many protective factors for these young adults come from their community's culture. "Access to cultural resources combined with the ability to use them is what helps lower suicide risk," says Dr. James Allen from the University of Minnesota.

Alaska Native Collaborative Hub for Research on Resilience (ANCHRR) is also looking at how the cultural and spiritual practices that Alaska Native communities harness work to protect youth against suicide and other risks they face.

CHOOSING YOUR TOOLS

The tools that best help you offset stress can differ from situation to situation, says Dr. Bergeman.

"Sometimes you have a stressor where you need to take action and solve the problem. But for other types of stressors, maybe you need emotional support," she says. "A way to think about resilience may be: How do you match what you need with the kinds of tools that you have?"

In a way, practice makes perfect, Dr. Bergeman says. Keep tabs on what felt helpful to you during stressful times. Ask yourself: How did you deal with it? Did you choose a healthy strategy? How might other people have helped you deal with it?

"That can prepare you for the next experience that may be more difficult," Dr. Bergeman says.[1]

---

[1] *NIH News in Health*, "Nurture Your Resilience: Bouncing Back from Difficult Times," National Institutes of Health (NIH), April 2022. Available online. URL: https://newsinhealth.nih.gov/2022/04/nurture-your-resilience. Accessed April 11, 2023.

WHAT CONTRIBUTES TO INDIVIDUAL RESILIENCE?

Individual resilience involves behaviors, thoughts, and actions that promote personal well-being and mental health. People can develop the ability to withstand, adapt to, and recover from stress and adversity—and maintain or return to a state of mental well-being—by using effective coping strategies.

A disaster can impair resilience due to stress, traumatic exposure, distressing psychological reactions, and disrupted social networks. Feelings of grief, sadness, and a range of other emotions are common after traumatic events. Resilient individuals, however, are able to work through the emotions and effects of stress and painful events and rebuild their lives.

People develop resilience by learning better skills and strategies for managing stress and better ways of thinking about life's challenges. To be resilient, one must tap into personal strengths and the support of family, friends, neighbors, and/or faith communities.

WHAT ARE THE CHARACTERISTICS THAT SUPPORT INDIVIDUAL RESILIENCE?

Age, gender, health, biology, education level, cultural beliefs and traditions, and economic resources can play important roles in psychological resilience. The following characteristics also contribute to individual resilience:

- **Social support and close relationships with family and friends**. People who have close social support and strong connections with family and friends are able to get help during tough times and also enjoy their relationships during everyday life.
- **The ability to manage strong feelings and impulses**. People who are able to manage strong emotions are less likely to get overwhelmed, frustrated, or aggressive. People who are able to manage feelings can still feel sadness or loss, but they are also able to find healthy ways to cope and heal.
- **Good problem-solving skills**. People problem-solve daily. Thinking, planning, and solving problems in an organized way are important skills. Problem-solving

Relationship between Psychological Resilience and Mental Health

skills contribute to feelings of independence and self-competence.
- **Feeling in control.** After the chaos of a disaster, it can be useful to engage in activities that help people regain a sense of control. This will help support the healing and recovery process.
- **Asking for help and seeking resources.** Resourceful people will get needed help more quickly if they know how to ask questions, are creative in their thinking about situations, are good problem solvers and communicators, and have a good social network to reach out to.
- **Seeing yourself as resilient.** After a disaster, many people may feel helpless and powerless, especially when there has been vast damage to the community. Being able to see yourself as resilient, rather than as helpless or as a victim, can help build psychological resilience.
- **Coping with stress in healthy ways.** People get feelings of pleasure and self-worth from doing things well. Strategies that use positive and meaningful ways to cope are better than those which can be harmful, such as drinking too much or smoking.
- **Helping others and finding positive meaning in life.** Positive emotions such as gratitude, joy, kindness, love, and contentment can come from helping others. Acts of generosity can add meaning and purpose to your life, even in the face of tragedy.

WHAT CAN RESILIENT INDIVIDUALS DO?
- Care for themselves and others day-to-day and during emergency situations.
- Actively support their neighborhoods, workplaces, and communities to recover after a disaster.
- Be confident and hopeful about overcoming present and future difficulties.
- Get needed resources more effectively and quickly.

- Be physically and mentally healthier and have overall lower recovery expenses and service needs.
- Miss fewer days of work.
- Maintain stable family and social connections.
- Reestablish routines more quickly, which helps children and adults alike.[2]

Section 56.2 | Building Resilience in Children and Youth Dealing with Trauma

All youth face difficulties, which can range from traumatic losses to everyday disappointments. The ability to cope and recover (or "bounce back") after a setback is important to their success. Experts call this "childhood resilience," and it is a skill that can be learned.

HOW PARENTS CAN HELP CHILDREN IN BUILDING RESILIENCE

You can help your children develop resilience by taking the following steps:

- **Model a positive outlook**. Children will learn from your ability to bounce back from difficulties. When faced with a challenge yourself, model an "I can do it" attitude. Remind yourself and your child that the current problem is temporary and "things will get better."
- **Build confidence**. Comment frequently on what your child does well. Point out when he or she demonstrates qualities such as kindness, persistence, and integrity.
- **Build connections**. Create a strong, loving family and encourage your child to make good friends. This will help ensure that he or she has plenty of support in times of trouble.

---

[2] Office of the Assistant Secretary for Preparedness and Response (ASPR), "Individual Resilience," U.S. Department of Health and Human Services (HHS), September 8, 2020. Available online. URL: https://aspr.hhs.gov/at-risk/Pages/individual_resilience.aspx. Accessed March 15, 2023.

Relationship between Psychological Resilience and Mental Health

- **Encourage goal-setting.** Teach children to set realistic goals and work toward them one step at a time. Even small steps can build confidence and resilience.
- **See challenges as learning opportunities.** Tough times are often when we learn the most. Resist the urge to solve your child's problem for him or her—this can send a message that you do not believe he or she can handle it. Instead, offer love and support and show faith in his or her ability to cope. Remind him or her of times when he or she has solved problems successfully in the past.
- **Teach self-care.** Many challenges are easier to face when we eat well and get enough exercise and rest. Self-care can also mean taking a break from worrying about relaxing or having some fun.
- **Help others.** Empower your child by giving him or her opportunities to help out at home or do age-appropriate volunteer work for his or her school, neighborhood, or place of worship.[3]

FACTORS THAT CONTRIBUTE TO CHILDHOOD RESILIENCE

While many factors contribute to resilience, the following three stand out:
- cognitive development/problem-solving skills
- self-regulation
- relationships with caring adults

Cognitive Development/Problem-Solving Skills

As a species, we have been solving problems since the beginning of time. Watch a child play, and you will see that his or her problem-solving skills are nearly always at work. Infants attempt to soothe themselves by figuring out how to put their thumbs in their mouths or crying for a caregiver. Toddlers try to fit shapes

---

[3] Child Welfare Information Gateway, "Building Resilience in Children and Teens," U.S. Department of Health and Human Services (HHS), April 18, 2016. Available online. URL: www.childwelfare.gov/pubPDFs/resilience_ts.pdf. Accessed March 15, 2023.

into shape sorters. As children mature, the problems they solve get more complex. Solving problems engages our prefrontal cortex, sometimes called the "thinking brain," which is the seat of our executive function. During times of stress and trauma, this part of our brain is typically shut down so that our body can respond to the threats it is facing. By helping children engage in problem-solving activities, they not only gain a sense of self-efficacy and mastery but also reengage the parts of their brain that may have been offline. Because the neural pathways of young brains are still being wired, the more we can engage and reinforce healthy pathways, the better. Developing problem-solving skills also helps children with self-regulation skills, another key quality that fosters resilience.

Self-Regulation

Self-regulation is the ability to control oneself in a variety of ways. Infants develop regular sleep–wake patterns. Schoolchildren learn to raise their hands and wait patiently to be called on rather than shouting out an answer. College students concentrate for hours on a research paper, delaying the gratification that might come with being outdoors on a sunny day. Self-regulation has been identified as "the cornerstone" of child development. In the seminal publication *From Neurons to Neighborhoods*, experts conclude, "Development may be viewed as an increased capacity for self-regulation, seen particularly in the child's ability to function more independently in a personal and social context." It involves working memory, the ability to focus on a goal, tolerance for frustration, and controlling and expressing one's emotions appropriately and in context. Self-regulation is key for academic and social success and plays a significant role in mental health outcomes—all things that can be a challenge for children experiencing homelessness and other stressors.

Relationships with Caring Adults

Ideally, we form close attachment relationships with our primary caregiver(s) beginning at birth. As we get older, those relationships extend to teachers, neighbors, family, friends, coaches, and others. Disrupted attachment relationships can be devastating for young children because they are still developing an internal working model of what relationships look like and because they rely so intensively on their caregivers to get their basic needs met.

By developing relationships with caring adults, whether they be parents, family members, coaches, teachers, or neighbors, children learn about healthy relationships—ones that are consistent, predictable, and safe. They receive guidance, comfort, and mentoring.

PLAY: A KEY STRATEGY FOR DEVELOPING RESILIENCE

What strategies can we use to draw out children's resilience? The short answer is playing. We can create play experiences for children of all ages that give them ways to engage in solving problems, develop self-regulation skills, and form relationships. Here are some ideas:

- "Simon Says" helps children practice several self-regulation skills (e.g., working memory and inhibitory control).
- LEGO, blocks, and other tactile toys give children opportunities to solve problems and focus on a goal ("I want to build a tower. How can I build the tower really high without it falling?"). If they are playing with an adult (especially one who lets the child direct the play), they are also building a relationship.
- Doing one or more of the following activities can also be helpful:
  - breathing exercises and bodywork (yoga or stretching)
  - reading books, playing games, and having conversations about identifying emotions
  - letting children talk aloud (and/or hear you talk aloud) about solving a problem
  - dancing, singing, listening to music, and playing musical instruments and experimenting with speed (fast song, slow song), volume (sing loudly, sing quietly), and breath (play your instrument and hold

the note as long as you can and now try making short, staccato notes)
- any activity that strengthens the relationship between the child and her/his primary caregiver

Trauma can undermine resilience because it challenges the very things that make us strong. By helping children restore and enhance their sense of control, connection, and meaning—through the skills described above and in many other ways—you can give them opportunities to persevere and thrive.[4]

---

[4] "Childhood Resilience," Substance Abuse and Mental Health Services Administration (SAMHSA), November 22, 2021. Available online. URL: www.samhsa.gov/homelessness-programs-resources/hpr-resources/childhood-resilience. Accessed March 15, 2023.

Chapter 57 | Building a Healthy Body Image and Self-Esteem

Chapter Contents
Section 57.1—Healthy Body Image 447
Section 57.2—How to Improve Your Self-Esteem 450

Section 57.1 | Healthy Body Image

WHAT IS BODY IMAGE?
Your body image is what you think and how you feel when you look in the mirror or when you picture yourself in your mind. This includes how you feel about your appearance; what you think about your body itself, such as your height and weight; and how you feel within your own skin. Body image also includes how you behave as a result of your thoughts and feelings. You may have a positive or negative body image. Body image is not always related to your weight or size.

WHY ARE WOMEN SO FOCUSED ON BODY IMAGE?
In the United States, girls and women hear and see messages about how they look from the first moments they are alive, throughout much of their childhood, and into adulthood. Young girls and teens are more likely to be praised for how they look than for their thoughts or actions. The media focuses on showing women who are thin, attractive, and young. Images of these women are often edited using computer technology. As a result, girls and young women often try to reach beauty and body ideals that do not exist in the real world.

WHAT CAUSES A NEGATIVE BODY IMAGE?
Past events and circumstances can cause you to have a negative body image, including:
- being teased or bullied as a child for how you looked
- being told you are ugly, too fat, or too thin or having other aspects of your appearance criticized
- seeing images or messages in the media (including social media) that make you feel bad about how you look
- having underweight, overweight, or obesity

In rare cases, people can have such a distorted view of their bodies that they have a mental health condition called "body dysmorphic disorder" (BDD). BDD is a serious illness in which a person is preoccupied with minor or imaginary physical flaws.

ARE SOME PEOPLE LIKELY TO DEVELOP A NEGATIVE BODY IMAGE?

Yes. Girls are more likely than boys to have a negative body image. This may be because many women in the United States feel pressured to measure up to strict and unrealistic social and cultural beauty ideals, which can lead to a negative body image.

White girls and young women are slightly more likely to have a negative body image than African American or Hispanic girls and young women. However, cultural beauty ideals change over time, and it can be difficult to correctly measure a complicated idea such as body image among women from different backgrounds. Children of parents who diet or who have a negative body image are also likely to develop unhealthy thoughts about their own bodies.

HOW DOES OVERWEIGHT OR OBESITY AFFECT BODY IMAGE?

People who have obesity are likely to have a negative body image, but not all who have obesity or overweight are dissatisfied with their bodies. Those with a healthy weight can also have a negative body image although obesity can make a person's negative body image more severe.

Weight is not the only part of a person's body that determines body image. Self-esteem, past history, daily habits such as grooming, and the particular shape of your body all contribute to body image. Weight is an important part of body image, but it is not the only part.

HOW DOES UNDERWEIGHT AFFECT BODY IMAGE?

People who are underweight due to a health condition such as an eating disorder, cancer, or Crohn disease may have a negative body image due to the effects of their condition. People who are underweight without another health condition may also have a negative body image if others comment negatively on their weight or express other negative attitudes.

Building a Healthy Body Image and Self-Esteem

WHAT IS A HEALTHY BODY IMAGE?

A healthy body image means you feel comfortable in your body and you feel good about the way you look. This includes what you think and feel about your appearance and how you judge your own self-worth. A negative body image can put you at higher risk of certain mental health conditions, such as eating disorders and depression.

WHY IS A HEALTHY BODY IMAGE IMPORTANT?

People with a positive body image are more likely to have good physical and mental health. People with negative thoughts and feelings about their bodies are likely to develop certain mental health conditions, such as eating disorders and depression. Researchers think dissatisfaction with their bodies may be part of the reason more women than men have depression.

A negative body image may also lead to low self-esteem, which can affect many areas of your life. You may not want to be around other people or may constantly obsess about what you eat or how much you exercise. But you can take steps to develop a healthier body image.

HOW CAN YOU HAVE A HEALTHY BODY IMAGE?

Research shows that if you have overweight or obesity, your body image may improve if you participate in a weight loss program, even if you do not lose as much weight as you hoped. The weight loss program should include a focus on healthy eating and physical activity.

If you are underweight and have a negative body image, you can work with a doctor or nurse to gain weight in a healthy way and treat any other health problems you have. If you are eating healthy and getting enough exercise, your weight may matter less in your body image.

The more you practice thinking positive thoughts about yourself and the fewer negative thoughts you have about your body, the better you will feel about who you are and how you look. While very few people are 100 percent positive about every aspect of their body, it can help focus on the things you do like. Also, most people realize as they get older that how they look is only one part of who they are. Working on accepting how you look is healthier than constantly working to change how you look.[1]

Section 57.2 | How to Improve Your Self-Esteem

Self-worth is an essential component of our well-being. The American Psychological Association (APA) defines self-worth as "your evaluation of yourself as a capable and valuable human being deserving of consideration and respect. It is an internal sense of being worthy of love." Self-worth is valuing yourself and the unique qualities that define who you are. It is an internal feeling of worth and not to be based on external validation. When we intrinsically feel we are worthy, our self-image and self-esteem are not dependent on other people's perceptions; in fact, we are able to have healthier relationships because we do not require validation from another to feel good about ourselves. When we have high self-worth, we are more resilient; we have internal protections from rejection and failure; and we are less vulnerable to anxiety.

While self-worth is your overall feeling of worthiness, self-confidence is feeling competent in specific areas of your life. You can have high self-worth and feel less confident in a specific domain (work, relationships, hobbies, etc.); therefore, it is not necessary to feel confident in all domains of your life to have positive self-worth.

Our thoughts, feelings, and behaviors are often a direct result of our self-worth. For example, if you continually internally judge yourself harshly, this may be an indicator of more self-reflection around your feelings of worth. Another example is if you push positive relationships away, you may not feel worthy of a healthy relationship. The good news is we can develop new mental habits that create new neural pathways and alter our self-worth. Psychologist

---

[1] Office on Women's Health (OWH), "Body Image," U.S. Department of Health and Human Services (HHS), February 17, 2021. Available online. URL: www.womenshealth.gov/mental-health/body-image-and-mental-health/body-image. Accessed March 15, 2023.

Building a Healthy Body Image and Self-Esteem

Rick Hanson, senior fellow of the Greater Good Science Center at the University of California, Berkeley, calls this intentional adaptation of positive mental habits "self-directed neuroplasticity." Below are some skills that, if practiced regularly, can boost your self-worth:

- **Challenge your inner critic.** The first step in building self-worth is knowing your thoughts and challenging your inner critic. Negative thoughts reinforce low self-worth. However, metacognition, or the capacity to be aware of your thoughts, can be difficult. Often it is helpful to notice how you are feeling or behaving and investigate the thoughts that preceded the feeling or behavior. If you observe a negative inner dialogue, this is an opportunity to ask yourself the question: "Is this thought true?" We often believe whatever our thoughts are telling us without challenging them. You can also practice saying, "My thoughts are not who I am." Once you are in tune with your thoughts, you can talk to yourself as a compassionate coach would, one who wants you to be the best version of yourself.
- **Self-compassion.** It is the ability to comfort yourself, to be kind to yourself, and to treat yourself with the same compassion that you would offer to others during a difficult time. Self-compassion comes from self-reflection, recognizing those times when you are being hard on yourself and then choosing to be kind. A tool that can help you practice self-compassion is to stop yourself when you are being self-flagellating and ask, "What would I say to a child going through the same thing?" and speak to yourself with that same compassion. It does not mean to dismiss faults or mistakes but to recognize that you are human, and if you make a mistake or experience rejection, you are still a good person who is worthy of love, especially love from yourself.

  Self-compassion is also the care you give yourself. When you are taking care of yourself, you are doing so because you are worth this care. Daily healthy habits such as exercise, eating healthfully, setting healthy boundaries, creating a sleep hygiene routine, self-care behaviors, and so on are all ways that you tell yourself "You are important." You do not have to practice these behaviors all at once but try to incorporate at least one self-care routine daily at first and add in others over time.

- **Focus on strengths/gratitude/acceptance**. If you are experiencing negative self-worth, highlighting your strengths can shift your mindset from a negative self-image to a more holistic image with strengths and challenges. A tool that can boost your self-worth is to write out specific domains in your life that are meaningful to you and list your strengths within that domains. These strengths are not based on accomplishments, such as good grades or outcome-oriented but rather your unique traits in that area. An example of this may look like:
  - **Work**. I am on time, I am dedicated, I can write concisely and informatively, I am supportive of my colleagues, I am collaborative, I follow up when needed, I ask for help, and so on.
  - **Relationships**. I am a good listener, I am supportive and caring, I reach out and check in often, I accept responsibility for my actions, and so on. If you do this for all meaningful areas in your life, you can review these strengths when needed. Allow yourself to feel grateful for these strengths. "I am grateful that I ask for help when I need it. By asking for help, I am demonstrating that I want to learn and increase my ability to do my job more efficiently." Appreciation for your strengths over time can build your self-worth.
- **Engage in activities that align with your values**. Values are our internal compasses and our deep-rooted beliefs about what is important to us. When you align your activities to your values, you are naturally building your self-worth because you are being authentic to your core beliefs. For example, if you value helping others and engage in helping activities, this has a positive

Building a Healthy Body Image and Self-Esteem

effect on how you feel about yourself. Taking inventory of your values can help inform this practice. Make a list of your values and brainstorm ways to actively engage in behaviors or activities that align with those values.

Cultivating self-worth is a practice, and changes may take time, but remember you are worth it.[2]

---

[2] "Accountability and Self: Addressing Self-Esteem, Self-Worth and Self-Image," National Institutes of Health (NIH), March 6, 2023. Available online. URL: https://oitecareersblog.od.nih.gov/2023/03/06/accountability-and-self-addressing-self-esteem-self-worth-and-self-image/. Accessed April 27, 2023.

Chapter 58 | Dealing with the Effects of Trauma

WHAT IS TRAUMA?
"Most people associate posttraumatic stress symptoms with veterans and combat situations," says Dr. Amit Etkin, a mental health expert funded by the National Institutes of Health (NIH) at Stanford University. "However, all sorts of trauma happen during one's life that can lead to posttraumatic stress disorder (PTSD) and PTSD-like symptoms."

This includes people who have been through physical or sexual assault, abuse, an accident, a disaster, or many other serious events.

Anyone can develop PTSD at any age. According to the National Center for Posttraumatic Stress Disorder (NCPTSD), about 7 or 8 out of every 100 people will experience PTSD at some point in their lives.

"We don't have a blood test that would tell you or a question you can ask somebody to know if they're in the highest risk group for developing PTSD," says Dr. Farris Tuma, Sc.D., chief of the Traumatic Stress Research Program of the National Institute of Mental Health (NIMH). "But we do know that there are some things that increase risk in general and some things that protect against it."

COPING WITH TRAUMA
How you react when something traumatic happens, and shortly afterward, can help or delay your recovery.

"It's important to have a coping strategy for getting through the bad feelings of a traumatic event," Dr. Tuma says. A good coping strategy, he explains, is finding somebody to talk with about your feelings. A bad coping strategy would be turning to alcohol or drugs.

Having a positive coping strategy and learning something from the situation can help you recover from a traumatic event. So you can seek support from friends, family, or a support group.

Talking with a mental health professional can help someone with posttraumatic stress symptoms learn to cope. It is important for anyone with PTSD-like symptoms to be treated by a mental health professional who is trained in trauma-focused therapy.

"For those who start therapy and go through it, a large percentage of those will get better and will get some relief," Dr. Tuma says. Some medications can help treat certain symptoms, too.

PTSD affects people differently, so a treatment that works for one person may not work for another. Some people with PTSD need to try different treatments to find what works for their symptoms.

FINDING TREATMENTS

"While we currently diagnose this as one disorder in psychiatry, in truth, there's a lot of variation between people and the kinds of symptoms that they have," Dr. Etkin says.

These differences can make it difficult to find a treatment that works. Dr. Etkin's team is trying to understand why some people's brains respond to treatment and others do not.

"PTSD is very common. But the variety of ways that it manifests in the brain is vast," Dr. Etkin explains. "We don't know how many underlying conditions there are, or distinct brain problems there are, that lead to PTSD. So we are trying to figure that part out."

His team has identified brain circuits that show when therapy is working. They have found a separate brain circuit that can predict who will respond to treatment.

His group is now testing a technique called "noninvasive brain stimulation" for people who do not respond to treatment. They hope that stimulating certain brain circuits will make therapy more effective.

Most people recover naturally from trauma. But it can take time. If you are having symptoms for too long—or that are too intense—talk with your health-care provider or mental health professional.

Dealing with the Effects of Trauma

In times of crisis, call the National Suicide Prevention Lifeline at 800-273-TALK (800-273-8255) or visit the emergency room.

"PTSD is real. This is not a weakness in any way," Dr. Tuma explains. "People shouldn't struggle alone and in silence."[1]

---

[1] *NIH News in Health*, "Dealing with Trauma," National Institutes of Health (NIH), June 2018. Available online. URL: https://newsinhealth.nih.gov/2018/06/dealing-trauma. Accessed March 15, 2023.

Chapter 59 | Stress in Disaster Responders and Recovery Workers

Chapter Contents
Section 59.1—Depression and First Responders 461
Section 59.2—Compassion Fatigue 464
Section 59.3—Tips for Families of Returning
　　　　　　　Disaster Responders 468

Section 59.1 | Depression and First Responders

Research into behavioral health conditions in emergency medical services (EMS) personnel reveals that one of the core risk factors for first responders is the pace of their work. First responders are always on the front line facing highly stressful and risky calls. This tempo can lead to an inability to integrate work experiences. For instance, according to a study, 69 percent of EMS professionals have never had enough time to recover between traumatic events. As a result, depression, stress and posttraumatic stress symptoms, suicidal ideation, and a host of other functional and relational conditions have been reported.

Depression is commonly reported in first responders, and rates of depression as well as severity vary across studies. For instance, in a case–control study of certified EMS professionals, depression was reported in 6.8 percent, with mild depression being the most common type (3.5%). Among medical team workers responding to the great East Japan earthquake, 21.4 percent were diagnosed with clinical depression. In a study in Germany, 3.1 percent of emergency physicians had clinical depression.

DEPRESSION AND FIREFIGHTERS

The nature of the work of firefighters, including repeated exposure to painful and provocative experiences and erratic sleep schedules, can pose significant risks to firefighters' mental health. To add to that risk, firefighters face many barriers to seeking help, including stigma and the cost of treatment. For instance, according to a study, volunteer firefighters have greater structural barriers to the use of mental health services (including cost, inadequate transportation, difficulty getting time off from work, and availability of resources) than career firefighters and the general population.

As with EMS professionals, depression is commonly reported in firefighters, and studies have found various rates and severity of depression. One study found that volunteer firefighters reported markedly elevated levels of depression as compared to career firefighters (with an odds ratio for volunteer firefighters of 16.85 and for career firefighters of 13.06). The researchers observed that greater structural barriers to mental health care (such as cost and availability of resources) might explain the increased levels of depression observed among volunteer firefighters. Additionally, competing demands for volunteer firefighters (having a separate job) create stress vulnerabilities that contribute to the development or exacerbation of behavioral health conditions. Organizational factors (such as more systematic and stringent recruitment and screening within career departments relative to volunteer departments) may contribute to the difference in the levels of behavioral health symptoms. In another study, 22.2 percent of female career firefighters were at risk of depression, while 38.5 percent of female volunteer firefighters were at risk of depression. This could be attributed to social pressures associated with working in a male-dominated profession. Additionally, although women firefighters reported similar job stressors to men, they also reported experiencing significantly more occupational discrimination than their male peers.

DEPRESSION AND POLICE OFFICERS

Police officers are at increased risk of negative mental health consequences due to the dangerous nature of their jobs as well as the greater likelihood that they experience critical incidents, environmental hazards, and traumatic events. In a study, about three-fourths of the surveyed officers reported having experienced a traumatic event, but less than half of them had told their agency about it. Additionally, about half of the officers reported personally knowing one or more law enforcement officers who changed after experiencing a traumatic event, and about half reported knowing an officer in their agency or another agency who had committed suicide. Depression in police officers after the 9/11 attacks was found at 24.7 percent prevalence and at 47.7 percent prevalence of both depression and anxiety.

BEHAVIORAL HEALTH OF FIRST RESPONDERS

First responders are always at the forefront of each incident or disaster, and they ensure the safety and well-being of the population.

Stress in Disaster Responders and Recovery Workers

They are, however, in great danger of being exposed to potentially traumatic situations that pose a risk of harm to them or the people under their care. This constitutes a great risk for the behavioral health of first responders, putting them at risk for stress, posttraumatic stress disorder (PTSD), depression, substance use, and suicide ideation and attempts. Both natural and technological disasters were found to be associated with increased risk of these conditions, as were factors such as resiliency, trust in self and team, duration on the disaster scene, individual coping style, and postdisaster mental health support.

To improve the behavioral health of the first responders, a cooperative effort is needed between organizational leadership and coworkers to establish a work environment that provides adequate training and ensures the resiliency and health of first responders by protecting them from overwork and excessive stress and supporting them in seeking help when needed. First responders carry the weight of their own safety and well-being as well as those they serve, and thus, making programmatic changes to educate them, offering them support, and protecting their health and well-being would reduce the risk of burnout, fatigue, or other behavioral health issues associated with being overworked, uncertain, or stressed. Behavioral and public health agencies can help prevent or alleviate behavioral health issues in first responders through preventive training on resiliency and behavioral health prior to disasters or other events, interventions to address burnout, and peer support programs. As noted, such efforts and programs are a cultural shift in fields in which professionals sometimes have coped with disastrous and traumatic experiences on the job by trying to disregard their reactions or using other maladaptive techniques, such as substance misuse. As more first responders discover the resilience they can access through others and particularly their peers, they become better able to maintain their own behavioral health while addressing the myriad challenges of disaster response.[1]

---

[1] "First Responders: Behavioral Health Concerns, Emergency Response, and Trauma," Substance Abuse and Mental Health Services Administration (SAMHSA), May 2018. Available online. URL: www.samhsa.gov/sites/default/files/dtac/supplementalresearchbulletin-firstresponders-may2018.pdf. Accessed March 15, 2023.

Section 59.2 | Compassion Fatigue

Disaster behavioral health response work can be very satisfying but can also take its toll on you. Research indicates that compassion fatigue (CF) is made up of two main components: burnout and secondary traumatic stress. When experiencing burnout, you may feel exhausted and overwhelmed, such as nothing you do will help make the situation better. For some responders, the negative effects of this work can make them feel like the trauma of the people they are helping is happening to them or the people they love. This is called "secondary traumatic stress." When these feelings go on for a long time, they can develop into "vicarious trauma." This type of trauma is rare but can be so distressing that the way a person views the world changes for the worse.

SIGNS OF BURNOUT AND SECONDARY TRAUMATIC STRESS

It is important to acknowledge the limitations of your skills and your own personal risks (such as a history of trauma) and other negative aspects of the disaster response experience (e.g., gruesome scenes or intense grieving) so that you recognize how they may be affecting your feelings as well as your behavior. Some responders may experience several of the following signs of burnout and the more serious component of CF, secondary traumatic stress. Remember, not all disaster behavioral health responders will experience every symptom.

When you experience burnout, a symptom of CF, you may have some of the following feelings:
- as if nothing you can do will help
- tired—even exhausted—and overwhelmed
- like a failure
- as though you are not doing your job well
- frustrated
- cynical
- disconnected from others, lacking feelings, and indifferent

Stress in Disaster Responders and Recovery Workers

- depressed
- as if you need to use alcohol or other mind-altering substances to cope

Signs of secondary traumatic stress, a more serious component of CF, may include the following:
- fear in situations that others would not think were frightening
- excessive worry that something bad will happen to you, your loved ones, or colleagues
- easily startled, feeling "jumpy" or "on guard" all of the time
- wary of every situation, expecting a traumatic outcome
- physical signs such as a racing heart, shortness of breath, and increased tension headaches
- sense of being haunted by the troubles you see and hear from others and not being able to make them go away
- the feeling that others' trauma is yours

If you are experiencing any of these signs of stress, talk with a friend or colleague, seek wise counsel from a trusted mentor, or ask your supervisor to help you determine a course of action. You may also consider seeking help from a qualified mental health professional.

RISKS OF BEING A DISASTER BEHAVIORAL HEALTH RESPONDER

Willingness to be in the trenches when responding to a disaster is one of the things that makes you credible and trustworthy to survivors. This usually means you live in conditions similar to those of disaster survivors. For example, you may have trouble finding enough food, let alone nutritious food. You may struggle with a lack of personal space and privacy. You are likely to experience disruptions in sleep due to hectic work schedules or surrounding noise. These things can wear you down behaviorally, cognitively, physically, spiritually, and emotionally. You may also become more vulnerable to feeling acute traumatic stress, sorrow, and anger of the people you help. You may even experience feelings of guilt for surviving the disaster. When this happens, you may have trouble understanding the risks to your own health and safety.

COPING WITH COMPASSION FATIGUE

Traditionally, disaster workers have been trained to screen survivors for negative behavioral health effects. More recently, the field is also focusing on identifying survivor resilience, fostering strengths, and encouraging self-care. Just as you assist survivors in this process, you can apply this approach to yourself on a routine basis—even when not on a disaster assignment—to avoid CF. By focusing on building your strengths and carrying out self-care activities, you are contributing to your behavioral, cognitive, physical, spiritual, and emotional resilience. The following strategies can help you do just that:

- Focus on the four core components of resilience: adequate sleep, good nutrition, regular physical activity, and active relaxation (e.g., yoga or meditation).
- Get enough sleep or at least rest. This is of great importance, as it affects all other aspects of your work—your physical strength, your decision-making, and your temperament.
- Drink enough fluids to stay hydrated and eat the best quality food that you can access.
- Complete basic hygiene tasks such as combing your hair, brushing your teeth, and changing clothes when possible. Wearing clean clothes can make you feel better.
- Try to wash up, even just your hands and face, after you leave your work shift. Think of it as a symbolic "washing away" of the hardness of the day.
- Make time to learn about the people with whom you work. Taking time for conversations will help foster feelings of positive regard toward yourself and others.
- Engage with your fellow workers to celebrate successes and mourn sorrows as a group.

Stress in Disaster Responders and Recovery Workers

- Take time to be alone so you can think, meditate, and rest.
- Practice your spiritual beliefs or reach out to a faith leader for support.
- Take time away from work when possible. Removing yourself from the disaster area can help you remember that not every place is so troubled.
- Try to find things to look forward to.
- Communicate with friends and family as best you can. If you do not have Internet or cell phone access or ways to mail letters, write to loved ones anyway and send the letters later.
- Create individual ceremonies or rituals. For example, write down something that bothers you and then burn it as a symbolic goodbye. Focus your thoughts on letting go of stress or anger or on honoring the memory, depending on the situation.

PREVENTION OF COMPASSION FATIGUE

When combined, the self-care practices mentioned above can help prevent the development of CF. Once you begin to routinely practice these healthy habits, they become part of your overall prevention plan. Not only do healthy habits strengthen your ability to cope while in the moment, they can help your body remember how to bounce back to a healthier state. Remember, prevention is part of a good preparedness plan.[2]

---

[2] "Tips for Disaster Responders—Understanding Compassion Fatigue," Substance Abuse and Mental Health Services Administration (SAMHSA), 2014. Available online. URL: https://store.samhsa.gov/sites/default/files/d7/priv/sma14-4869.pdf. Accessed March 15, 2023.

Section 59.3 | Tips for Families of Returning Disaster Responders

Increasing attention is being paid to the challenges that emergency and disaster responders face as they perform their work and then return to their loved ones and normal routine. As the family member of a response worker, you have faced your own challenges in keeping your household functioning while your loved one was away.

SIGNS OF STRESS IN DISASTER RESPONDERS

These are normal reactions to working in stressful situations, but if they persist for more than two weeks or worsen, professional help may be needed. Contact your primary care physician or seek assistance from a trusted mental health professional. Below is a list of some of the common signs of stress to look for in your returning loved one:
- anxiety, restlessness, or fear
- insomnia or other sleep problems
- fatigue
- recurring dreams or nightmares or intrusive thoughts
- stomach or gastrointestinal upset/appetite change
- heart palpitations/fluttering
- preoccupation with the disaster events or people they helped
- sadness and crying easily, hopelessness, or despair
- hypervigilance, easily startled
- irritability, anger, resentment, increased conflicts with friends/family
- overly critical and blaming others or self
- grief, guilt, or self-doubt
- increased use of alcohol or other drugs or misuse of prescription medication
- isolation or social withdrawal
- morbid humor
- decision-making difficulties

- confusion between trivial and major issues
- concentration problems or distractibility
- job- or school-related problems
- decreased libido/sexual interest
- decreased immune response (e.g., frequent colds, coughs, and other illnesses)

RETURNING HOME

Reunions following disaster assignments away from home are usually eagerly anticipated by all. While they can sometimes be harder than we expect, they can be effectively managed. When welcoming a loved one who is returning from disaster response work, keep the following in mind:
- Homecoming is more than an event; it is a process of reconnection for you and all those connected to your loved one.
- Even though coming home represents a return to safety, security, and "normality" for your loved one, the routines and pace at home are markedly different from life in a disaster zone.
- In your loved one's absence, you and other household members have likely assumed many roles and functions that may now need to change. Be patient during this period and recognize that many routines may not return—at least immediately—to what they were like previously.
- It may be helpful to take time to reconnect with your returning loved one before inviting your larger social circle to visit. Take the time you need first.

ADJUSTING TO LIFE AT HOME

Some other things to keep in mind while adjusting to the return of a loved one include the following:
- Celebrating a homecoming is important and should reflect your own style, preferences, and traditions.
- Asking your returning loved one to refrain from discussing graphic, gruesome, and highly distressing

details will help avoid upsetting or traumatizing others. This is especially important when discussing the experience with, or in the presence of, children. Consider sharing the more positive aspects of your experience.
- Talking about disaster experiences is a personal and delicate subject for both you and your loved one. Many people prefer to limit sharing such experiences with only a coworker or close friend. Often the need or desire to talk about the disaster experience will vary over time. Let your returning loved one take the lead. Listening rather than asking questions is the guiding rule. You might feel abandonment or anger about your loved one having been away, which might make it hard for you to listen actively and with empathy. These feelings are natural and will likely go away over time.
- Keeping your social calendar fairly free and flexible for the first few weeks after the homecoming is important. Respect the need for time alone and time with significant others, especially children. Explain to those who may feel slighted that this is a strong recommendation for returning disaster responders.
- Allowing your loved one an adjustment period will help him or her adapt physically to the local time zone as well as to environmental changes, such as temperature, continuous noise, or interruptions.
- Engaging in activities you enjoyed doing together, such as playing games, shopping for food, sharing favorite meals, and other activities, can help you reconnect.
- Knowing that your children's reactions may not be what you or your returning loved one may have expected or desired is important. Very often, children will act shy at first. They may withdraw or act angry as a response to their parent's absence. Be patient and understanding concerning these reactions and give children time to get reacquainted.

- Being flexible with your homecoming expectations will allow you to share time without placing too much pressure on anyone. It is normal to experience some disappointment or letdown when the homecoming is not what you had hoped. The reality of homecomings and reunions seldom matches one's ideas or desires.

MULTIPLE DISASTER RESPONSE ASSIGNMENTS

Responders may be called to another disaster assignment after only a short time at home. This can be challenging and stressful for everybody. It is natural to feel sad, even to cry. You have reconnected once again and begun to establish routines. Try to understand if your loved one distances herself or himself physically or emotionally in preparation for leaving. At the time of departure, it is important that you let your loved one know how proud you are of his or her sacrifice and commitment. Expressing pride while saying goodbye is positive and can help strengthen everyone.[3]

---

[3] "Adjusting to Life at Home," Substance Abuse and Mental Health Services Administration (SAMHSA), 2014. Available online. URL: https://store.samhsa.gov/sites/default/files/d7/priv/sma14-4872.pdf. Accessed March 15, 2023.

Chapter 60 | Grief, Bereavement, and Coping with Loss

WHAT IS GRIEF?

Grief is a normal response to a loss during or after a disaster or other traumatic events. Grief can happen in response to the loss of life, as well as to drastic changes to daily routines and ways of life that usually bring us comfort and a feeling of stability. Common grief reactions include the following:
- shock, disbelief, or denial
- anxiety
- distress
- anger
- periods of sadness
- loss of sleep and loss of appetite

Some people may experience multiple losses during a disaster or large-scale emergency event. Sometimes, you might be unable to be with a loved one when they die or unable to mourn someone's death in person with friends and family. Other types of loss include unemployment or not making enough money, loss or reduction in support services, and other changes in your lifestyle. These losses can happen at the same time, which can complicate or prolong grief and delay a person's ability to adapt, heal, and recover.[1]

---

[1] "Grief and Loss," Centers for Disease Control and Prevention (CDC), September 6, 2022. Available online. URL: www.cdc.gov/mentalhealth/stress-coping/grief-loss/index.html. Accessed March 15, 2023.

TYPES OF GRIEF

About 10 percent of bereaved people experience complicated grief, a condition that makes it harder for some people to adapt to the loss of a loved one. People with this prolonged, intense grief tend to get caught up in certain kinds of thinking, says psychiatrist Dr. M. Katherine Shear at Columbia University, who studies complicated grief. They may think the death did not have to happen or happened in the way that it did. They might also judge their grief—questioning if it is too little or too much—and focus on avoiding reminders of the loss.

"It can be very discouraging to experience complicated grief, but it's important not to be judgmental about your grief and not to let other people judge you," Dr. Shear explains.

Dr. Shear and her research team created and tested a specialized therapy for complicated grief in three studies funded by the National Institutes of Health (NIH). The therapy aimed to help people identify the thoughts, feelings, and actions that can get in the way of adapting to the loss. They also focused on strengthening one's natural process of adapting to the loss. The studies showed that 70 percent of people taking part in the therapy reported improved symptoms. In comparison, only 30 percent of people who received the standard treatment for depression had improved symptoms.

You may begin to feel the loss of your loved one even before their death. This is called "anticipatory grief." It is common among people who are long-term caregivers. You might feel sad about the changes you are going through and the losses you are going to have. Some studies have found that when patients, doctors, and family members directly address the prospect of death before the loss happens, it helps survivors cope after death.[2]

IF YOU FEEL DISTRESSED FROM OTHER TYPES OF LOSS OR CHANGE

Sometimes, you may feel grief due to the loss of a job; the inability to connect in person with friends, family, or religious organizations; missing special events and milestones (such as graduations,

---

[2] *NIH News in Health*, "Coping with Grief," National Institutes of Health (NIH), October 2017. Available online. URL: https://newsinhealth.nih.gov/2017/10/coping-grief. Accessed March 15, 2023.

Grief, Bereavement, and Coping with Loss

weddings, and vacations); and experiencing drastic changes to daily routines and ways of life that bring comfort. You may also feel a sense of guilt for grieving over losses that seem less important than the loss of life. Grief is a universal emotion; there is no right or wrong way to experience it, and all losses are significant.

Here are some ways to cope with feelings of grief:
- Acknowledge your losses and your feelings of grief.
  - Find ways to express your grief. Some people express grief and find comfort through art, writing, talking to friends or family, cooking, music, gardening, or other creative practices.
- Consider developing new rituals in your daily routine to stay connected with your loved ones to replace those that have been lost.
  - People who live together may consider playing board games and exercising together outdoors.
  - People who live alone or are separated from their loved ones may consider interacting through phone calls and apps that allow for playing games together virtually.
- If you are worried about future losses, try to stay in the present and focus on aspects of your life that you have control over right now.

HELPING CHILDREN COPE WITH GRIEF

Children may show grief differently than adults. Children may have a particularly hard time understanding and coping with the loss of a loved one. Sometimes, children appear sad and talk about missing the person or act out. Other times, they play, interact with friends, and do their usual activities. As a result of measures taken to limit the spread of COVID-19, they may also grieve over the loss of routines such as going to school and playing with friends. Parents and other caregivers play an important role in helping children process their grief.

To support a child who may be experiencing grief, do the following:
- Ask questions to determine the child's emotional state and better understand their perceptions of the event.

- Give children permission to grieve by allowing time for children to talk or express thoughts or feelings in creative ways.
- Provide age and developmentally appropriate answers.
- Practice calming and coping strategies with your child.
- Take care of yourself and model coping strategies for your child.
- Maintain routines as much as possible.
- Spend time with your child reading, coloring, or doing other activities they enjoy.

Signs that children may need additional assistance include changes in their behavior (such as acting out, not being interested in daily activities, changes in eating and sleeping habits, persistent anxiety, sadness, or depression). Speak to your child's health-care provider if troubling reactions seem to go on too long and interfere with school or relationships with friends or family if you are unsure of or concerned about how your child is doing.[3]

LIFE AFTER LOSS

Losing someone you love can change your world. You miss the person who died and want them back. You may feel sad, alone, or even angry. You might have trouble concentrating or sleeping. If you were a busy caregiver, you might feel lost when you are suddenly faced with lots of unscheduled time. These feelings are normal. There is no right or wrong way to mourn. Scientists have been studying how we process grief and are learning more about healthy ways to cope with loss.

The death of a loved one can affect how you feel, how you act, and what you think. Together, these reactions are called "grief." It is a natural response to loss. Grieving does not mean that you have to feel certain emotions. People can grieve in very different ways.

Cultural beliefs and traditions can influence how someone expresses grief and mourns. For example, in some cultures, grief is expressed quietly and privately. In others, it can be loud and out in the open. Culture also shapes how long family members are expected to grieve.

---
[3] See footnote [1]

Grief, Bereavement, and Coping with Loss

"People often believe they should feel a certain way," says Dr. Wendy Lichtenthal, a psychologist at Memorial Sloan-Kettering Cancer Center (MSKCC). "But such 'shoulds' can lead to feeling badly about feeling badly. It is hugely important to give yourself permission to grieve and allow yourself to feel whatever you are feeling. People can be quite hard on themselves and critical of what they are feeling. Be compassionate and kind to yourself."

ADAPTING TO LOSS

Experts say you should let yourself grieve in your own way and time. People have unique ways of expressing emotions. For example, some might express their feelings by doing things rather than talking about them. They may feel better going on a walk or swimming or doing something creative such as writing or painting. For others, it may be more helpful to talk with family and friends about the person who is gone or with a counselor.

"Though people don't often associate them with grief, laughing and smiling are also healthy responses to loss and can be protective," explains Dr. George Bonanno, who studies how people cope with loss and trauma at Columbia University. He has found that people who express flexibility in their emotions often cope well with loss and are healthier over time.

"It's not about whether you should express or suppress emotions, but that you can do this when the situation calls for it," he says. For instance, a person with emotional flexibility can show positive feelings, such as joy, when sharing a happy memory of the person they lost and then switch to expressing sadness or anger when recalling more negative memories, such as an argument with that person.

Grief is a process of letting go and learning to accept and live with loss. The amount of time it takes to do this varies with each person. "Usually people experience a strong acute grief reaction when someone dies and at the same time they begin the gradual process of adapting to the loss," explains Dr. Shear. "To adapt to a loss, a person needs to accept its finality and understand what it means to them. They also have to find a way to reenvision their life with possibilities for happiness and for honoring their enduring connection to the person who died."

Researchers like Dr. Lichtenthal have found that finding meaning in life after loss can help you adapt. Connecting to those things that are most important, including the relationship with the person who died, can help you coexist with the pain of grief.

LIFE BEYOND LOSS

Scientists funded by the National Institutes of Health (NIH) continue to study different aspects of the grieving process. They hope their findings will suggest ways to help people cope with the loss of a loved one.

Although the death of a loved one can feel overwhelming, many people make it through the grieving process with the support of family and friends. Take care of yourself, accept offers of help from those around you, and be sure to get counseling if you need it.

"We believe grief is a form of love and it needs to find a place in your life after you lose someone close," Dr. Shear says. "If you are having trouble moving forward in your own life, you may need professional help. Please don't lose hope. We have some good ways to help you."[4]

---

[4] See footnote [2].

Chapter 61 | Coping with the Holiday Blues

During the holiday season, the need for a trauma-informed approach is critical. Everywhere we turn, we are reminded that it is supposed to be "the most wonderful time of the year." While for some that may be true, for others the holiday season is wrought with triggers such as songs, scents, and rituals. Then there is pressure to conform to particular social and familial expectations, the increased presence of alcohol, and more interactions with family and friends. For those experiencing homelessness, the holidays may also serve as a reminder of what does not exist—a home in which to celebrate, cook, decorate, and rejoice. Loss, loneliness, and shame are powerful triggers.[1]

WHAT YOU CAN DO
Spend Time with People You Care About
Sometimes, staying at home is the more appealing option. But spending time with those you care about can help you feel connected to others. Reach out to the people with whom you can be yourself for one-on-one or small group gatherings. If the people you love do not live nearby, schedule a time for a video call. Just seeing a loved one's smiling face can make a big difference in your mood.

---

[1] "Recognizing Holiday Triggers of Trauma," Substance Abuse and Mental Health Services Administration (SAMHSA), June 4, 2022. Available online. URL: www.samhsa.gov/homelessness-programs-resources/hpr-resources/recognizing-holiday-triggers. Accessed May 4, 2023.

Give Back

If you are feeling isolated or lonely, try volunteering in your community. Stock shelves at the local food bank, help out at a nursing home, or spend time at a nearby animal shelter. It feels good to help others, and you might find you have a skill that your community really needs. Plus, volunteering is a great way to surround yourself with other people and take your mind off of your worries for a while.

Do Not Compare Yourself to Others

An article encouraged people to avoid looking at social media during the holidays. Pictures can be misleading and make it look like people are having a lot more fun than they actually are. Social media allows people to share their best moments, which are not always an accurate representation of everyday life. Try to remember that your friend with the "perfect" life has bad times, too—they just do not share those pictures.

Sweat It Out

You probably see exercise as a must-do on every health-related list you ever read. It is there for a reason. Exercise has a long list of benefits, including helping you deal with stress and anxiety. If it is too cold in your area to enjoy a walk or run, now is a good time to see what workout DVDs are available at your local library. There are smartphone apps that can also guide you through a workout.

Get Some Sun

For some people, the winter season means seasonal affective disorder (SAD) brought on by a lack of sunlight. People with SAD experience many of the same symptoms as people with depression. If you find that you have these kinds of symptoms every year or for months at a time over the winter season, talk to your doctor. People with light-to-moderate SAD may find relief by spending extra hours outdoors, while people with moderate-to-severe SAD often benefit from light therapy and/or antidepressants.

Have Fun without Overdoing It

Enjoying good food and drink is part of what the holidays are all about, but set limits for yourself, especially with alcohol. At the moment, it may seem like a stress reliever, but alcohol is only putting any feelings of stress or anxiety on hold. It does not solve any problems, and it can make things worse.

Be Honest about How You Are Feeling

Sometimes, the hardest part of this season is thinking you should feel a certain way, even when you do not. Do not force it. When friends or family ask how you are doing, be honest. You never know who else might be feeling the same way.

Ask for Help

If there is something your friends and family can do to make the holidays more enjoyable for you, tell them. No one but you know what you need. But, if you feel like you have tried everything and still feel down, consider getting help from a professional. Talking to a therapist, even for a few weeks, might be just the boost you need to get over your holiday blues and feel yourself again.[2]

---

[2] Office on Women's Health (OWH), "Beat the Holiday Blues," U.S. Department of Health and Human Services (HHS), December 10, 2015. Available online. URL: www.womenshealth.gov/blog/beat-holiday-blues. Accessed March 15, 2023.

Chapter 62 | **Peer Support and Social Inclusion**

WHAT IS PEER SUPPORT?
Peer support encompasses a range of activities and interactions between people who have shared similar experiences of being diagnosed with mental health conditions. This mutuality—often called "peerness"—between a peer worker and person using services promotes connection and inspires hope.

Peer support offers a level of acceptance, understanding, and validation not found in many other professional relationships. "I am an expert at not being an expert, and that takes a lot of expertise," said one (anonymous) peer worker, highlighting the supportive rather than directive nature of the peer relationship. By sharing their own lived experience and practical guidance, peer workers help people develop their own goals, create strategies for self-empowerment, and take concrete steps toward building fulfilling, self-determined lives for themselves.

WHAT DOES A PEER SUPPORT SPECIALIST DO?
Support the Recovery of Individuals
Peer workers offer encouragement, practical assistance, guidance, and understanding to support recovery. Peer support workers walk alongside people in recovery, offering individualized support and demonstrating that recovery is possible. They share their own lived experience of moving from hopelessness to hope. They share tools that can complement or replace clinical support by providing strategies for self-empowerment and achieving a self-determined life.

They support people in recovery to connect with their own inner strength, motivation, and desire to move forward in life, even when experiencing challenges. Peer workers offer different types of support, including:
- emotional support (empathy and camaraderie)
- informational support (connections to information and referrals to community resources that support health and wellness)
- instrumental support (concrete supports such as housing or employment)
- affiliational support (connections to community supports, activities, and events)

Improve Mental Health Systems

Peer support is valuable not only for the person receiving services but also for behavioral health professionals and the systems in which they work. Peer workers educate their colleagues and advance the field by sharing their perspectives and experience in order to increase understanding of how practices and policies may be improved to promote wellness and resiliency. This is particularly important in mental health systems, where historical oppression, violence, and discrimination present significant barriers to recovery for many people. Peer workers play vital roles in moving behavioral health professionals and systems toward recovery orientation.

IS PEER RECOVERY SUPPORT EFFECTIVE FOR PEOPLE WITH MENTAL HEALTH CONDITIONS?

The research on peer support in mental health systems is still emerging, but the findings are promising. The research to date suggests that peer recovery support may result in the following:
- increased empowerment and hope
- increased social functioning
- increased engagement and activation in the treatment
- increased community engagement
- increased quality of life and life satisfaction
- reduced use of inpatient services

- decreased self-stigma
- decreased costs to the mental health system
- decreased hospitalization[1]

SOCIAL INCLUSION

Social inclusion of people experiencing homelessness through peer support and consumer involvement or social connections is a key component of recovery.

People experiencing homelessness have lost the protection of a home and their community. They are often marginalized and isolated within the larger society. Also, people with mental and/or substance use disorders frequently face challenges in building and maintaining social connections. They may fail to seek out treatment for fear of discrimination or feel unworthy of help. Helping people experiencing homelessness overcome these beliefs and participate in treatment is a key step in recovery.

Social inclusion offers opportunities to reengage with the community and form positive relationships. Consumer involvement is the practice of integrating people with lived experience of homelessness into staff and leadership roles at homeless service agencies. Consumers may provide peer support as role models and resources for other services. Peer support creates a sense of belonging for both the individual providing the service and those receiving the support.[2]

---

[1] "Value of Peers, 2017," Substance Abuse and Mental Health Services Administration (SAMHSA), November 17, 2017. Available online. URL: www.samhsa.gov/sites/default/files/programs_campaigns/brss_tacs/value-of-peers-2017.pdf. Accessed March 15, 2023.

[2] "Social Inclusion," Substance Abuse and Mental Health Services Administration (SAMHSA), August 12, 2019. Available online. URL: www.samhsa.gov/homelessness-programs-resources/hpr-resources/social-inclusion. Accessed March 15, 2023.

Chapter 63 | Helping a Family Member or Friend with Depression

SUPPORTING A FRIEND OR FAMILY MEMBER WITH MENTAL HEALTH PROBLEMS

You can help your friend or family member by recognizing the signs of mental health problems and connecting them to professional help.

Talking to friends and family about mental health problems can be an opportunity to provide information, support, and guidance. Learning about mental health issues can lead to the following:
- improved recognition of early signs of mental health problems
- earlier treatment
- greater understanding and compassion

If a friend or family member is showing signs of a mental health problem or reaching out to you for help, offer support by:
- finding out if the person is getting the care that they need and want—if not, connect them to help
- expressing your concern and support
- reminding your friend or family member that help is available and that mental health problems can be treated
- asking questions, listening to ideas, and being responsive when the topic of mental health problems comes up

- reassuring your friend or family member that you care about them
- offering to help your friend or family member with everyday tasks
- including your friend or family member in your plans—continue to invite them without being overbearing, even if your friend or family member resists your invitations
- educating other people so they understand the facts about mental health problems and do not discriminate
- treating people with mental health problems with respect, compassion, and empathy

HOW TO TALK ABOUT MENTAL HEALTH

Do you need help starting a conversation about mental health? Try leading with the following questions and make sure to actively listen to your friend or family member's response:
- I have been worried about you. Can we talk about what you are experiencing? If not, who are you comfortable talking to?
- What can I do to help you to talk about issues with your parents or someone else who is responsible and cares about you?
- What else can I help you with?
- I am someone who cares and wants to listen. What do you want me to know how you are feeling?
- Who or what has helped you deal with similar issues in the past?
- Sometimes, talking to someone who has dealt with a similar experience helps. Do you know of others who have experienced these types of problems who you can talk with?
- It seems like you are going through a difficult time. How can I help you find support?
- How can I help you find more information about mental health problems?
- I am concerned about your safety. Have you thought about harming yourself or others?

Helping a Family Member or Friend with Depression

When talking about mental health problems, do the following:
- Know how to connect people to help.
- Communicate in a straightforward manner.
- Speak at a level appropriate to a person's age and development level (preschool children need fewer details as compared to teenagers).
- Discuss the topic at the time and place where the person feels safe and comfortable.
- Watch for reactions during the discussion and slow down or back up if the person becomes confused or looks upset.

Sometimes, it is helpful to make a comparison to a physical illness. For example, many people get sick with a cold or the flu, but only a few get really sick with something serious such as pneumonia. People who have a cold are usually able to do their normal activities. However, if they get pneumonia, they will have to take medicine and may have to go to the hospital.

Similarly, feelings of sadness, anxiety, worry, irritability, or sleep problems are common for most people. However, when these feelings get very intense, last for a long period of time, and begin to interfere with school, work, and relationships, it may be a sign of a mental health problem. And, just like people need to take medicine and get professional help for physical conditions, someone with a mental health problem may need to take medicine and/or participate in therapy to get better.[1]

HOW CAN YOU TAKE CARE OF YOURSELF?

You may have your own feelings of fear and anger about the trauma. You may feel guilty because you wish your family member would just forget all the problems and get on with life. You may feel confused or frustrated because your loved one has changed, and you may worry that your family life will never get back to normal. All

---

[1] "For Friends and Family Members," Substance Abuse and Mental Health Services Administration (SAMHSA), April 24, 2023. Available online. URL: www.samhsa.gov/mental-health/how-to-talk/friends-and-family-members. Accessed April 25, 2023.

of this can drain you. It can affect your health and make it hard for you to help your loved one. If you are not careful, you may get sick yourself, become depressed, or burn out and stop helping your loved one. To help yourself, you need to take care of yourself and have other people help you.

Tips to Care for Yourself
- Do not feel guilty or feel that you should know it all. Remind yourself that nobody has all the answers. It is normal to feel helpless at times.
- Do not feel bad if things change slowly. You cannot change anyone. People must change themselves.
- Take care of your physical and mental health. If you feel yourself getting sick or often feel sad and hopeless, see your doctor.
- Do not give up your outside life. Make time for activities and hobbies you enjoy. Continue to see your friends.
- Take time to be by yourself. Find a quiet place to gather your thoughts and "recharge."
- Get regular exercise, even just a few minutes a day. Exercise is a healthy way to deal with stress.
- Eat healthy foods. When you are busy, it may seem easier to eat fast food than to prepare healthy meals. But healthy foods will give you more energy to carry you through the day.
- Remember the good things. It is easy to get weighed down by worry and stress. But do not forget to see and celebrate the good things that happen to you and your family.

WHERE CAN YOU GO FOR HELP?
During difficult times, it is important to have people in your life who you can depend on. These people are your support network. They can help you with everyday jobs or by giving you love and understanding.

Helping a Family Member or Friend with Depression

You may get support from:
- family members
- friends, coworkers, and neighbors
- members of your religious or spiritual group
- support groups
- doctors and other health professionals[2]

---

[2] National Center for Posttraumatic Stress Disorder (NCPTSD), "Helping a Family Member Who Has PTSD," U.S. Department of Veterans Affairs (VA), November 8, 2022. Available online. URL: www.ptsd.va.gov/family/how_family_member.asp. Accessed March 16, 2023.

Part 8 | Depression and Suicide

Chapter 64 | Understanding Suicide

WHAT IS SUICIDE?
Suicide is when people harm themselves with the goal of ending their life and they die as a result. A suicide attempt is when people harm themselves with the goal of ending their life, but they do not die. Avoid using terms such as "committing suicide," "successful suicide," or "failed suicide" when referring to suicide and suicide attempts, as these terms often carry negative meanings.

WHAT ARE THE WARNING SIGNS OF SUICIDE?
Warning signs that someone may be at immediate risk for attempting suicide include the following:
- talking about wanting to die or wanting to kill themselves
- talking about feeling empty or hopeless or having no reason to live
- talking about feeling trapped or feeling that there are no solutions
- feeling unbearable emotional or physical pain
- talking about being a burden to others
- withdrawing from family and friends
- giving away important possessions
- saying goodbye to friends and family
- putting affairs in order, such as making a will
- taking great risks that could lead to death, such as driving extremely fast
- talking or thinking about death often

Other serious warning signs that someone may be at risk for attempting suicide include the following:
- displaying extreme mood swings, suddenly changing from very sad to very calm or happy
- making a plan or looking for ways to kill themselves, such as searching for lethal methods online, stockpiling pills, or buying a gun
- talking about feeling great guilt or shame
- using alcohol or drugs more often
- acting anxious or agitated
- changing eating or sleeping habits
- showing rage or talking about seeking revenge

WHO IS AT RISK FOR SUICIDE?

People of all genders, ages, and ethnicities can be at risk for suicide. The main risk factors for suicide are:
- a history of suicide attempts
- depression, other mental disorders, or substance use disorder (SUD)
- chronic pain
- family history of a mental disorder or substance use
- family history of suicide
- exposure to family violence, including physical or sexual abuse
- presence of guns or other firearms in the home
- having recently been released from prison or jail
- exposure, either directly or indirectly, to others' suicidal behavior, such as that of family members, peers, or celebrities

Most people who have risk factors for suicide will not attempt suicide, and it is difficult to tell who will act on suicidal thoughts. Although risk factors for suicide are important to keep in mind, someone who is showing warning signs of suicide may be at higher risk for danger and need immediate attention.

Stressful life events (such as the loss of a loved one, legal troubles, or financial difficulties) and interpersonal stressors (such as shame, harassment, bullying, discrimination, or relationship troubles) may contribute to suicide risk, especially when they occur along with suicide risk factors.

DOES ASKING SOMEONE ABOUT SUICIDE PUT THE IDEA IN THEIR HEAD?

No. Studies have shown that asking people about suicidal thoughts and behaviors does not cause or increase such thoughts. Asking someone directly, "Are you thinking of killing yourself?" can be the best way to identify someone at risk for suicide.

DO CERTAIN GROUPS OF PEOPLE HAVE HIGHER RATES OF SUICIDE?

According to the Centers for Disease Control and Prevention (CDC), women are more likely to attempt suicide than men, but men are more likely to die by suicide than women. This may be because men are more likely to attempt suicide using very lethal methods, such as a firearm or suffocation (e.g., hanging), and women are more likely to attempt suicide by poisoning, including overdosing on prescribed or unprescribed prescription drugs. However, recent CDC data suggest that the leading means of suicide for women may be shifting toward more lethal methods.

The CDC data also show that suicide rates vary by race, ethnicity, age, and gender. American Indian and Alaska Native men have the highest rates of suicide, followed by non-Hispanic White males.

Although the rate of suicide death among preteens and younger teens is lower than that of older adolescents and adults, it has increased over time. Suicide now ranks as the second leading cause of death for youth aged 10–14. For children under the age of 12, research indicates that Black children have a higher rate of suicide death than White children.

DO PEOPLE "THREATEN" SUICIDE TO GET ATTENTION?

Suicidal thoughts or actions are a sign of extreme distress and an indicator that someone needs help. Talking about wanting to die by suicide is not a typical response to stress. All talk of suicide should be taken seriously and requires immediate attention.

WHAT SHOULD YOU DO IF YOU ARE IN CRISIS OR SOMEONE YOU KNOW IS CONSIDERING SUICIDE?

If you notice warning signs of suicide—especially a change in behavior or new, concerning behavior—get help as soon as possible.

Family and friends are often the first to recognize the warning signs of suicide, and they can take the first step toward helping a loved one find mental health treatment.

If someone tells you that they are going to kill themselves, do not leave them alone. Do not promise that you will keep their suicidal thoughts a secret—tell a trusted friend, family member, or other trusted adult.

Call 911 if there is immediate danger or go to the nearest emergency room.

You can also contact:
- **988 Suicide & Crisis Lifeline**. The lifeline provides 24-hour, confidential support to anyone in suicidal crisis or emotional distress.
- **Call or text 988**. This number connects you with a trained crisis counselor. Support is also available via live chat.

WHAT IF YOU SEE SUICIDAL MESSAGES ON SOCIAL MEDIA?

Knowing how to get help when someone posts suicidal messages can help save a life. Many social media sites have a process to get help for the person posting the message.

Contact social media outlets directly if you are concerned about a friend's social media updates or dial 911 in an emergency.[1]

---

[1] "Frequently Asked Questions about Suicide," National Institute of Mental Health (NIMH), 2021. Available online. URL: www.nimh.nih.gov/health/publications/suicide-faq. Accessed March 15, 2023.

Chapter 65 | Suicide in the United States

Suicide is a major public health concern. It is among the leading causes of death in the United States. Suicide is defined as death caused by a nonfatal, self-directed injurious behavior with the intent to die as a result of the behavior. A suicide attempt might not result in injury. Suicidal ideation refers to thinking about, considering, or planning suicide.

SUICIDE IS A LEADING CAUSE OF DEATH IN THE UNITED STATES

According to the Leading Causes of Death Reports of the WISQARS™ of the Centers for Disease Control and Prevention (CDC) in 2020:
- suicide was the twelfth leading cause of death overall in the United States, claiming the lives of over 45,900 people
- suicide was the second leading cause of death among individuals between the ages of 10–14 and 25–34, the third leading cause of death among individuals between the ages of 15–24, and the fourth leading cause of death among individuals between the ages of 35 and 44
- there were nearly two times as many suicides (45,979) in the United States as there were homicides (24,576)

SUICIDE RATES
Trends over Time
- Suicide rates are based on the number of people who have died by suicide per 100,000 population. When comparing

rates from one year to another year, "age-adjusted" rates allow for differences in population age distributions and changes in population size over time to be taken into account.
- Figure 65.1 shows age-adjusted suicide rates in the United States for each year from 2000 through 2020 for the total population and for males and females separately.
  - The total age-adjusted suicide rate in the United States increased 35.2 percent from 10.4 per 100,000 in 2000 to 14.2 per 100,000 in 2018, before declining to 13.9 per 100,000 in 2019 and declining again to 13.5 per 100,000 in 2020.
  - In 2020, the suicide rate among males was four times higher (22.0 per 100,000) than among females (5.5 per 100,000).

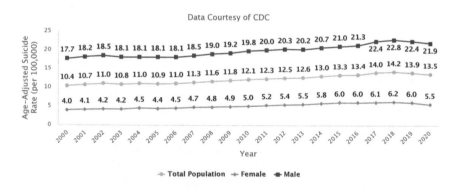

Figure 65.1. Suicide Rates in the United States (2000–2020)
National Institute of Mental Health (NIMH)

Demographics
- Crude suicide rate calculations take population size within subgroups in any given year or time frame into

Suicide in the United States

account. They can be a useful tool for understanding the relative proportion of people affected within different demographic groups.
- Figure 65.2 shows the crude rates of suicide within sex and age categories in 2020.
  - Among females, the suicide rate was highest for those aged 45–64 (7.9 per 100,000).
  - Among males, the suicide rate was highest for those aged 75 and older (40.5 per 100,000).

Figure 65.3 shows the age-adjusted rates of suicide for race/ethnicity groups in 2020. The rates of suicide were highest for American Indian, non-Hispanic males (37.4 per 100,000), followed by White, non-Hispanic males (27.0 per 100,000). Among females, the rates of suicide were highest for American Indian, non-Hispanic females (10.8 per 100,000) and White, non-Hispanic females (6.9 per 100,000).

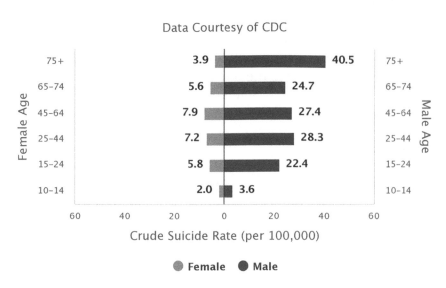

Figure 65.2. Suicide Rates by Age Group (2020)

National Institute of Mental Health (NIMH)

Depression Sourcebook, Sixth Edition

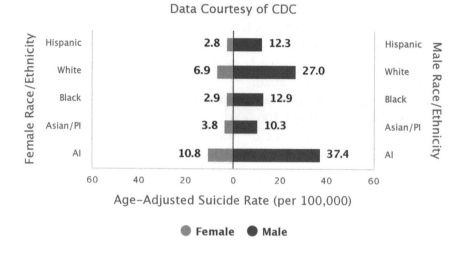

Figure 65.3. Suicide Rates by Race/Ethnicity (2020)

National Institute of Mental Health (NIMH)

SUICIDE BY METHOD
Number of Suicide Deaths by Method

Table 65.1 includes information on the total number of suicides by the most common methods.

In 2020, firearms were the most common method used in suicide deaths in the United States, accounting for over half of all suicide deaths (24,292).

Table 65.1. Suicide by Method (2020)

Suicide Method	Number of Deaths
Total	45,979
Firearms	24,292
Suffocation	12,495
Poisoning	5,528
Other	3,664

Suicide in the United States

Percentage of Suicide Deaths by Method

Figure 65.4 shows the percentages of suicide deaths by method among females and males in 2020. Among females, the most common methods of suicide were firearms (33.0%), suffocation (29.1%), and poisoning (28.6%). Among males, the most common methods of suicide were firearms (57.9%), followed by suffocation (26.7%).

SUICIDAL THOUGHTS AND BEHAVIORS AMONG U.S. ADULTS

Figure 65.5 shows that 4.9 percent of adults aged 18 and older in the United States had serious thoughts about suicide in 2020.

Among adults across all age groups, the prevalence of serious suicidal thoughts was highest among young adults aged 18–25 (11.3%).

The prevalence of serious suicidal thoughts was highest among adults aged 18 and older who reported having multiple (two or more) races (11.0%).

Figure 65.6 shows that in 2020, 0.5 percent of adults aged 18 and older in the United States reported they attempted suicide in the past year.

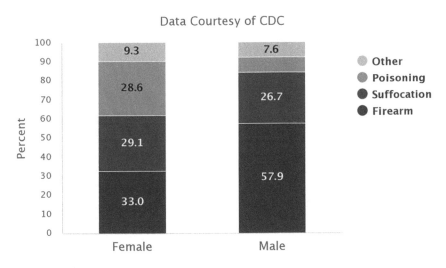

Figure 65.4. Percentage of Suicide Deaths by Method in the United States (2020)
National Institute of Mental Health (NIMH)

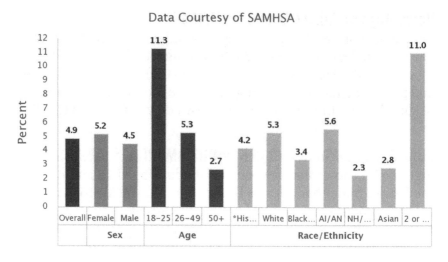

Figure 65.5. Past Year Prevalence of Suicidal Thoughts among U.S. Adults (2020)
National Institute of Mental Health (NIMH)

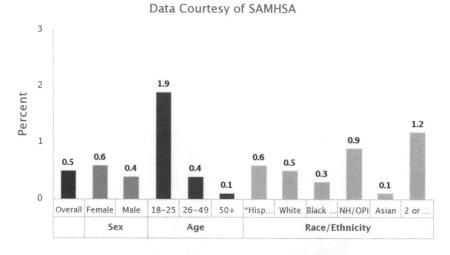

Figure 65.6. Past Year Prevalence of Suicide Attempts among U.S. Adults (2020)
National Institute of Mental Health (NIMH)

Among adults across all age groups, the prevalence of suicide attempts in the past year was highest among young adults aged 18–25 (1.9%).

Suicide in the United States

Among adults aged 18 and older, the prevalence of suicide attempts in the past year was highest among those who report having multiple (two or more) races (1.2%).[1]

---

[1] "Suicide," National Institute of Mental Health (NIMH), June 2022. Available online. URL: www.nimh.nih.gov/health/statistics/suicide. Accessed March 20, 2023.

Chapter 66 | Suicidal Behavior, Risk, and Protective Factors

Suicide causes immeasurable pain, suffering, and loss to individuals, families, and communities nationwide. On average, nearly 130 Americans die by suicide each day, that is, one death every 11 minutes. Suicide is the second leading cause for people aged 10–14 and 25–34, and more than 12.2 million adults in the United States had serious thoughts of suicide within the past 12 months. But suicide is preventable, so it is important to know what to do.[1]

FACTORS CONTRIBUTING TO SUICIDE RISK

Suicide is rarely caused by a single circumstance or event. Instead, a range of factors—at the individual, relationship, community, and societal levels—can increase risk. These risk factors are situations or problems that can increase the possibility that a person will attempt suicide.

Individual Risk Factors

The following are a few personal factors that contribute to risk:
- previous suicide attempt
- history of depression and other mental illnesses
- serious illness such as chronic pain

---

[1] MentalHealth.gov, "Suicidal Behavior," U.S. Department of Health and Human Services (HHS), December 5, 2022. Available online. URL: www.mentalhealth.gov/what-to-look-for/suicidal-behavior. Accessed March 21, 2023.

- criminal/legal problems
- job/financial problems or loss
- impulsive or aggressive tendencies
- substance use
- current or prior history of adverse childhood experiences
- sense of hopelessness
- violence victimization and/or perpetration

Relationship Risk Factors

The following are a few harmful or hurtful experiences within relationships that contribute to risk:
- bullying
- family/loved one's history of suicide
- loss of relationships
- high conflict or violent relationships
- social isolation

Community Risk Factors

The following are a few challenging issues within a person's community that contribute to risk:
- lack of access to health care
- suicide cluster in the community
- stress of acculturation
- community violence
- historical trauma
- discrimination

Societal Risk Factors

The following are a few cultural and environmental factors within the larger society that contribute to risk:
- the stigma associated with help-seeking and mental illness
- easy access to lethal means of suicide among people at risk
- unsafe media portrayals of suicide

Suicidal Behavior, Risk, and Protective Factors

FACTORS PROTECTING AGAINST SUICIDE RISK
Many factors can reduce the risk of suicide. Similar to risk factors, a range of factors at the individual, relationship, community, and societal levels can protect people from suicide. Everyone can help prevent suicide. We can take action in communities and as a society to support people and help protect them from suicidal thoughts and behavior.

Individual Protective Factors
The following are a few personal factors that protect against suicide risk:
- effective coping and problem-solving skills
- reasons for living (e.g., family, friends, pets, etc.)
- strong sense of cultural identity

Relationship Protective Factors
The following are a few healthy relationship experiences that protect against suicide risk:
- support from partners, friends, and family
- feeling connected to others

Community Protective Factors
The following are a few supportive community experiences that protect against suicide risk:
- feeling connected to school, community, and other social institutions
- availability of consistent and high-quality physical and behavioral health care

Societal Protective Factors
The following are a few cultural and environmental factors within the larger society that protect against suicide risk:
- reduced access to lethal means of suicide among people at risk
- cultural, religious, or moral objections to suicide

Suicide is connected to other forms of injury and violence. For example, people who have experienced violence, including child abuse, bullying, or sexual violence, have a higher suicide risk.[2]

---

[2] "Risk and Protective Factors," Centers for Disease Control and Prevention (CDC), November 2, 2022. Available online. URL: www.cdc.gov/suicide/factors/index.html?CDC_AA_refVal=https%3A%2F%2Fwww.cdc.gov%2Fviolenceprevention%2Fsuicide%2Friskprotectivefactors.html. Accessed March 21, 2023.

Chapter 67 | Suicide among Youth and Older Adults

Chapter Contents

Section 67.1—Teen Suicide 513
Section 67.2—Suicide among Young Adults 516
Section 67.3—Older Adults: Depression and
                Suicide Facts 518

Section 67.1 | Teen Suicide

Teenagers have their whole lives ahead of them, they are often told. The idea that a teen could be thinking about ending that life might be hard for their friends, families, or other people in their community to believe.

But the risk of suicide should be on the radar of anyone who interacts with teens, says Dr. Jane Pearson, a mental health expert at the National Institutes of Health (NIH).

The rate of teen suicide has increased over the last decade. Suicide is now the second leading cause of death for teens and young adults in the United States.

Experts do not know why this rate has been rising. But the NIH-funded researchers are working on better ways to find and help teens who are thinking of suicide.

"There are some very effective treatments for youth who are suicidal," Dr. Pearson explains. "We are trying to figure out how to make those treatments more accessible for more youth."

WHO IS AT RISK?

Many things can increase the risk of suicide in teenagers. One major risk factor is experiencing a mental health issue such as depression, anxiety, or trauma. Most people who die by suicide have struggled with a mental health condition.

Other risk factors include a family history of suicide, violence, or substance abuse. Teens also experience many stressful life events for the first time. These can include a breakup with a romantic partner, trouble at school, violence, or conflicts with friends.

"Teens do not have the life experience to know that these things will be temporary, that they will get through it," Dr. Pearson says. And they might think they would rather be dead than feel the way they do at that moment in time, she adds.

Persistent misunderstandings about suicide can also keep teens from getting the help they need, adds Dr. Pearson.

"Many people think that a teen talking about or attempting suicide are so-called gestures, or cries for attention," Dr. Pearson explains. They do not think that the teen is in real danger.

"That is definitely a myth," says Dr. Cheryl King, a suicide-prevention researcher at the University of Michigan. "If someone has been repeatedly suicidal or talking about it for a long time, that should have us more concerned rather than less concerned."

KNOWING WHEN TEENS NEED HELP

Some of the warning signs that a teen is thinking about suicide are talking about wanting to die, feeling hopeless, or being trapped or in unbearable pain.

If you are concerned about a teen who may be thinking about suicide, start a conversation, says Dr. Joan Asarnow, a suicide-prevention researcher and clinical psychologist at the University of California, Los Angeles.

"A conversation can just start with 'Are you OK?' or 'Is there something that feels like it is too big of a problem?'" Dr. Asarnow explains.

Pearson recommends that people start these conversations early when they first start to feel that something is wrong with a teen. "It is going to be easier to help somebody before they have really decided on a course of action to kill themselves," she says.

But many teens have suicidal thoughts that go unrecognized. Dr. King and other NIH-funded researchers are studying ways to better identify teens at risk of suicide.

Dr. King is testing a new method to screen teens who come into hospital emergency rooms for suicide risk. While most teens do not see a mental health specialist, she says, "roughly one in five goes to the emergency department at least once a year. So, it is a particularly good place for suicide-risk screening."

This is especially true because risk-taking behaviors such as substance abuse and dangerous driving can land teens in the emergency room, Dr. King explains. And teens who engage in such behaviors are at higher risk of suicide.

Other researchers are looking at ways to use technology to identify when teens already known to be at risk of suicide are most vulnerable. For example, one team is testing whether smartwatches can detect when teens' emotions are affecting their body before the teens themselves feel distressed.

"New technologies may provide us with a way to intervene at the moment where the kids really need it, without depending on them to reach out on their own," Dr. Asarnow explains.

KEEPING TEENS SAFE

Treatments are available that can help teens at risk of suicide. "Underlying mental health issues like depression and trauma are treatable conditions, and there are ways we can help youths with these troubles once we know about them," says Dr. King. Talk therapy and medications can both be effective for many people.

The NIH-funded researchers have also developed therapies that can help very high-risk teens—those who have already attempted suicide, sometimes more than once.

Asarnow and her colleagues recently showed that types of intensive counseling for teens and their families could reduce the risk of another suicide attempt by about a third. This counseling, based on treatments called "cognitive-behavioral therapy" (CBT) and "dialectical behavior therapy" (DBT), teaches coping strategies and life skills.

Involving the family in suicide prevention seems to be more effective than just treating the teen, Dr. Asarnow says. Her program counsels and teaches parents as well as the teens in their care.

One thing any family can do to help protect a teen thinking of suicide is to talk with a health-care provider about putting together a safety plan, she adds. A safety plan is a document the teen and trusted adults create together. It includes coping strategies and contact information for people who have agreed to help in times of crisis.

A safety plan also includes commitments from the family to keeping the teen's environment safe, such as limiting access to medications and firearms.

The decision to harm oneself is often made in a split second. A safety plan "makes the best decisions and the easy things to do," Dr. Pearson explains. "The family wants that, and the teen wants that."

If you or someone you know is thinking about suicide, you can call the National Suicide Prevention Lifeline at 1-800-273-TALK.

You can also text "HOME" to the Crisis Text Line at 741741. Experts recommend both parents and teens store these numbers on their smartphones.[1]

Section 67.2 | Suicide among Young Adults

Developmentally, the years between childhood and adulthood represent a critical period of transition and significant cognitive, mental, emotional, and social change. While adolescence is a time of tremendous growth and potential, navigating new milestones in preparation for adult roles involving education, employment, relationships, and living circumstances can be difficult. These transitions can lead to various mental health challenges that can be associated with an increased risk of suicide.

Suicide is the second leading cause of death among youth aged 15–24. Approximately 1 out of every 15 high school students reports attempting suicide each year. One out of every 53 high school students reports having made a suicide attempt that was serious enough to be treated by a doctor or a nurse. For each suicide death among young people, there may be as many as 100–200 suicide attempts. For some groups of youth—including those who are involved in the child welfare and juvenile justice systems; lesbian, gay, bisexual, and transgender (LGBT); American Indian/Alaska Native; and military service members—the incidence of suicidal behavior is even higher.

Despite how common suicidal thoughts and attempts (as well as mental health disorders that can be associated with increased risk for suicide) are among youth, there is a great deal known about prevention as well as caring for youth and communities after an attempt or death. Parents, guardians, family members, friends, teachers, school administrators, coaches and extracurricular

---

[1] "Teen Suicide," National Institutes of Health (NIH), September 2019. Available online. URL: https://newsinhealth.nih.gov/2019/09/teen-suicide. Accessed March 16, 2023.

activity leaders, mentors, service providers, and many others can play a role in preventing suicide and supporting youth.[2]

PREVENTING YOUTH SUICIDE

Suicide is a serious public health problem that can have lasting, significant effects on youth, families, peers, and communities. The causes of suicide among youth are complex and involve many factors. Reducing risk factors and increasing protective factors and resilience are critical.

Knowing the warning signs is also critical. Warning signs for those at risk of suicide include talking about wanting to die, feeling hopeless, having no reason to live, feeling trapped or in unbearable pain, seeking revenge, and being a burden on others; looking for methods and making plans such as searching online or buying a gun; increasing use of alcohol or drugs; acting anxious or agitated; behaving recklessly; sleeping too little or too much; withdrawal or isolation; and displaying rage and extreme mood swings. The risk of suicide is greater if a behavior is new or has increased and if it seems related to a painful event, loss, or change. Paying attention to warning signs for mental health challenges that can be associated with increased risk for suicide is also important.

No one person (parent, teacher, counselor, administrator, mentor, etc.) can implement suicide prevention efforts on their own. The participation, support, and active involvement of families, schools, and communities are essential. Youth-focused suicide prevention strategies are available. Promotion and prevention services are also available to address mental health issues. Schools, where youth spend the majority of their time, are a natural setting to support mental health.[3]

---

[2] "Suicide Prevention," Youth.gov, September 10, 2014. Available online. URL: https://youth.gov/youth-topics/youth-suicide-prevention. Accessed March 17, 2023.

[3] "Preventing Youth Suicide," Youth.gov, September 11, 2014. Available online. URL: https://youth.gov/youth-topics/youth-suicide-prevention/preventing-youth-suicide. Accessed March 17, 2023.

Section 67.3 | Older Adults: Depression and Suicide Facts

Older men die by suicide at a rate that is more than seven times higher than that of older women. The incidence of suicide is particularly high among older, White males (30.3 suicides per 100,000). Notably, the rate of suicide in the oldest group of White males (aged 85 and over) is over four times higher than the nation's overall rate of suicide.

There are several important risk factors for suicide in older adults. These include, among others:
- depression
- prior suicide attempts
- marked feelings of hopelessness
- comorbid general medical conditions that significantly limit functioning or life expectancy
- pain and declining role function (e.g., loss of independence or a sense of purpose)
- social isolation
- family discord or losses (e.g., the recent death of a loved one)
- inflexible personality or marked difficulty adapting to change
- access to lethal means (e.g., firearms)
- alcohol or medication misuse or abuse
- impulsivity in the context of cognitive impairment

Suicide attempts are often more lethal in older adults than in younger adults. Older people who attempt suicide are often more frail, more isolated, more likely to have a plan, and more determined than younger adults. These factors suggest that older adults are less likely to be rescued and are more likely to die from a suicide attempt than younger adults. Firearms are the most common means of suicide in older adults (67%), followed by poisoning (14%) and suffocation (12%). Of note, older adults are nearly twice as likely to use firearms as a means of suicide than people under age 60. The lethality of older adult suicide attempts suggests that interventions must be aggressive and that multiple prevention methods should be used.

Suicide among Youth and Older Adults

Prevention of suicide in older adults requires many different strategies. Multilayered prevention initiatives that combine universal, selective, and indicated prevention strategies may provide the greatest benefit in reducing suicide in older adults.

Universal prevention focuses on the entire population. These strategies try to reduce risk factors for suicide and improve older adult health. They are usually done by providing information and improving the skills of older people and their caregivers. Selected recommendations include the following:
- implementing depression screenings
- providing education on factors associated with increased suicide risk and protective factors
- providing education on suicide prevention, "hotlines," and local crisis team referral
- limiting access to means of suicide, such as firearms

SELECTIVE PREVENTION

It targets people who are at increased risk for suicide but who may not display suicidal thoughts or behavior. Examples include older adults who experience life transitions (e.g., retirement, moving from home) or losses (e.g., death of a spouse/partner, painful chronic illness) that make them vulnerable to depression and suicide. Selective prevention efforts try to reduce risk factors for suicide or improve resilience. Some examples include the following:
- Focus services on reducing disability and enhancing independent functioning.
- Increase provider awareness of the losses that are important to older people, such as retirement, loss of driver's license, and loss of important body functions (e.g., vision, mobility).
- Increase provider awareness of substance abuse and mental health problems in older adults.
- Make systematic screening tools available to staff in medical and nonmedical settings and train staff to screen for suicide risk.
- Address social isolation and lack of access to social support for at-risk older adults.

INDICATED PREVENTION

Indicated prevention efforts aim to prevent suicide among older adults who have survived a suicide attempt or are at high risk for suicide. Because of the close association between depression and suicide, the detection and effective treatment of depression are keys to reducing suicides. Routine screening for depression can be done with many instruments, such as the PHQ-9 (www.phqscreeners.com) and the Geriatric Depression Scale (GDS; www.stanford.edu/~yesavage/GDS.html). A variety of psychotherapy and antidepressant medications are effective at treating symptoms of depression and can reduce suicidal ideation in some older adults. Selected recommendations include the following:

- training professionals to detect, intervene, and manage depression and suicide risk
- implementing practice guidelines for the detection and management of suicide in later life
- reassuring the depressed or hopeless older adult that his or her existence is meaningful and appreciated and that his or her well-being is important (e.g., home visits, regular postcards or phone calls, and connection to the alarm central for immediate help when needed, such as TeleHelpTeleCheck)
- taking action to ensure the safety and effective treatment of older adults who are at imminent risk for suicide

ASSESSING AND ACTING UPON SUICIDE RISK

Aging services, behavioral health, and primary care providers can play an important role in preventing suicide by identifying at-risk older adults and taking appropriate follow-up actions. The goal of assessing suicide risk in an older person is to help determine the most appropriate actions to keep the older person safe.

Suicidal thoughts are often a symptom of depression and should always be taken seriously. Passive suicidal thoughts (also termed "death ideation") include thoughts of being better off dead. They are not necessarily associated with an increased risk for suicide but are a sign of significant distress and should be addressed clinically.

Suicide among Youth and Older Adults

The extent to which death ideation increases suicide risk is not known, and more research is needed. In contrast, active suicidal thoughts include thoughts of taking action toward hurting oneself. These thoughts are of immediate concern and require further assessment and intervention. The last question of the PHQ-9, a depression scale commonly used in many health-care settings, asks: "In the past two weeks, have you had any thoughts of hurting or killing yourself?" If an older adult responds positively to a question about thoughts of self-harm, he or she is considered to have "active suicidal ideation":

- **Past suicide attempt.** "Have you ever attempted to harm yourself in the past?"
- **Suicide plan.** "Have you had thoughts about how you might actually hurt yourself?" (This could include thoughts of timing, location, lethality, availability of means, and preparatory acts.)
- **Probability (perceived).** "How likely do you think it is that you will act on these thoughts about hurting yourself or ending your life sometime over the next month?"
- **Preventive factors.** "Is there anything that would prevent or keep you from harming yourself?"

Positive answers to any of these questions should be discussed with a qualified mental health professional to determine the degree of urgency and steps for further assessment and intervention. Older adults who have thoughts about killing themselves with a plan and intent to act should not be left alone but should be supervised for their safety until emergency services are in place.

Timely and appropriate responses to active suicidal thoughts can prevent suicide in older adults. Different levels of action should be taken for any endorsement of suicidal ideation.

- Using the algorithm of the "P4 Screener," for an older adult showing low risk (i.e., suicidal thoughts without the endorsement of "past suicide attempt" or "suicide plan"), suggested actions include expressing concern, getting "buy-in" to inform the older adult's primary care provider, urging that the older adult remove

means, consulting a supervisor within 24–48 hours, and identifying possible coping strategies.
- For an older adult with a moderate risk of suicide (i.e., active suicidal thoughts with either a "suicide plan" or a "past suicide attempt"), the previously mentioned actions should be taken; consultation/supervision should be sought; and interventions such as phone check-ins and repeat assessments should be considered.
- For an older adult at high risk of suicide (i.e., active suicidal thoughts with a "past suicide attempt" or "suicide plan" as well as the endorsement of "probability" of acting or intent and/or lack of "preventive factors"), a supervisor/consultant should be called immediately without leaving the older adult alone, and emergency services should be considered (e.g., emergency room, mobile crisis, or 911).[4]

RECOGNIZE AND RESPOND TO SUICIDE RISK

Senior centers can play an important role in preventing suicide by identifying older adults who may be at immediate risk, taking appropriate follow-up actions to keep them safe, and connecting them to the help they need. Since suicidal behavior is closely linked to mental disorders and substance misuse, it is important to recognize and respond to depression and misuse of alcohol and medications among older adults.

Senior center staff and volunteers should be able to recognize the warning signs of suicide and know how to respond immediately if someone displays any of them.

What Senior Center Staff Can Do

Designate someone at your senior center to serve as the point person for addressing concerns related to suicide risk. For example,

---

[4] "Older Americans Behavioral Health Issue Brief 4: Preventing Suicide in Older Adults," Administration for Community Living (ACL), 2012. Available online. URL: https://acl.gov/sites/default/files/programs/2016-11/Issue%20Brief%204%20Preventing%20Suicide.pdf. Accessed April 27, 2023.

Suicide among Youth and Older Adults

you could designate the senior center director, a social worker, or other appropriate staff member to serve in this capacity.

Identify a mental health professional in the community who will be your contact for advice and referrals. Contact local behavioral health providers to identify one or more mental health professionals who can provide this assistance to your senior center and its participants.

Develop a written protocol for recognizing and immediately responding to the warning signs of suicide. The protocol should include information on how to recognize warning signs and behaviors. It should also indicate the senior center point person to notify and the community mental health provider to contact for assistance.[5]

---

[5] "Promoting Emotional Health And Preventing Suicide," Substance Abuse and Mental Health Services Administration (SAMHSA), March 23, 2020. Available online. URL: https://store.samhsa.gov/sites/default/files/d7/priv/sma15-4416.pdf. Accessed April 27, 2023.

Chapter 68 | Warning Signs of Suicide and How to Deal with It

Chapter Contents
Section 68.1—Suicide Risk Screening 527
Section 68.2—Treating People with Suicidal Thoughts............. 532
Section 68.3—Preventing Suicide 535
Section 68.4—Taking Care of a Family Member after
 a Suicide Attempt 537

Section 68.1 | Suicide Risk Screening

Warning signs are observations that signal an increase in the probability that a person intends to engage in suicidal behavior in the immediate future (i.e., minutes and days). Warning signs present tangible evidence to the clinician that a person is at heightened risk of suicide in the short term. Warning signs may be experienced in the absence of risk factors.

DIRECT WARNING SIGNS
- **Suicidal communication.** Writing or talking about suicide, wishing to die (threatening to hurt or kill themselves), or intention to act on those ideas.
- **Preparations for suicide.** Evidence or expression of suicide intent and/or taking steps toward implementation of a plan. Making arrangements to divest responsibility for dependent others (children, pets, or elders), making other preparations such as updating wills, making financial arrangements for paying bills, saying goodbye to loved ones, and so on.
- **Seeking access or recent use of lethal means.** Owning or planning to acquire weapons, medications, toxins, or other lethal means.

INDIRECT WARNING SIGNS
- **Substance abuse.** Increasing or excessive substance use (alcohol, drugs, smoking).
- **Hopelessness.** Expresses the feeling that nothing can be done to improve the situation.
- **Purposelessness.** Express no sense of purpose, no reason for living, and decreased self-esteem.
- **Anger.** Rage or seeking revenge.
- **Recklessness.** Engaging impulsively in risky behavior.

- **Feeling trapped.** Expressing feelings of being trapped with no way out.
- **Social withdrawal.** Withdrawing from family, friends, and society.
- **Anxiety.** Agitation, irritability, angry outbursts, and feeling like they want to "jump out of their skin."
- **Mood changes.** Dramatic changes in mood or lack of interest in usual activities/friends.
- **Sleep.** Insomnia, inability to sleep, or sleeping all the time.
- **Guilt or shame.** Expressing overwhelming self-blame or remorse.[1]

WHAT IS A SUICIDE RISK SCREENING?

Every year, nearly 800,000 people around the world take their own lives. Many more attempt suicide. In the United States, it is the tenth leading cause of death overall and the second leading cause of death in people aged 10–34. Suicide has a lasting impact on those left behind and on the community at large.

Although suicide is a major health problem, it can often be prevented. A suicide risk screening can help find out how likely it is that someone will try to take their own life. During most screenings, a provider will ask some questions about behavior and feelings. There are specific questions and guidelines that providers can use. These are known as "suicide risk assessment tools." If you or a loved one is found to be at risk for suicide, you can get medical, psychological, and emotional support that may help avoid a tragic outcome.

WHAT IS IT USED FOR?

A suicide risk screening is used to find out if someone is at risk for trying to take their own life.

---

[1] "Assessment and Management of Patients at Risk for Suicide," U.S. Department of Veterans Affairs (VA), February 2014. Available online. URL: www.healthquality.va.gov/guidelines/MH/srb/VASuicidePreventionPocketGuidePRINT508FINAL.pdf. Accessed April 27, 2023.

Warning Signs of Suicide and How to Deal with It

WHY DO YOU NEED A SUICIDE RISK SCREENING?
You or a loved one may need a suicide risk screening if you notice any of the following warning signs:
- feeling hopeless and/or trapped
- talking about being a burden to others
- increased use of alcohol or drugs
- having extreme mood swings
- withdrawing from social situations or wanting to be alone
- a change in eating and/or sleeping habits

You may also need a screening if you have certain risk factors. You may be likely to try to harm yourself if you have:
- tried to kill yourself before
- depression or other mood disorder
- a history of suicide in your family
- a history of trauma or abuse
- a chronic illness and/or chronic pain

A suicide risk screening can be very helpful for people with these warning signs and risk factors. Other warning signs may need to be addressed immediately. These include:
- talking about suicide or wanting to die
- searching online for ways to kill yourself, getting a gun, or stockpiling medicines such as sleeping pills or pain medicines
- talking about having no reason to live

If you or a loved one has any of these warning signs, seek help right away. Call 911 or the National Suicide Prevention Lifeline at 1-800-273-TALK (8255).

WHAT HAPPENS DURING A SUICIDE RISK SCREENING?
A screening may be done by your primary care provider or a mental health provider. A mental health provider is a health-care professional who specializes in diagnosing and treating mental health problems.

Your primary care provider may give you a physical exam and ask you about your use of drugs and alcohol, changes in eating and sleeping habits, and mood swings. These could have many different causes. He or she may ask you about any prescription drugs you are taking. In some cases, antidepressants can increase suicidal thoughts, especially in children, teenagers, and young adults (under the age of 25). You may also get a blood test or other tests to see if a physical disorder is causing your suicidal symptoms.

During a blood test, a health-care professional will take a blood sample from a vein in your arm using a small needle. After the needle is inserted, a small amount of blood will be collected into a test tube or vial. You may feel a little sting when the needle goes in or out. This usually takes less than five minutes.

Your primary care provider or a mental health provider may also use one or more suicide risk assessment tools. A suicide risk assessment tool is a type of questionnaire or guideline for providers. These tools help providers evaluate your behavior, feelings, and suicidal thoughts. The most commonly used assessment tools include the following:

- **Patient Health Questionnaire-9 (PHQ9).** This tool is made up of nine questions about suicidal thoughts and behaviors.
- **Ask Suicide-Screening Questions.** This includes four questions and is geared toward people aged 10–24.
- **SAFE-T.** This is a test that focuses on five areas of suicide risk, as well as suggested treatment options.
- **The Columbia-Suicide Severity Rating Scale (C-SSRS).** This is a suicide risk assessment scale that measures four different areas of suicide risk.

WILL YOU NEED TO DO ANYTHING TO PREPARE FOR A SUICIDE RISK SCREENING?

You do not need any special preparations for this screening.

ARE THERE ANY RISKS IN SCREENING?

There is no risk in having a physical exam or a questionnaire. There is very little risk in having a blood test. You may have slight pain or bruising at the spot where the needle was put in, but most symptoms go away quickly.

WHAT DO THE RESULTS MEAN?
If the results of your physical exam or blood test show a physical disorder or a problem with a medicine, your provider may provide treatment and change or adjust your medicines as necessary.

The results of a suicide risk assessment tool or suicide risk assessment scale can show how likely it is you will attempt suicide. Your treatment will depend on your risk level. If you are at very high risk, you may be admitted to a hospital. If your risk is more moderate, your provider may recommend one or more of the following:
- psychological counseling from a mental health professional
- medicines, such as antidepressants (But younger people on antidepressants should be closely monitored. The medicines sometimes increase suicide risk in children and young adults.)
- treatment for addiction to alcohol or drugs[2]

WHAT YOU CAN DO
If you believe someone is at risk of suicide:
- Ask them if they are thinking about killing themselves. (This will not put the idea into their heads or make it likely that they will attempt suicide.)
- Call the U.S. National Suicide Prevention Lifeline at 800-273-TALK (8255).
- Take the person to an emergency room or seek help from a medical or mental health professional.
- Remove any objects that could be used in a suicide attempt.
- If possible, do not leave the person alone.[3]

---

[2] MedlinePlus, "Suicide Risk Screening," National Institutes of Health (NIH), September 14, 2021. Available online. URL: https://medlineplus.gov/lab-tests/suicide-risk-screening. Accessed May 5, 2023.
[3] "How You Can Play a Role in Preventing Suicide," U.S. Department of Health and Human Services (HHS), September 10, 2012. Available online. URL: www.hhs.gov/sites/default/files/national-strategy-for-suicide-prevention-factsheet.pdf. Accessed March 17, 2023.

Section 68.2 | Treating People with Suicidal Thoughts

Evidence-based treatment approaches for people who present with suicidal ideation or who have made a suicide attempt aim to reduce the frequency and intensity of suicidal ideation and prevent the recurrence of self-harm behaviors and premature death. Most effective treatments are conducted by a licensed mental health professional (e.g., psychologist, psychiatrist, clinical social worker, or marriage and family therapist) and take place over multiple sessions. Treatment may occur in a variety of settings, primarily as outpatient, intensive outpatient, and partial hospital programs. In some cases, treatment is initiated in an emergency department or psychiatric hospital following a suicide attempt and continues on an outpatient basis following discharge.

Interventions may primarily focus on treating suicidal thoughts and behaviors directly but should also address self-harm as a potential symptom of one of the disorders that commonly co-occur with suicidal thoughts and behaviors (e.g., depression, borderline personality disorder). When self-harm behavior or suicide risk is associated with a mental illness, providers need to identify that condition and modify treatment plans to specifically address the risk of suicide.[4]

TREATMENTS AND THERAPIES

Effective, evidence-based interventions are available to help people who are at risk for suicide.

Brief Interventions
- **Safety planning.** Personalized safety planning has been shown to help reduce suicidal thoughts and actions. Patients work with a caregiver to develop a plan that describes ways to limit access to lethal means, such as

---

[4] "Treatment for Suicidal Ideation, Self-Harm, and Suicide Attempts among Youth," Substance Abuse and Mental Health Service Administration (SAMHSA), 2020. Available online. URL: https://store.samhsa.gov/sites/default/files/pep20-06-01-002.pdf. Accessed May 4, 2023.

firearms, pills, or poisons. The plan also lists coping strategies and people and resources that can help in a crisis.
- **Follow-up phone calls.** Research has shown that when at-risk patients receive further screening, a safety plan intervention, and a series of supportive phone calls, their risk of suicide goes down.

Psychotherapies

Multiple types of psychosocial interventions, including the following, have been found to help individuals who have attempted suicide. These types of interventions may prevent someone from making another attempt.
- **Cognitive-behavioral therapy (CBT).** This type of therapy can help people learn new ways of dealing with stressful experiences. CBT helps individuals recognize their thought patterns and consider alternative actions when thoughts of suicide arise.
- **Dialectical behavior therapy (DBT).** This therapy has been shown to reduce suicidal behavior in adolescents. DBT has also been shown to reduce the rate of suicide in adults with borderline personality disorder, a mental illness characterized by an ongoing pattern of varying moods, self-image, and behavior that often results in impulsive actions and problems in relationships. A therapist trained in DBT can help a person recognize when their feelings or actions are disruptive or unhealthy and teach the person skills that can help them cope more effectively with upsetting situations.

Medication

Some individuals at risk for suicide might benefit from medication. Health-care providers and patients can work together to find the best medication or medication combination, as well as the right dose. Because many individuals at risk for suicide often have mental illnesses or substance use problems, individuals might benefit from medication along with psychosocial intervention.

Clozapine is an antipsychotic medication used primarily to treat individuals with schizophrenia. To date, it is the only medication with a specific U.S. Food and Drug Administration (FDA) indication for reducing the risk of recurrent suicidal behavior in patients with schizophrenia or schizoaffective disorder.

If you are prescribed a medication, be sure you do the following:
- Talk with your health-care provider or a pharmacist to make sure you understand the risks and benefits of the medications you are taking.
- Do not stop taking medication without talking to your health-care provider first. Suddenly stopping a medication may lead to a "rebound" or worsening of symptoms. Other uncomfortable or potentially dangerous withdrawal effects are also possible.
- Report any concerns about side effects to your health-care provider right away. You may need a change in the dose or a different medication.
- Report serious side effects to the FDA MedWatch Adverse Event Reporting program online or by phone at 1-800-332-1088. You or your health-care provider may send a report.

Collaborative Care

Collaborative care is a team-based approach to mental health care. A behavioral health-care manager will work with the person, their primary health-care provider, and mental health specialists to develop a treatment plan. Collaborative care has been shown to be an effective way to treat depression and reduce suicidal thoughts.[5]

---

[5] "Suicide Prevention," National Institute of Mental Health (NIMH), July 15, 2019. Available online. URL: www.nimh.nih.gov/health/topics/suicide-prevention. Accessed March 8, 2023.

Warning Signs of Suicide and How to Deal with It

Section 68.3 | Preventing Suicide

Suicide is a serious public health problem in the United States. It contributes to premature death, long-term disability, lost productivity, and significant health-care costs.

Suicide deaths reflect only a portion of the problem. Every year, millions of Americans seriously think about suicide or plan or attempt suicide. Suicide and suicide attempts can contribute to lasting impacts on individuals, families, and communities. The good news is that suicide is preventable. The vision of the National Center for Injury Prevention and Control of the Centers for Disease Control and Prevention (CDC) of "no lives lost to suicide" relies on implementing a comprehensive public health approach to prevention. This approach:

- uses data to drive decision-making
- implements and evaluates multiple prevention strategies that enhance resilience and improve well-being based on the best available evidence
- works to prevent people from becoming suicidal

PREVENTING SUICIDE IS A PRIORITY

The CDC's Suicide Prevention Resource for Action (Prevention Resource) details the strategies with the best available evidence to reduce suicide. The Prevention Resource can help states and communities prioritize suicide prevention activities most likely to have an impact. The programs, practices, and policies in the Prevention Resource can be tailored to the needs of populations and communities.

The Prevention Resource has the following three components states and communities can use to inform their suicide prevention efforts:

- Strategies are the actions to achieve the goal of preventing suicide.
- Approaches are the specific ways to advance each strategy.
- Policies, programs, and practices included have evidence of impact on suicide, suicide attempts, or risk and protective factors.

STRATEGIES FOR ACTION

The Prevention Resource represents a select group of strategies based on the best available evidence to help communities and states focus on activities with the greatest potential to prevent suicide. These strategies focus on preventing the risk of suicide before it occurs and reducing the immediate and long-term harms of suicidal behavior for individuals, families, communities, and society:

- strengthening economic support
- creating protective environments
- improving access and delivery of suicide care
- promoting healthy connections
- teaching coping and problem-solving skills
- identifying and supporting people at risk
- lessening harm and preventing future risk

NEED HELP? KNOW SOMEONE WHO DOES?

Contact the 988 Suicide & Crisis Lifeline if you are experiencing mental-health-related distress or are worried about a loved one who may need crisis support.

- Call or text 988.
- Chat at 988lifeline.org.

Connect with a trained crisis counselor. 988 is confidential, free, and available 24/7/365.

Visit the 988 Suicide & Crisis Lifeline for more information at 988lifeline.org.[6]

---

[6] "Suicide Prevention Resource for Action," Centers for Disease Control and Prevention (CDC), October 26, 2022. Available online. URL: www.cdc.gov/suicide/resources/prevention.html. Accessed March 17, 2023.

Warning Signs of Suicide and How to Deal with It

Section 68.4 | Taking Care of a Family Member after a Suicide Attempt

Suicidal thoughts and actions generate conflicting feelings in family members who love the person who wishes to take his or her own life. This section discusses some important points on how to take care of yourself and your family member following a suicide attempt and to help you move forward.

WHAT HAPPENS IN THE EMERGENCY DEPARTMENT?
Goal

The goal of an emergency department visit is to get the best outcome for the person at a time of crisis—resolving the crisis, stabilizing the patient medically and emotionally, and making recommendations and referrals for follow-up care or treatment. There are several steps in the process, and they all take time.

When someone is admitted to an emergency department for a suicide attempt, a doctor will evaluate the person's physical and mental health. Emergency department staff should look for underlying physical problems that may have contributed to the suicidal behavior, such as side effects from medications, untreated medical conditions, or the presence of street drugs that can cause emotional distress. While emergency department staff prefer to assess people who are sober, they should not dismiss things people say or do when intoxicated, especially comments about how they might harm themselves or others.

Assessment

After emergency department staff evaluate your family member's physical health, a mental health assessment should be performed, and the physician doing the exam should put your relative's suicidal behavior into context. The assessment will generally focus on the following three areas:
- What psychiatric or medical conditions are present? Are they being or have they been treated? Are the

suicidal thoughts and behavior a result of a recent change, or are they a longstanding condition?
- What did the person do to harm herself or himself? Have there been previous attempts? Why did the person act, and why now? What current stressors, including financial or relationship losses, may have contributed to this decision? Does the person regret surviving the suicide attempt? Is the person angry with someone? Is the person trying to reunite with someone who has died? What is the person's perspective on death?
- What support systems are there? Who is providing treatment? What treatment programs are a good match for the person? What do the individual and the family feel comfortable with?

Finally, a doctor may assess in more detail the actual suicide attempt that brought your relative into the emergency department. Information that the treatment team should look for includes the presence of a suicide note, the seriousness of the attempt, or a history of previous suicide attempts.

WHAT THE EMERGENCY DEPARTMENT NEEDS TO KNOW: HOW YOU CAN HELP

Inform the emergency department personnel if your relative has:
- access to a gun, lethal doses of medications, or other means of suicide
- stopped taking prescribed medicines
- stopped seeing a mental health provider or physician
- written a suicide note or will
- given possessions away
- been in or is currently in an abusive relationship
- an upcoming anniversary of a loss
- started abusing alcohol or drugs
- recovered well from a previous suicidal crisis following a certain type of intervention

Warning Signs of Suicide and How to Deal with It

Confidentiality and Information Sharing
Family members are a source of history and are often key to the discharge plan.

Provide as much information as possible to the emergency department staff. Even if confidentiality laws prevent the medical staff from giving you information about your relative, you can always give them information. Find out who is doing the evaluation and talk with that person. You can offer information that may influence the decisions made for your relative.

If you ever again have to accompany your relative to the emergency department after an attempt, remember to bring all medications, suspected causes of overdose, and any names and phone numbers of providers who may have information. Emergency department personnel should try to contact the medical professionals who know the situation best before making decisions.

Other important information about your relative's history to share with the emergency department staff includes the following:

- **A family history of actual suicide**. Mental health professionals are taught to pay attention to this because there is an increased risk in families with a history of suicide.
- **Details about your relative's treatment team**. Information such as a recent change in medication, the therapist being on vacation, and so on is relevant for emergency department staff because, if they do not feel hospitalization is best, they need to discharge your family member to a professional's care.
- **Advance directives**. If the person has an advance directive, review this with the emergency department treatment team. If you have a guardianship, let them know that as well.

You may want to get permission from the staff and your relative to sit in on your relative's evaluation in the emergency department to listen and add information as needed. Your role is to balance the emergency department staff's training and the interview of the patient with your perspective. The best emergency department decisions are made with all the relevant information.

If your relative has a hearing impairment or does not speak English, he or she may have to wait for someone who knows American Sign Language or an interpreter. It is generally not a good idea to use a family member to interpret in a medical situation.

NEXT STEPS AFTER THE EMERGENCY DEPARTMENT

After your relative's physical and mental health are thoroughly examined, the emergency department personnel will decide if your relative needs to be hospitalized—either voluntarily or by a commitment. If hospitalization is necessary, you can begin to work with the receiving hospital to offer information and support and to develop a plan for the next steps in your relative's care. If involuntary hospitalization is necessary, the hospital staff should explain this legal procedure to your relative and you so that you both have a clear understanding of what will take place over the next 3–10 days while a court decides on the next steps for treatment.

If the emergency department's treatment team, the patient, and you do not feel hospitalization is necessary, then you should all be a part of developing a follow-up treatment plan. In developing a plan, consider the questions about the treatment plan shown in Table 68.1.

Table 68.1. Questions Family and Friends Should Ask about the Follow-up Treatment Plan

Ask Your Family Member (Be Honest and Direct with Your Questions and Concerns)	Ask the Treatment Team (Including Doctor, Therapist, Nurse, Social Worker, and So On)
Do you feel safe to leave the hospital, and are you comfortable with the discharge plan?	Do you believe professionally that my family member is ready to leave the hospital?
How is your relationship with your doctor, and when is your next appointment?	Why did you make the decision(s) that you did about my family member's care or treatment?
What has changed since your suicidal feelings or actions began?	Is there a follow-up appointment scheduled? Can it be moved to an earlier date?

Warning Signs of Suicide and How to Deal with It

Table 68.1. Continued

Ask Your Family Member (Be Honest and Direct with Your Questions and Concerns)	Ask the Treatment Team (Including Doctor, Therapist, Nurse, Social Worker, and So On)
What else can I/we do to help you after you leave the emergency department?	What is my role as a family member in the safety plan?
Will you agree to talk with me/us if your suicidal feelings return? If not, is there someone else you can talk to?	What should we look for, and when should we seek more help, such as returning to the emergency department or contacting other local resources and providers?
Remember: It is critical for the patient to schedule a follow-up appointment as soon as possible after discharge from the emergency department.	

WHAT YOU NEED TO KNOW

Make safety a priority for your relative recovering from a suicide attempt. Research has shown that a person who has attempted to end his or her life has a much higher risk of later dying by suicide. Safety is ultimately an individual's responsibility, but often a person who feels suicidal has a difficult time making good choices. As a family member, you can help your loved one make a better choice while reducing the risk.

Reduce the Risk at Home

To help reduce the risk of self-harm or suicide at home, here are some things to consider:
- Guns are high-risk and the leading means of death for suicidal people. They should be taken out of the home and secured.
- Overdoses are common and can be lethal. If it is necessary to keep pain relievers such as aspirin, Advil, and Tylenol in the home, only keep small quantities or consider keeping medications in a locked container. Remove unused or expired medicine from the home.
- Alcohol use or abuse can decrease inhibitions and cause people to act more freely on their feelings. As with pain relievers, keep only small quantities of alcohol in the home or none at all.

Create a Safety Plan
Following a suicide attempt, a safety plan should be created to help prevent another attempt. The plan should be a joint effort between your relative and his or her doctor, therapist, or the emergency department staff and you. As a family member, you should know your relative's safety plan and understand your role in it, including:
- knowing your family member's "triggers," such as an anniversary of a loss, alcohol, or stress from relationships
- building support for your family member with mental health professionals, family, friends, and community resources
- working with your family member's strengths to promote his or her safety
- promoting communication and honesty in your relationship with your family member

Remember that safety cannot be guaranteed by anyone—the goal is to reduce the risks and build support for everyone in the family. However, it is important for you to believe that the safety plan can help keep your relative safe. If you do not feel that it can, let the emergency department staff know before you leave.

Maintain Hope and Self-Care
Families commonly provide a safety net and a vision of hope for their suicidal relative, and that can be emotionally exhausting. Never try to handle this situation alone—get support from friends, relatives, and organizations such as the National Alliance on Mental Illness (NAMI) and get professional input whenever possible.

MOVING FORWARD
Emergency department care is by nature short-term and crisis-oriented, but some longer-term interventions have been shown to help reduce suicidal behavior and thoughts. You and your relative can talk to the doctor about various treatments for mental illnesses that may help reduce the risk of suicide for people diagnosed with

Warning Signs of Suicide and How to Deal with It

illnesses such as schizophrenia, bipolar disorder, or depression. Often, these illnesses require multiple types of interventions, and your relative may benefit from a second opinion from a specialist.

If your relative abuses alcohol or other drugs, it is also important to seek help for this problem, along with suicidal behavior. Seek out a substance abuse specialist. Contact your local substance abuse treatment provider by calling 800-662-4357 or visiting www.findtreatment.samhsa.gov, or contact groups such as Alcoholics Anonymous (AA) or Narcotics Anonymous (NA) to help your loved one; Al-Anon may be a good resource for you as a family member. If it is available in your area, an integrated treatment program such as assertive community treatment (ACT) may provide better outcomes than traditional care for some severely ill individuals.

Ultimately, please reach out for help in supporting your family member and yourself through this crisis.

Remember that the emergency department is open 24 hours a day, 365 days a year, to treat your family member if the problem continues and if your family member's medical team is unavailable to provide the needed care.[7]

---

[7] "After an Attempt," Substance Abuse and Mental Health Services Administration (SAMHSA), 2018. Available online. URL: https://store.samhsa.gov/sites/default/files/d7/priv/sma18-4357eng.pdf. Accessed Marc`h 17, 2023.

Chapter 69 | Recovering from a Suicide Attempt

The time right after your suicide attempt can be the most confusing and emotional part of your entire life. In some ways, it may even be more difficult than the time preceding your attempt. Not only are you still facing the thoughts and feelings that led you to consider suicide, but now you may also be struggling to figure out what to do since you survived.

It is likely that your decision to try to kill yourself did not come out of the blue. It probably developed over time, perhaps from overwhelming feelings that seemed too much to bear. Experiencing these emotions might have been especially difficult if you had to deal with them alone. A variety of stressful situations can lead to suicidal feelings, including the loss of a loved one, relationship issues, financial difficulties, health problems, trauma, depression, or other mental health concerns. It is possible that you were experiencing some of these problems when you started to think about suicide.

While the events that lead to a suicide attempt can vary from person to person, a common theme that many suicide attempt survivors report is the need to feel relief. At desperate moments, when it feels like nothing else is working, suicide may seem like the only way to get relief from unbearable emotional pain.

Just as it took time for the pain that led to your suicide attempt to become unbearable, it may also take some time for it to subside. That is okay. The important thing is that you are still here; you are alive, which means you have time to find healthier and more effective ways to cope with your pain.

WHAT ARE YOU FEELING RIGHT NOW?

Right now, you are probably experiencing many conflicting emotions. You may be thinking:

- "Why am I still here? I wish I were dead. I could not even do this right."
- "I do not know if I can get through this. I do not even have the energy to try."
- "I cannot do this alone."
- "How do I tell anyone about this? What do I say to them? What will they think of me?"
- "Maybe someone will pay attention to me now; maybe someone will help me."
- "Maybe there is a reason I survived. How do I figure out what that reason is?"

Right after a suicide attempt, many survivors have said that the pain that led them to harm themselves was still present. Some felt angry that they had survived their attempts. Others felt embarrassed, ashamed, or guilty that they put their family and friends through a difficult situation. Most felt alone and said they had no idea how to go on living. They did not know what to expect and even questioned whether they had the strength to stay alive. Still, others felt that if they survived their attempt, there must be some reason they were still alive, and they wanted to discover why.

You are probably experiencing some of the same feelings and may be wondering how others have faced these challenges.

ARE YOU THE ONLY ONE WHO FEELS THIS WAY?

Knowing how others made it through can help you learn ways to recover from your own suicide attempt.

It is estimated that more than 1 million people attempt suicide each year in the United States from all parts of society. In other words, you are not alone. However, it can be hard to know how other survivors recovered because suicide is a personal topic that often is not discussed openly and honestly. This can leave those affected feeling like they do not know where to turn.

Recovering from a Suicide Attempt

Shame, dreading the reaction of others, and fear of being hospitalized are some of the reasons that prevent people from talking about suicide. This is unfortunate because direct and open communication about suicide can help prevent people from acting on suicidal thoughts.

It is okay if you feel conflicting emotions right now. Other suicide attempt survivors know that what they are experiencing is normal. They understand that your concerns are real. Going on will not be easy, and finding a way to ease your emotional pain may be challenging, but this can be a time to start down a new path toward a better life—to start your journey toward help and hope.

Those who have recovered from a suicide attempt want you to know the following:

- You are not alone. You matter. Life can get better. It may be difficult, but the effort you invest in your recovery will be worth it.
- Right now, moving forward may seem impossible. And, while it probably will not be easy, many other survivors will tell you that they are glad they held on and worked for a better life. By taking a few steps now and then a few more when you are ready, you can regain your strength.
- Sometimes, it can be helpful just to take a few steps forward, even when you do not feel like it. In fact, you might start to remember that others care about you. You might discover that suicide is not the only way to relieve your pain. You may find that your feelings will change, either on your own or by working with a counselor.

TAKING THE FIRST STEPS

Making big changes right now might be out of the question for you. You may not even know where to begin. That is okay. Recovery is a process, and it is important that you move at your own pace. There are a few things you might want to do to ease your transition back to everyday life:

- First, it might be less stressful to decide in advance how to deal with others' questions about your suicide

attempt. The people around you may be surprised by your suicide attempt and have questions or comments about what happened. Thinking about what you might say in advance can help you prepare for their reactions.
- Second, reestablishing connections may help you feel better. Often, the stress or depression that leads to a suicide attempt can cause people to disconnect from others who care about them or the things they used to enjoy doing. Reconnecting with the people and things you love or loved can help instill hope.
- Third, because suicidal thoughts might return, you will want to be prepared with a plan to stay safe. A safety plan is a tool that can help you identify triggers (such as events or experiences) that lead to suicidal thoughts and can help you cope if the pain that led to your suicide attempt returns.
- Fourth, finding and working with a counselor can help you start to recover. Unlike friends or family, a counselor is an unbiased listener who will not be personally affected by your suicide attempt. The counselor's role is to help you sort through your feelings and find ways to feel better. A counselor can be a peer supporter, a psychiatrist, a social worker, a psychologist, or other skilled people. If counseling is not possible, there are also ways you can help yourself, but remember that you do not have to go through this alone.

TALKING WITH OTHERS ABOUT YOUR ATTEMPT

One of the most difficult tasks you might face will be responding to the questions people ask about your suicide attempt. The shame, guilt, confusion, and other emotions that might follow an attempt can make it tough to speak about it with others, especially if people respond in a way that does not feel supportive.

Often, those closest to you may be feeling lots of emotions about your attempt. They may be scared, confused, or angry about what happened, causing them to focus on their own feelings rather than being as supportive as you need them to be. Their reactions might hurt you, whether they mean to or not.

To make it easier, here are some suggestions that can be helpful.

It Is Your Story to Tell, or Not

The details of your experience are personal, and it is up to you to determine what you want to share and with whom. Sharing what happened with your doctors, nurses, counselors, or peer supporters can help them give you the right kind of support. In most cases, they are required to keep the details of what you share confidential.

You may want to share some of the details and your feelings about what happened with other people you trust, such as family or friends. How much you share or the details you decide to give are up to you and what you feel comfortable with.

People Do Not Always Say the Right Things

It is difficult to predict how people will respond when they learn that you tried to kill yourself. Some people might change the subject or avoid the topic altogether because of their fear of death or suicide. Others who are close to you may be confused, hurt, or angry about what has happened. They may judge or blame you. They may feel betrayed or be wondering what they could have done to prevent you from attempting suicide.

Often, those who care the most about you have the strongest reactions to your suicide attempt because they cannot imagine life without you. It is helpful to remember that a strong reaction may reflect your family's or friends' depth of concern about you.

Sometimes, you may feel that they are overly controlling. It may seem like they are watching everything you do or will not leave you alone because they are afraid you may attempt suicide again. This can be very frustrating when you are trying to recover from an attempt.

It can take time to repair the trust in your relationships. If you can show that you are committed to safety, it might allow those close to you to feel more comfortable giving you the space you need.

Learning more about suicide can help the people who care about you be more supportive. If they better understand what led to your suicide attempt, they might be better able to give you what you need, especially if you communicate your needs in a clear and direct way.

Direct Communication May Help You Get What You Need

While it may be hard for you to talk about what happened, it is also important for you to try your best to be direct in communicating what you need. It may seem obvious to you, but others may not understand or know the best way to support you. This period can be challenging because you might want to ask people for help, but you do not want to scare anyone if you are still struggling. This is especially true if you are concerned that people might overreact and insist on care in a hospital when you believe you just need more support and understanding.

A system for monitoring the intensity of your suicidal thoughts, should you have them, can help you notice if things are getting better or worse. It can also help you communicate how much assistance you need from those supporting you. Using a scale from one to five (with one being minimal distress or no thoughts of suicide and five being extreme distress and thoughts of imminent suicide) can make it easier to express how you are feeling. Take note of not only what is going on around you and through your mind when you are at a "four" or a "five" but also when you are at a "one" or a "two." These may be situations, people, or strengths that will help you get through the hard days.

Support Can Make Things Easier

It might be hard at first, but having someone you feel comfortable talking to after your attempt is very important. You may face some challenges as you move forward; knowing there is at least one person you can turn to will make the road to recovery less daunting. Being alone with suicidal thoughts can be dangerous. Having supportive people around you and educating them on how to help you can be a crucial part of staying safe.

Recovering from a Suicide Attempt

Ask Yourself, "What Do I Need from a Support Person?"
Different people need different things after a suicide attempt, so make sure the person you choose meets your unique needs. Maybe you need someone who will listen to you without judgment, or maybe you need someone who will come and be with you when you are feeling alone. Perhaps it would be helpful to have someone close to you who can go with you to appointments, or perhaps you want to schedule regular phone calls with a trusted friend. No matter what kind of assistance you need, it is helpful to have at least one person with whom you can share your thoughts of suicide—someone who will stay calm and help you when you need support. Once you know what you need, it may be easier to find someone to help. And remember, because you might not get everything you need from one person, it can be helpful to have a variety of people available to support you, if possible.

REESTABLISHING CONNECTIONS
It is likely that the overwhelming life events, stress, and depression that led to your suicide attempt affected your ability to enjoy life. Struggling with suicidal thoughts can be exhausting and leave you with little energy to do the things you once loved. It can also put stress on your relationships with friends and family. The irony of depression and suicidal thinking is that they may cause you to give up the things in life that help you feel better just when you need them the most.

Even up until the moment of their attempts, many suicide attempt survivors report that there was an internal struggle going on inside them. One side argued that suicide was the best way to end the pain they were experiencing. The other side struggled to find another way to feel better. To put it another way, most people with suicidal thoughts had reasons for dying and reasons for living.

Before your suicide attempt, you might have lost connections to your reasons for living, but it is important to reestablish those connections because they can help instill hope. They can remind you about the things you love in life. Personalizing this can help remind you of where you were before you started to feel suicidal and where you would like to be again.

PLANNING TO STAY SAFE

You might still have thoughts of suicide after your attempt, even if you have decided that you want to stay alive. Perhaps the pain that led to your suicide attempt is still there. It is okay to have suicidal thoughts. Everyone needs to feel relief from unbearable pain, and suicidal thoughts may be one of the ways you have learned to cope. What is important is that you do not act on those thoughts and that you try to find other safer ways to ease your pain. A safety plan can help you do this.

MOVING TOWARD A HOPEFUL FUTURE

After you have taken your first steps back into daily life, it might be time to consider taking on a few more challenges. You have already made it through the toughest part. Now it is time to think about doing some things that can give you a greater sense of well-being and happiness.[1]

---

[1] "A Journey toward Health and Hope," Substance Abuse and Mental Health Services Administration (SAMHSA), 2015. Available online. URL: https://store.samhsa.gov/sites/default/files/d7/priv/sma15-4419.pdf. Accessed March 16, 2023.

Part 9 | Additional Help and Information

Chapter 70 | Glossary of Terms Related to Depression

agitation: A condition in which a person is unable to relax and be still. The person may be very tense and irritable and become easily annoyed by small things.

Alzheimer disease (AD): A brain disorder that slowly destroys memory and thinking skills and, eventually, the ability to carry out the simplest tasks. It is the most common cause of dementia among older adults.

anticonvulsant: A drug or other substance used to prevent or stop seizures or convulsions. Also called "antiepileptic."

antidepressant: Medication used to treat depression and other mood and anxiety disorders.

antipsychotic: Medication used to treat psychosis.

anxiety: An abnormal sense of fear, nervousness, and apprehension about something that might happen in the future.

anxiety disorder: Any of a group of illnesses that fill people's lives with overwhelming anxieties and fears that are chronic and unremitting. Anxiety disorders include panic disorder, obsessive-compulsive disorder (OCD), posttraumatic stress disorder (PTSD), phobias, and generalized anxiety disorder (GAD).

avoidance: One of the symptoms of posttraumatic stress disorder (PTSD). Those with PTSD avoid situations and reminders of their trauma.

behavioral therapy: This therapy focuses on a person's actions and aims to change unhealthy behavior patterns.

This glossary contains terms excerpted from documents produced by several sources deemed reliable.

benzodiazepine: A type of central nervous system (CNS) depressant prescribed to relieve anxiety and sleep problems. Valium and Xanax are among the most widely prescribed medications.

bipolar disorder: A depressive disorder in which a person alternates between episodes of major depression and mania (periods of abnormally and persistently elevated mood). Also referred to as manic depression.

cognition: Conscious mental activities (such as thinking, communicating, understanding, solving problems, processing information, and remembering) that are associated with gaining knowledge and understanding.

cognitive-behavioral therapy (CBT): This therapy helps people focus on how to solve their current problems. The therapist helps the patient learn how to identify distorted or unhelpful thinking patterns, recognize and change inaccurate beliefs, relate to others in more positive ways, and change behaviors accordingly.

deep brain stimulation: A neurosurgical treatment utilizing a neurostimulator placed in the brain to deliver electrical signals to specific parts of the brain to help control unwanted movements such as in Parkinson disease (PD) or regulate the firing of neurons in the brain to help control the symptoms of disorders such as epilepsy or depression.

delusions: Beliefs that have no basis in reality.

dementia: Loss of brain function that occurs with certain diseases. It affects memory, thinking, language, judgment, and behavior.

depression: A mental condition marked by ongoing feelings of sadness, despair, loss of energy, and difficulty dealing with normal daily life. Other symptoms of depression include feelings of worthlessness and hopelessness, loss of pleasure in activities, changes in eating or sleeping habits, and thoughts of death or suicide.

dysthymia: A depressive disorder that is less severe than major depressive disorder but is more persistent.

eating disorder: Eating disorders, such as anorexia nervosa (AN), bulimia nervosa (BN), and binge eating disorder (BED), involve serious problems with eating. This could include an extreme decrease of food or severe overeating, as well as feelings of distress and concern about body shape or weight.

electroconvulsive therapy (ECT): A treatment for severe depression that is usually used only when people do not respond to medications and

Glossary of Terms Related to Depression

psychotherapy. ECT involves passing a low-voltage electric current through the brain. The person is under anesthesia at the time of treatment.

emotional distress: Feelings of depression, fear, and anxiety that can happen after being diagnosed with cancer.

fibromyalgia: A disorder that causes aches and pain all over the body and involves tender points on specific places on the neck, shoulders, back, hips, arms, and legs that hurt when pressure is put on them.

hallucinations: Hearing, seeing, touching, smelling, or tasting things that are not real.

hypertension: Also called "high blood pressure," it is having blood pressure greater than 0 over 90 millimeters of mercury (mmHg). Long-term high blood pressure can damage blood vessels and organs, including the heart, kidneys, eyes, and brain.

insomnia: Not being able to sleep.

interpersonal therapy (IPT): This therapy is based on the idea that improving communication patterns and the ways people relate to others will effectively treat depression. IPT helps identify how a person interacts with other people. When a behavior is causing problems, IPT guides the person to change the behavior.

ischemia: Lack of blood supply to a part of the body. Ischemia may cause tissue damage due to the lack of oxygen and nutrients.

light therapy: This type of therapy is used to treat seasonal affective disorder (SAD), a form of depression that usually occurs during the autumn and winter months when the amount of natural sunlight decreases. During light therapy, a person sits in front of a "light box" for periods of time, usually in the morning. The box emits a full spectrum light, and sitting in front of it appears to help reset the body's daily rhythms.

major depressive disorder (MDD): Also called "major depression," this is a combination of symptoms that interfere with a person's ability to work, sleep, study, eat, and enjoy once-pleasurable activities.

mania: Feelings of intense mental and physical hyperactivity, elevated mood, and agitation.

meditation: It is a type of mind and body practice. There are many types of meditation, most of which originated in ancient religious and spiritual traditions. Some forms of meditation instruct the practitioner to become mindful of thoughts, feelings, and sensations and to observe them in a nonjudgmental way.

mental health: A state of successful performance of mental function, resulting in productive activities, fulfilling relationships with other people, and the ability to adapt to change and to cope with adversity. Mental health is indispensable to personal well-being, family and interpersonal relationships, and contribution to the community or society.

mental illness: A health condition that changes a person's thinking, feelings, or behavior (or all three) and that causes the person distress and difficulty in functioning.

migraine: Headaches that are usually pulsing or throbbing and occur on one or both sides of the head. They are moderate to severe in intensity, associated with nausea, vomiting, sensitivity to light and noise, and worsen with routine physical activity.

mood disorders: Mental disorders primarily affecting a person's mood.

obsessive-compulsive disorder (OCD): An anxiety disorder in which a person suffers from obsessive thoughts and compulsive actions, such as cleaning, checking, counting, or hoarding. The person becomes trapped in a pattern of repetitive thoughts and behaviors that are senseless and distressing but very hard to stop.

panic disorder: An anxiety disorder in which a person suffers from sudden attacks of fear and panic. The attacks may occur without a known reason, but many times, they are triggered by events or thoughts that produce fear in the person, such as taking an elevator or driving.

phobia: An anxiety disorder in which a person suffers from an unusual amount of fear of a certain activity or situation.

physical therapy: Therapy aimed to restore movement, balance, and coordination.

postpartum depression: This type of depression is experienced when a new mother has a major depressive episode within one month after delivery.

posttraumatic stress disorder (PTSD): An anxiety disorder that can occur after you have been through a traumatic event.

premenstrual dysphoric disorder (PMDD): A severe form of premenstrual syndrome, which causes feelings of sadness or despair, or even thoughts of suicide, feelings of tension or anxiety, panic attacks, mood swings or frequent crying, and other severe symptoms.

Glossary of Terms Related to Depression

psychiatrist: A doctor who treats mental illness. Psychiatrists must receive additional training and serve a supervised residency in their specialty. They can prescribe medications.

psychoeducation: Learning about mental illness and ways to communicate, solve problems, and cope.

psychosis: Conditions that affect the mind, where there has been some loss of contact with reality. When someone becomes ill in this way, it is called a "psychotic episode."

psychotherapy: A treatment method for mental illness in which a mental health professional (psychiatrist, psychologist, counselor) and a patient discuss problems and feelings to find solutions. Psychotherapy can help individuals change their thought or behavior patterns or understand how past experiences affect current behaviors.

resilience: The ability to successfully adapt to stressors, maintaining psychological well-being in the face of adversity. It is the ability to "bounce back" from difficult experiences.

schizoaffective disorder: A mental condition that causes both a loss of contact with reality (psychosis) and mood problems (depression or mania).

schizophrenia: A severe mental disorder that appears in late adolescence or early adulthood. People with schizophrenia may have hallucinations, delusions, loss of personality, confusion, agitation, social withdrawal, psychosis, and/or extremely odd behavior.

seasonal affective disorder (SAD): A depression during the winter months when there is less natural sunlight.

serotonin syndrome: This syndrome usually occurs when older antidepressants are combined with selective serotonin reuptake inhibitors. A person with serotonin syndrome may be agitated, have hallucinations (see or hear things that are not real), have a high temperature, or have unusual blood pressure changes.

social phobia: A strong fear of being judged by others and of being embarrassed. This fear can be so strong that it gets in the way of going to work or school or doing other everyday things.

St. John's wort: A plant with yellow flowers that has been used for centuries for health purposes, including depression and anxiety.

stimulants: A class of drugs that enhance the activity of monamines (such as dopamine) in the brain, increasing arousal, heart rate, blood pressure, and respiration, and decreasing appetite; they include some medications used to treat attention deficit hyperactivity disorder (ADHD; e.g., methylphenidate and amphetamines), as well as cocaine and methamphetamine.

suicide: Death caused by self-directed injurious behavior with any intent to die as a result of the behavior.

tolerance: A condition in which higher doses of a drug are required to produce the same effect achieved during initial use; often associated with physical dependence.

trauma: A life-threatening event, such as military combat, natural disasters, terrorist incidents, serious accidents, or physical or sexual assault in adult or childhood.

yoga: An ancient system of practices used to balance the mind and body through exercise, meditation (focusing thoughts), and control of breathing and emotions.

Chapter 71 | Directory of Organizations That Help People with Depression and Suicidal Thoughts

GOVERNMENT AGENCIES

Agency for Healthcare Research and Quality (AHRQ)
5600 Fishers Ln.
7th Fl.
Rockville, MD 20857
Phone: 301-427-1104
Website: www.ahrq.gov

Centers for Disease Control and Prevention (CDC)
1600 Clifton Rd.
Atlanta, GA 30329-4027
Toll-Free: 800-CDC-INFO
(800-232-4636)
Toll-Free TTY: 888-232-6348
Website: www.cdc.gov

Child Welfare Information Gateway
330 C St., S.W.
Washington, DC 20201
Toll-Free: 800-394-3366
Website: www.childwelfare.gov
Email: info@childwelfare.gov

girlshealth.gov
200 Independence Ave., S.W.
Rm. 712E
Washington, DC 20201
Toll-Free: 800-994-9662
Website: www.girlshealth.gov

Resources in this chapter were compiled from several sources deemed reliable; all contact information was verified and updated in May 2023.

Globalchange.gov
1800 G St., N.W., Ste. 9100
Washington, DC 20006
Phone: 202-223-6262
Fax: 202-223-3065
Website: www.globalchange.gov

HealthCare.gov
Toll-Free: 800-318-2596
Toll-Free TTY: 855-889-4325
Website: www.healthcare.gov

healthfinder.gov
1101 Wootton Pkwy., Ste. 420
Rockville, MD 20852
Website: www.healthfinder.gov

Health Resources and Services Administration (HRSA)
5600 Fishers Ln.
Rockville, MD 20857
Toll-Free: 877-464-4772
Toll-Free TTY: 877-897-9910
Website: www.hrsa.gov

National Cancer Institute (NCI)
9609 Medical Center Dr.
BG 9609, MSC 9760
Bethesda, MD 20892-9760
Phone: 240-276-6600
Toll-Free: 800-4-CANCER
(800-422-6237)
Website: www.cancer.gov
Email: NCIinfo@nih.gov

National Center for Complementary and Integrative Health (NCCIH)
9000 Rockville Pike
Bethesda, MD 20892
Toll-Free: 888-644-6226
Toll-Free TTY: 866-464-3615
Website: www.nccih.nih.gov
Email: info@nccih.nih.gov

National Center for Health Statistics (NCHS)
3311 Toledo Rd.
Hyattsville, MD 20782-2064
Phone: 301-458-4901
Website: www.cdc.gov/nchs
Email: nhis@cdc.gov

National Center for Posttraumatic Stress Disorder (NCPTSD)
215 N. Main St.
White River Junction, VT 05009
Phone: 802-296-6300
Fax: 802-296-5135
Website: www.ptsd.va.gov
Email: ncptsd@va.gov

National Institute of Mental Health (NIMH)
6001 Executive Blvd.
Rm. 6200, MSC 9663
Bethesda, MD 20892-9663
Phone: 301-443-4513
Toll-Free: 866-615-6464
TTY: 301-443-8431
Toll-Free TTY: 866-415-8051
Fax: 301-443-4279
Website: www.nimh.nih.gov
Email: nimhinfo@nih.gov

Directory of Organizations

National Institute on Aging (NIA)
31 Center Dr.
Bldg. 31C
Bethesda, MD 20894
Toll-Free: 800-222-2225
Toll-Free TTY: 800-222-4225
Website: www.nia.nih.gov
Email: niaic@nia.nih.gov

National Institutes of Health (NIH)
9000 Rockville Pike
Bethesda, MD 20892
Phone: 301-496-4000
TTY: 301-402-9612
Website: www.nih.gov

Office of Disability Employment Policy (ODEP)
200 Constitution Ave., N.W.
Washington, DC 20210
Phone: 202-693-7880
Toll-Free: 866-ODEP-DOL
(866-633-7365)
Website: www.dol.gov/odep
Email: odep@dol.gov

Office of Minority Health (OMH) Resource Center
1101 Wootton Pkwy., Ste. 100
Tower Oaks Bldg.
Rockville, MD 20852
Toll-Free: 800-444-6472
TDD: 301-251-1432
Fax: 301-251-2160
Website: minorityhealth.hhs.gov
Email: info@minorityhealth.hhs.gov

Substance Abuse and Mental Health Services Administration (SAMHSA)
5600 Fishers Ln.
Rockville, MD 20857
Toll-Free: 877-SAMHSA-7
(877-726-4727)
Toll-Free TTY: 800-487-4889
Website: www.samhsa.gov
Email: SAMHSAInfo@samhsa.hhs.gov

U.S. Department of Education (ED)
400 Maryland Ave., S.W.
Washington, DC 20202
Phone: 202-401-2000
Toll-Free: 800-USA-LEARN
(800-872-5327)
Website: www.ed.gov

U.S. Department of Health and Human Services (HHS)
200 Independence Ave., S.W.
Hubert H. Humphrey Bldg.
Washington, DC 20201
Toll-Free: 877-696-6775
Website: www.hhs.gov

U.S. Equal Employment Opportunity Commission (EEOC)
131 M St., N.E.
Washington, DC 20507
Toll-Free: 800-669-4000
Toll-Free TTY: 800-669-6820
Website: www.eeoc.gov
Email: info@eeoc.gov

U.S. Food and Drug Administration (FDA)
10903 New Hampshire Ave.
Silver Spring, MD 20993-0002
Phone: 301-796-8240
Toll-Free: 888-INFO-FDA (888-463-6332)
Toll-Free TTY: 866-300-4374
Website: www.fda.gov

U.S. National Library of Medicine (NLM)
8600 Rockville Pike
Bethesda, MD 20894
Phone: 301-594-5983
Toll-Free: 888-FIND-NLM (888-346-3656)
Website: www.nlm.nih.gov
Email: NLMCommunications@nih.gov

PRIVATE AGENCIES

Alzheimer's Association
225 N. Michigan Ave.
17th Fl.
Chicago, IL 60601
Toll-Free: 800-272-3900
Website: www.alz.org

American Academy of Child and Adolescent Psychiatry (AACAP)
3615 Wisconsin Ave., N.W.
Washington, DC 20016-3007
Phone: 202-966-7300
Fax: 202-464-0131
Website: www.aacap.org
Email: executive@aacap.org

American Academy of Family Physicians (AAFP)
11400 Tomahawk Creek Pkwy.
Leawood, KS 66211
Toll-Free: 800-274-2237
Website: www.aafp.org
Email: aafp@aafp.org

American Academy of Pediatrics (AAP)
345 Park Blvd.
Itasca, IL 60143
Toll-Free: 800-433-9016
Fax: 847-434-8000
Website: www.aap.org

American Art Therapy Association (AATA)
4875 Eisenhower Ave., Ste. 240
Alexandria, VA 22304
Phone: 703-548-5860
Toll-Free: 888-290-0878
Fax: 703-783-8468
Website: www.arttherapy.org
Email: info@arttherapy.org

American Association for Geriatric Psychiatry (AAGP)
6728 Old McLean Village Dr.
McLean, VA 22101
Phone: 703-884-9453
Fax: 703-556-8729
Website: www.aagponline.org
Email: info@aagponline.org

Directory of Organizations

American Association for Marriage and Family Therapy (AAMFT)
277 S. Washington St., Ste. 210
Alexandria, VA 22314
Phone: 703-838-9808
Fax: 703-838-9805
Website: www.aamft.org
Email: central@aamft.org

American Association of Suicidology (AAS)
448 Walton Ave., Ste. 790
Hummelstown, PA 17036
Toll-Free: 888-977-3836
Website: www.suicidology.org
Email: Info@suicidology.org

American College Health Association (ACHA)
8455 Colesville Rd., Ste. 740
Silver Spring, MD 20910
Phone: 410-859-1500
Fax: 410-859-1510
Website: www.acha.org
Email: contact@acha.org

American Foundation for Suicide Prevention (AFSP)
199 Water St.
11th Fl.
New York, NY 10038
Phone: 212-363-3500
Toll-Free: 888-333-AFSP
(888-333-2377)
Fax: 646-435-0978
Website: www.afsp.org
Email: info@afsp.org

American Medical Association (AMA)
330 N. Wabash Ave., Ste. 39300
AMA Plaza
Chicago, IL 60611-5885
Phone: 312-464-4782
Toll-Free: 800-262-3211
Website: www.ama-assn.org

American Psychiatric Association (APA)
800 Maine Ave., S.W., Ste. 900
Washington, DC 20024
Phone: 202-559-3900
Toll-Free: 888-35-PSYCH
(888-357-7924)
Website: www.psychiatry.org
Email: apa@psych.org

American Psychological Association (APA)
750 1st St., N.E.
Washington, DC 20002-4242
Phone: 202-336-5500
Toll-Free: 800-374-2721
TDD/TTY: 202-336-6123
Website: www.apa.org

American Psychotherapy Association
2750 E. Sunshine St.
Springfield, MO 65804
Phone: 417-823-0173
Toll-Free: 800-205-9165
Website: www.americanpsychotherapy.com

Anxiety and Depression Association of America (ADAA)
8701 Georgia Ave., Ste. 412
Silver Spring, MD 20910
Toll-Free: 800-273-TALK
(800-273-8255)
Website: www.adaa.org
Email: information@adaa.org

Arthritis Foundation
1355 Peachtree St., N.E., Ste. 6
Atlanta, GA 30309
Toll-Free: 800-283-7800
Website: www.arthritis.org
Email: corporate@arthritis.org

Association for Behavioral and Cognitive Therapies (ABCT)
305 7th Ave.
16th Fl.
New York, NY 10001
Phone: 212-647-1890
Fax: 212-647-1865
Website: www.abct.org

Beacon Tree Foundation
9201 Arboretum Pkwy., Ste. 140
N. Chesterfield, VA 23236
Toll-Free: 800-414-6427
Website: www.beacontree.org
Email: info@beacontree.org

Brain and Behavior Research Foundation
747 3rd Ave.
33rd Fl.
New York, NY 10017
Phone: 646-681-4888
Toll-Free: 800-829-8289
Website: www.bbrfoundation.org
Email: info@bbrfoundation.org

Brain Injury Association of America (BIAA)
3057 Nutley St. 805
Fairfax, VA 22031-1931
Phone: 703-761-0750
Toll-Free: 800-444-6443
Fax: 703-761-0755
Website: www.biausa.org
Email: info@biausa.org

Caring.com
P.O. Box 32217
Charlotte, NC 28232
Toll-Free: 800-973-1540
Website: www.caring.com

Center for Anxiety™
200 W. 57th St., Ste. 1008
New York, NY 10019
Phone: 646-837-5557
Toll-Free: 888-837-7473
Fax: 646-837-5495
Website: www.centerforanxiety.org
Email: info@centerforanxiety.org

Directory of Organizations

Cleveland Clinic
9500 Euclid Ave.
Cleveland, OH 44195
Phone: 216-444-2200
Toll-Free: 800-223-2273
Website: my.clevelandclinic.org

The Dana Foundation
1270 Avenue of the Americas
12th Fl.
New York, NY 10020
Phone: 212-223-4040
Fax: 212-317-8721
Website: www.dana.org
Email: danainfo@dana.org

Depressed Anonymous (DA)
P.O. Box 17414
Louisville, KY 40214
Phone: 502-569-1989
Website: www.depressedanon.com

Depression and Bipolar Support Alliance (DBSA)
55 E. Jackson Blvd., Ste. 490
Chicago, IL 60604
Toll-Free: 800-826-3632
Fax: 312-642-7243
Website: www.dbsalliance.org
Email: info@DBSAlliance.org

Family Caregiver Alliance (FCA)
235 Montgomery St., Ste. 930
San Francisco, CA 94104
Phone: 415-434-3388
Toll-Free: 800-445-8106
Website: www.caregiver.org
Email: info@caregiver.org

Geriatric Mental Health Foundation (GMHF)
6728 Old McLean Village Dr.
McLean, VA 22101
Phone: 703-884-9453
Fax: 703-556-8729
Website: www.gmhfonline.org

International Foundation for Research and Education on Depression (iFred)
P.O. Box 17598
Baltimore, MD 21297
Fax: 443-782-0739
Website: www.ifred.org
Email: info@ifred.org

International OCD Foundation (IOCDF)
P.O. Box 961029
Boston, MA 02196
Phone: 617-973-5801
Fax: 617-973-5801
Website: www.iocdf.org
Email: info@iocdf.org

Kristin Brooks Hope Center (KBHC)
Website: www.imalive.org/about-kbhc
Email: info@imalive.org

Mental Health America (MHA)
500 Montgomery St., Ste. 820
Alexandria, VA 22314
Phone: 703-684-7722
Toll-Free: 800-969-6642
Fax: 703-684-5968
Website: www.mentalhealthamerica.net

Multiple Sclerosis Association of America (MSAA)
375 Kings Hwy. N.
Cherry Hill, NJ 08034
Toll-Free: 800-532-7667
Fax: 856-661-9797
Website: www.mymsaa.org
Email: msaa@mymsaa.org

National Alliance on Mental Illness (NAMI)
4301 Wilson Blvd., Ste. 300
Arlington, VA 22203
Phone: 703-524-7600
Toll-Free: 800-950-NAMI
(800-950-6264)
Website: www.nami.org

National Association of Anorexia Nervosa and Associated Disorders (ANAD)
P.O. Box 409047
Chicago, IL 60640
Toll-Free: 888-375-7767
Website: www.anad.org
Email: hello@anad.org

National Association of School Psychologists (NASP)
4340 East-West Hwy., Ste. 402
Bethesda, MD 20814
Phone: 301-657-0270
Toll-Free: 866-331-NASP
(866-331-6277)
Fax: 301-657-0275
Website: www.nasponline.org

National Eating Disorders Association (NEDA)
333 Mamaroneck Ave., Ste. 214
White Plains, NY 10605
Phone: 212-575-6200
Toll-Free: 800-931-2237
Website: www.nationaleatingdisorders.org
Email: info@NationalEatingDisorders.org

National Federation of Families for Children's Mental Health (NFFCMH)
15800 Crabbs Branch Way, Ste. 300
Rockville, MD 20855
Phone: 240-403-1901
Website: www.ffcmh.org
Email: ffcmh@ffcmh.org

The Nemours Foundation
10140 Centurion Pkwy.
N. Jacksonville, FL 32256
Phone: 904-697-4100
Website: www.nemours.org

988 Suicide and Crisis Lifeline
Toll-Free: 800-273-8255
Website: 988lifeline.org

Parkinson's Foundation
1359 Bdwy., Ste. 1509
New York, NY 10018
Toll-Free: 800-4PD-INFO
(800-473-4636)
Website: www.parkinson.org
Email: contact@parkinson.org

Directory of Organizations

Postpartum Support International (PSI)
6706 S.W. 54th Ave.
Portland, OR 97219
Phone: 503-894-9453
Toll-Free: 800-944-4PPD (800-944-4773)
Fax: 503-894-9452
Website: www.postpartum.net
Email: psioffice@postpartum.net

Schizophrenia & Psychosis Action Alliance (S&PAA)
2308 Mount Vernon Ave., Ste. 207
Alexandria, VA 22301-1328
Phone: 240-423-9432
Toll-Free: 800-493-2094
Website: sczaction.org
Email: info@sczaction.org

Suicide Awareness Voices of Education (SAVE)
7900 Xerxes Ave., S., Ste. 810
Bloomington, MN 55431
Phone: 952-946-7998
Website: www.save.org
Email: save@save.org

Suicide Prevention Resource Center (SPRC)
1000 N.E., 13th St., Ste. 5900
Nicholson Twr.
Oklahoma City, OK 73104
Website: www.sprc.org

INDEX

INDEX

INDEX

Page numbers followed by "n" refer to citation information; by "t" indicate tables; and by "f" indicate figures.

A

abuse
    anxiety disorders 194
    depression and trauma 183
    mental illness 4
    posttraumatic stress disorder (PTSD) 455
    suicide 518
    teen depression 103
    treatment-resistant depression (TRD) 412
    women and depression 66
acceptance and commitment therapy (ACT), overview 337–339
ACEs *see* adverse childhood experiences
acquired immunodeficiency syndrome (AIDS), human immunodeficiency virus (HIV) 283
ACT *see* assertive community treatment
active relaxation, compassion fatigue (CF) 466
acupuncture, described 384
acute traumatic stress, disaster 465
AD *see* Alzheimer disease

addiction
    chronic pain and depression 239
    depression and older adults 118
    substance use disorder (SUD) 201
    suicide risk screening 531
ADHD *see* attention deficit hyperactivity disorder
adjunct therapy, acupuncture 384
Administration for Children and Families (ACF)
    publication
        interpersonal psychotherapy (IPT) 336n
advanced practice registered nurse (APRN), depression screening 326
adverse childhood experiences (ACEs), overview 185–189
Advil, suicide at home 541
African medicine, complementary health approaches 382
Agency for Healthcare Research and Quality (AHRQ), contact information 561
aging
    Alzheimer disease (AD) 296
    depression and women 66
    quality of life (QOL) 215
agitation
    antidepressants 113, 342
    postpartum depression 92
    seasonal affective disorder (SAD) 58
    warning signs 528

AIDS *see* acquired immunodeficiency syndrome
Alaska Natives, mental and behavioral health 125
alcohol
   climate change 220
   depression and epilepsy 306
   depression screening 324
   genetic and environmental risk 157
   human immunodeficiency virus (HIV) 286
   psychotherapy 330
   stress 172
   substance use disorder (SUD) 203
   traumatic brain injury (TBI) 258
alcohol abuse
   alcohol use disorder (AUD) 210
   cancer 271
   climate change 220
alcohol counseling, alcohol use disorder (AUD) 213
alcohol use disorder (AUD), overview 210–217
alcohol withdrawal
   acupuncture 385
   mutual-support groups 214
alcoholism
   cancer 262
   depression and older adults 118
Alzheimer disease (AD)
   chronic illnesses 236
   overview 295–297
Alzheimer's Association, contact information 564
American Academy of Child and Adolescent Psychiatry (AACAP), contact information 564
American Academy of Family Physicians (AAFP), contact information 564
American Academy of Pediatrics (AAP), contact information 564
American Art Therapy Association (AATA), contact information 564
American Association for Geriatric Psychiatry (AAGP), contact information 564
American Association for Marriage and Family Therapy (AAMFT), contact information 565
American Association of Suicidology (AAS), contact information 565
American College Health Association (ACHA), contact information 565
American Foundation for Suicide Prevention (AFSP), contact information 565
American Indians, mental and behavioral health 125
American Medical Association (AMA), contact information 565
American Psychiatric Association (APA), contact information 565
American Psychological Association (APA), contact information 565
American Psychotherapy Association, contact information 565
anemia
   cancer 263
   depression screening 325
   seasonal affective disorder (SAD) 365
ankylosing spondylitis (AS), fibromyalgia 244
anticipatory grief, depression management strategies 474
anticoagulants
   natural products 387t
   St. John's wort 398
anticonvulsant
   epilepsy 303
   mood stabilizers 346
   natural products 387t
antidepressants
   cancer patients 266

Index

antidepressants, *continued*
  combination treatment 351
  described 341
  disruptive mood dysregulation disorder (DMDD) 45
  epilepsy 303
  genes 372
  holiday blues 480
  major depression 28
  Medicare coverage 414
  natural products 387t
  persistent depressive disorder (PDD) 49
  postpartum depression 91
  posttraumatic stress disorder (PTSD) 374
  premenstrual dysphoric disorder (PMDD) 83
  premenstrual syndrome (PMS) 79
  St. John's wort 397
  suicide risk screening 530
  treatment-resistant depression (TRD) 410
antipsychotics
  bipolar disorder 38
  described 344
  disruptive mood dysregulation disorder (DMDD) 45
  Medicare coverage 414
antiretroviral therapy (ART), human immunodeficiency virus (HIV) 283
Anxiety and Depression Association of America (ADAA), contact information 566
anxiety disorders
  antidepressants 341
  bipolar disorder 37
  disruptive mood dysregulation disorder (DMDD) 44
  heart disease 277
  meditation and mindfulness 391
  overview 193–197
  premenstrual syndrome (PMS) 77
  psychotherapy 330
  substance use disorder (SUD) 203
  traumatic brain injury (TBI) 257
appetite
  antidepressants 342
  anxiety 248
  atypical depression 31
  cancer 261
  chronic illness 235
  cognitive-behavioral therapy for depression (CBT-D) 333
  depression and men 113
  depression and women 65
  depression screening 324
  disaster responders 468
  grief 473
  human immunodeficiency virus (HIV) 285
  major depression 23
  older adults 217
  premenstrual syndrome (PMS) 76
  seasonal affective disorder (SAD) 58, 365
  stroke 309
APRN *see* advanced practice registered nurse
ART *see* antiretroviral therapy
art therapy
  anxiety 200
  defined 290
arthritis
  caregiver stress 174
  fibromyalgia 245
  mental illness stigma 419
  overview 247–249
Arthritis Foundation, contact information 566
AS *see* ankylosing spondylitis
Asian Americans, racial and ethnic minorities 127
aspirin
  premenstrual dysphoric disorder (PMDD) 83

aspirin, *continued*
   premenstrual syndrome (PMS) 79
   suicide risk 541
assertive community treatment (ACT)
   major depression 29
   substance use disorder (SUD) 205
   suicide risk 543
Association for Behavioral and Cognitive Therapies (ABCT), contact information 566
atrial fibrillation (AF), heart disease 278
attention deficit hyperactivity disorder (ADHD)
   bipolar disorder 37
   depression and children 102
   depression and teens 104
   depression symptoms 13
   disruptive mood dysregulation disorder (DMDD) 44
   overview 251–253
   seasonal affective disorder (SAD) 59
   stimulants 344
   substance use disorder (SUD) 203
atypical antidepressants, major depression 28
atypical antipsychotics
   bipolar disorder 38
   mental health medications 345
atypical depression, overview 31–33
AUD *see* alcohol use disorder
autism, disruptive mood dysregulation disorder (DMDD) 45
Ayurvedic medicine, depression treatment 381

B

baby blues
   perinatal depression 67
   postpartum depression 86

back pain consortium (BACPAC), chronic illness 239
BACPAC *see* back pain consortium
balanced meals, self-management interventions 431
BDD *see* body dysmorphic disorder
Beacon Tree Foundation, contact information 566
behavioral disorders
   chronic illnesses 252
   myths and facts 10
behavioral problems, parenting stress 177
behavioral risk factor surveillance system (BRFSS), diabetes 275
behavioral therapy, major depression 28
benzodiazepines
   anxiety disorders 196
   cancer 268
   mental health medications 343
   natural products 387t
bereavement, depression management strategies 473
beta-blockers
   anxiety disorders 197
   mental health medications 343
bilateral ECT, brain stimulation therapies 357
binge eating
   mental illness stigma 421
   premenstrual dysphoric disorder (PMDD) 82
biofeedback, overview 377–378
bipolar depression
   antipsychotic medications 345
   treatment-resistant depression (TRD) 411
bipolar disorder
   antipsychotic 344
   atypical depression
   correctional facilities 149

Index

bipolar disorder, *continued*
  depression in men 111
  electroconvulsive therapy (ECT) 356
  epilepsy 302
  gender-diverse populations 134
  heart disease 277
  magnetic seizure therapy (MST) 362
  major depression 25
  mental illnesses 4
  natural products 387t
  overview 35–41
  postpartum depression 88
  psychosis 54
  seasonal affective disorder (SAD) 59
  St. John's wort 398
  substance use disorder (SUD) 203
  suicide risk 543
  traumatic brain injury (TBI) 257
BJMHS *see* Brief Jail Mental Health Screen
body dysmorphic disorder (BDD), negative body image 448
body image
  cancer 261
  overview 447–450
borderline personality disorder (BPD), dialectical behavior therapy (DBT) 533
BPD *see* borderline personality disorder
brain
  adverse childhood experiences (ACEs) 187
  attention deficit hyperactivity disorder (ADHD) 251
  bipolar disorder 36
  depression and older adults 121
  depression and women 65
  electroconvulsive therapy (ECT) 29
  meditation and mindfulness work 390
  mental illness 4
  multiple sclerosis (MS) 289
  Parkinson disease (PD) 298
  persistent depressive disorder (PDD) 47
  postpartum depression 87
  premenstrual dysphoric disorder (PMDD) 82
  rumination cycle 163
  stroke 307
  substance use disorder (SUD) 203
  teen depression 103
  trauma 456
Brain and Behavior Research Foundation, contact information 566
Brain Injury Association of America (BIAA), contact information 566
brain stimulation therapies, overview 355–364
breastfeeding
  human immunodeficiency virus (HIV) 283
  postpartum depression 91
brexanolone, postpartum depression 91
BRFSS *see* behavioral risk factor surveillance system
Brief Jail Mental Health Screen (BJMHS), depression and mental health 150
brief strategic family therapy (BSFT), substance use disorder (SUD) 205
bruising
  depression screening 325
  suicide risk screening 531
bruxism, brain biofeedback 377
BSFT *see* brief strategic family therapy

bullying
  LGBT youth 139
  suicide 497
  teen depression 103
bupropion
  antidepressants 267
  seasonal affective disorder (SAD) 61
buspirone, defined 343

C

CAM *see* complementary and alternative medicine
cancer
  body image 448
  chronic illnesses 235
  depression 65, 104, 261
  meditation and mindfulness 394
  mental illness 4
  nongenetic factors 158
  stress 174
cannabis *see* marijuana
cardiometabolic disease, mental health disorders 278
cardiovascular disease (CVD)
  depression and chronic illness 237
  movement therapies 386
  workplace stress 143
caregivers
  depression and Parkinson disease (PD) 301
  disruptive mood dysregulation disorder (DMDD) 44
  grief 474
  overview 172–176
  self-management 428
  suicide 519
caregiver stress
  depression in older adults 118
  overview 172–176
Caring.com, contact information 566

CAT *see* computerized axial tomography
catatonia
  bipolar disorder 40
  electroconvulsive therapy (ECT) 356
CBT *see* cognitive-behavioral therapy
Center for Anxiety ™, contact information 566
Centers for Disease Control and Prevention (CDC)
  contact information 561
  publications
    adverse childhood experiences (ACEs) 189n
    arthritis 249n
    attention deficit hyperactivity disorder (ADHD) 253n
    attitude toward mental illness 422n
    depression in children 103n
    depression in workers 276n
    diabetes 275n
    epilepsy 303n
    fibromyalgia 246n
    grief and loss 473n
    heart disease 280n
    LGBTQ+ youth 133n
    mental health 4n, 134n
    mental health conditions 157n
    mental health stigma 284n
    Parkinson disease (PD) 302n
    stroke 309n
    suicide prevention 536n
    suicide risk factors 510n
    well-being concepts 427n
    workplace mental health 148n
Centers for Medicare & Medicaid Services (CMS)
  publication
    Medicare 415n

Index

CER *see* comparative effectiveness research
certified nurse practitioners (CNPs), depression 326
CF *see* compassion fatigue
CFS *see* chronic fatigue syndrome
CHD *see* coronary heart disease
chemotherapeutic agents, St. John's wort (*Hypericum perforatum*) 398
chemotherapy, serotonin norepinephrine reuptake inhibitors (SNRIs) 267
child abuse
    mental illness 4
    suicide risk 510
Child Welfare Information Gateway
    contact information 561
    publication
        building resilience 441n
childbirth
    human immunodeficiency virus (HIV) 283
    meditation and mindfulness 393
    perinatal depression 68
    postpartum depression 86
childhood abuse
    multiple sclerosis (MS) 289
    nongenetic factors 158
childhood resilience, overview 440–444
childhood trauma, alcohol use disorder (AUD) 211
Chinese medicine, complementary health approaches 382
chronic disease
    adverse childhood experiences (ACEs) 186
    caregiver stress 174
    depression 237
    mental illness 421
    multiple sclerosis (MS) 287
    placebo effect 368

chronic fatigue syndrome (CFS), premenstrual syndrome (PMS) 77
chronic idiopathic constipation, biofeedback 377
chronic illness
    human immunodeficiency virus (HIV) 285
    overview 235–238
    persistent depressive disorder (PDD) 48
    self-management 428
    suicide 519
chronic pain
    acceptance and commitment therapy (ACT) 338
    arthritis 247
    depression 11
    genetic and environmental risk 157
    meditation and mindfulness 392
    multiple sclerosis (MS) 290
    overview 239–242
    placebo effect 368
    suicide 496
chronic stress
    depression and heart disease 278
    individual resilience 435
    parental burnout 177
    persistent depressive disorder (PDD) 47
    racial and ethnic minorities 130
citalopram
    cancer 267
    disruptive mood dysregulation disorder (DMDD) 45
Cleveland Clinic, contact information 567
clinical depression *see* major depressive disorder (MDD)
clinical nurse specialists (CNSs), depression screening 326
clinical social workers
    depression 120, 326
    suicide 532

clinical trials
    complementary health
        approaches 385
    mental health 394
    vagus nerve stimulation (VNS) 358
clozapine
    mental health 345
    suicide 534
CM *see* contingency management
CMHS *see* Correctional Mental Health Screen
CNPs *see* certified nurse practitioners
CNSs *see* clinical nurse specialists
cognition
    biofeedback 377
    major depression 288
cognitive development
    childhood resilience 441
    postpartum depression 94
cognitive problems, Parkinson disease (PD) 300
cognitive-behavioral therapy (CBT)
    anxiety disorders 196
    bipolar disorder 39
    cancer 266
    depression in children 102
    described 28
    fibromyalgia 245
    mental health 390
    older adults 120
    overview 333–334
    Parkinson disease (PD) 302
    seasonal affective disorder (SAD) 366
    suicide 515
combination treatment, overview 351–354
community violence, suicide 508
comorbidity, traumatic brain injury (TBI) 256
comparative effectiveness research (CER), combined therapy 354

compassion fatigue (CF), overview 464–467
complementary and alternative medicine (CAM)
    acupuncture 385
    multiple sclerosis (MS) 288
computerized axial tomography (CAT), major depression 27
constipation
    anxiety disorders 197
    depression 13
    fibromyalgia 243
    Parkinson disease (PD) 300
    premenstrual syndrome symptoms (PMS) 76
contingency management (CM), substance use disorder (SUD) 205
conventional medicine, complementary health approaches 381
coping strategies
    grief 476
    individual resilience 438
    mental health disorders 279
    psychotherapy 332
    suicide 515, 533
coronary heart disease (CHD)
    chronic illnesses 236
    mental health disorders 279
Correctional Mental Health Screen (CMHS), mental health 150
corticosteroids, depression and cancer 262
counseling
    anxiety disorders 196
    biofeedback 378
    caregiver stress 176
    depression and cancer 265
    depression in older adults 117
    depression in teens 105
    depression screening 326

Index

counseling, *continued*
    lesbian, gay, bisexual, and transgender (LGBT) 139
    mental health 9, 414
    multiple sclerosis (MS) 288
    persistent depressive disorder (PDD) 49
    pregnancy 85
    self-management 430
    suicide 515, 548
COVID-19
    grief 475
    lesbian, gay, bisexual, and transgender (LGBT) 135
cultural stereotypes, mental illness 419
CVD *see* cardiovascular disease
cyclosporine, St. John's wort (*Hypericum perforatum*) 398
cyclothymia *see* cyclothymic disorder
cyclothymic disorder, defined 36
CYP3A4 *see* cytochrome P450 3A4
cytochrome P450 3A4 (CYP3A4), St. John's wort (*Hypericum perforatum*) 398

D

The Dana Foundation, contact information 567
DBS *see* deep brain stimulation
DBT *see* dialectical behavior therapy
death ideation *see* suicide risk
deep brain stimulation (DBS), described 362
deep breathing
    complementary health approaches 383
    self-management interventions 431
    stress 171
delusions
    antipsychotics 345
    bipolar disorder 37

depression 12
depression in men 111
eating disorders 198
Parkinson disease (PD) 301
psychosis 54
dementia
    Alzheimer disease (AD) 296
    antipsychotics 344
    caregiver stress 172
deoxyribonucleic acid (DNA)
    Alzheimer disease (AD) 295
    antidepressants 373
Depressed Anonymous (DA), contact information 567
depression
    bipolar disorder 23
    body image 449
    chronic illness and mental health 242
    complementary health approaches 386
    environmental risk factors 157
    healthy lifestyle 101
    LGBT youth 139
    mental health 3, 413, 534
    neurological disorders 303
    overview 11–15
    pregnancy 348
    seasonal affective disorder (SAD) 61
    suicide risk 508
    trauma 184
    see also atypical depression; major depression
Depression and Bipolar Support Alliance (DBSA), contact information 567
depression screening
    arthritis 249
    mental health conditions 413
    older adults 519
    overview 323–326
    pregnancy 95

depression triggers, overview 225–230
depressive episodes
   bipolar disorder 35
   neurotransmitters 225
   seasonal affective disorder
      (SAD) 60
diabetes
   antianxiety medications 343
   high blood pressure (HBP) 392
   mental health 3, 215
   mental illness 419
   overview 273–276
   teen depression 104
dialectical behavior therapy (DBT)
   disruptive mood dysregulation
      disorder (DMDD) 44
   substance use disorder (SUD) 204
   suicide 515, 533
diarrhea
   depression 13
   herbs and supplements for
      depression 398
   premenstrual syndrome (PMS) 76
diet
   body image 448
   depression triggers 229
   mental health disorders 280
   persistent depressive disorder
      (PDD) 49
   treating depression 404
dietary supplement
   antidepressants 342
   chronic illnesses 238
   complementary health
      approaches 389
   premenstrual syndrome (PMS) 80
digoxin, St. John's wort (*Hypericum perforatum*) 398
disability
   behavioral or emotional
      challenges 407
   chronic pain 239

fibromyalgia 245
   mental health 8, 145
   older adults 117, 519
   Parkinson disease (PD) 301
disaster responders, stress 470
disasters
   climate change 219
   first responders 463
discrimination
   depression in children 406
   individual resilience 435
   LGBT youth 134
   mental health 217, 484
   suicide risk 508
disruptive mood dysregulation
   disorder (DMDD),
      overview 43–45
distractibility, disaster responders 469
distraction techniques, rumination
   cycle 163
diuretics, premenstrual syndrome
   (PMS) 79
divorce
   alcohol use disorder (AUD) 214
   depression triggers 227
   elements of psychotherapy 330
   major depression 24
   menopause 96
   nongenetic factors 158
DMDD *see* disruptive mood
   dysregulation disorder
DNA *see* deoxyribonucleic acid
dopamine
   cancer 267
   treatment-resistant depression
      (TRD) 410
drug abuse, cancer 262
drug dependency, traumatic brain
   injury (TBI) 258
drug interactions
   mental disorder 387t
   older adults 216, 347

Index

drug–gene interaction,
    antidepressants 373
drugs *see* medications
dysthymia
    depression types 11, 111
    see also persistent depressive
        disorder (PDD)

E

eating disorder
    bipolar disorder 37
    body image 448
    overview 198–200
    psychotherapy 330
    rumination 161
    teen depression 103
ECT *see* electroconvulsive therapy
Effective Health Care Program
    publication
        first-line therapy 354n
electroconvulsive therapy (ECT)
    brain stimulation therapies 355
    depression in older adults 121
    described 29
    epilepsy 303
emergency care, stroke 307
emergency department
    climate change and
        depression 222
    teen suicide 514
    traumatic brain injury (TBI) 255
emergency medical services (EMS),
    depression and first responders 461
emotional distress
    emergency department 537
    suicide 498
    traumatic brain injury (TBI) 258
emotional support
    individual resilience 437
    peer support 484
    psychotherapies 332

    stress 226
    suicide 528
employment
    assertive community treatment
        (ACT) 29
    human immunodeficiency virus
        (HIV) 284
    peer support 484
    psychosis 56
    stigma 420
    suicide 516
empty nest syndrome, described 227
EMS *see* emergency medical services
endorphins, electroconvulsive therapy
    (ECT) 29
environmental risk factors,
    overview 157–160
environmental stressor, climate change
    and depression 222
epilepsy
    depression and chronic illness 236
    mental illness stigma 419
    overview 302–306
    vagus nerve stimulation
        (VNS) 358
esketamine
    antidepressants 342
    postpartum depression 91
    treatment-resistant depression
        (TRD) 409
estrogen
    premenstrual syndrome (PMS) 75
    women and depression 65
Eunice Kennedy Shriver National
    Institute of Child Health and
    Human Development (NICHD)
    publication
        postpartum depression 95n
exercise
    acceptance and commitment
        therapy (ACT) 338
    bipolar disorder 41

exercise, *continued*
   complementary health
     approaches 385
   fibromyalgia 245
   holiday blues 480
   major depression 316
   men and depression 115
   menopause and depression 97
   multiple sclerosis (MS) 290
   racial and ethnic minorities 131
   self-esteem 451
   self-management 428
   smoking 210
   women and depression 70
   workplace stress 148

F

Family Caregiver Alliance (FCA),
   contact information 567
family counseling
   mental health services 413
   treatment option 406
family history
   alcohol use disorder (AUD) 211
   bipolar disorder 37
   depression in women 65
   depression screening 324
   depressive disorder 47
   fibromyalgia 243
   mental health problems 9
   premenstrual syndrome (PMS) 75
   suicide 496
family therapy
   attention deficit hyperactivity
     disorder (ADHD) 253
   behavioral therapies 205
   depression in children 102
   electroconvulsive therapy (ECT) 29
family violence, suicide 496
fast-acting antidepressant, placebo
   effect 369

fatigue
   behavioral health 463
   depression screening 323
   disaster responders 468
   fibromyalgia 243
   multiple sclerosis (MS) 288
   older adults 118
   perinatal depression 68
   premenstrual syndrome (PMS) 78
fear-avoidance physical therapy,
   mood-related disorders 240
fibromyalgia, overview 242–246
financial stress, depression triggers 226
firearms
   older adults 518
   suicide 496, 533
firefighters, described 461
first responders, overview 461–463
fluoxetine
   premenstrual dysphoric disorder
     (PMDD) 83
   selective serotonin reuptake
     inhibitors (SSRIs) 267
frontal lobes, traumatic brain injury
   (TBI) 256

G

GAD *see* generalized anxiety disorder
generalized anxiety disorder (GAD)
   depression 13
   gay and bisexual men 134
   see also anxiety disorder
genes
   Alzheimer disease (AD) 296
   bipolar disorder 37
   environmental risk factors 157
   mental health 9
   older adults 117
   pharmacogenomic testing 372
genetic factors
   depression in men 109

Index

genetic factors, *continued*
   mental health disorders 281
   see also environmental risk factors
genetics
   alcohol use disorder (AUD) 211
   anxiety disorders 194
   attention deficit hyperactivity disorder (ADHD) 252
   bipolar disorder 37
   depression 24
   teen depression 103
Geriatric Mental Health Foundation (GMHF), contact information 567
girlshealth.gov
   contact information 561
   publication
      psychotherapy 331n
Globalchange.gov
   contact information 562
   publication
      climate change and depression 224n
glutamate
   treatment-resistant depression (TRD) 410
   vagus nerve stimulation (VNS) 358
grief
   depression 13
   ectopic pregnancy 86
   extreme weather 220
   individual resilience 438
   overview 473–478
   talk therapy 106
   workplace stress 143
group therapy
   anxiety 200
   depression screening 326
   mental health 414
guilt
   anxiety 248
   compassion fatigue (CF) 466
   depression 12
   depression screening 323
   postpartum depression 89
   suicide risk screening 528
   trauma 183

H

hallucinations
   antipsychotic medications 344
   depression symptoms 27
   Parkinson disease (PD) 301
   psychotic depression 111
harassment
   LGBT youth 139
   stress 225
   suicide 497
HBP *see* high blood pressure
HDE *see* Humanitarian Device Exemption
head injuries, mental health disorders 259
headaches
   antidepressants 342
   biofeedback 377
   chronic illnesses 235
   compassion fatigue (CF) 465
   diabetes 274
   men and depression 110
   stress 169
   women and depression 67
   young children 403
health insurance
   finding a therapist 320
   workplace stress 146
health promotion
   diabetes 276
   well-being 425
Health Resources and Services Administration (HRSA), contact information 562
HealthCare.gov, contact information 562

healthfinder.gov, contact
    information 562
healthy body image, overview 447–450
heart attack
    mental health disorders 278
    panic disorder 195
    women and depression 66
heart disease
    adverse childhood experiences
        (ACEs) 186
    caregiver stress 173
    chronic illness 235
    diabetes 273
    mental illness stigma 419
    older adults 119
    overview 277–281
    women and depression 69
hepatic CYP450 enzymes, drug 372
hibernating, seasonal affective disorder
    (SAD) 58
high blood pressure (HBP)
    caregiver stress 173
    individual resilience 435
    meditation and mindfulness 392
    postpartum depression 93
    stroke 308
HIV *see* human immunodeficiency
    virus
holiday blues, overview 479–481
homelessness
    self-regulation 442
    social inclusion 485
homeopathy, complementary health
    approaches 382
homicide
    climate change 221
    mental health problems 7
    see also suicide
hopelessness
    anxiety 248
    depression symptoms 12
    disaster responders 468

multiple sclerosis (MS) 288
older adults 518
rumination cycle 161
suicide risk 508
teen depression 103
hormonal imbalance
    anxiety 199
    hormonal imbalances 229
hot flashes
    anxiety 194
    cancer 267
    hormone imbalance 228
    perimenopausal depression 68
human immunodeficiency virus
    (HIV), overview 283–286
Humanitarian Device Exemption
    (HDE), deep brain stimulation
    (DBS) 362
hyperphagia, older children and
    teens 13
hypersomnia
    atypical depression 32
    seasonal affective disorder (SAD) 58
hypertension
    ketamine 412
    meditation and mindfulness 392
    mental health disorders 279
hypomania, bipolar disorder 39
hypomanic episodes, bipolar disorder 39
hypotension *see* orthostatic
    hypotension
hypothyroidism
    atypical depression 32
    chronic illnesses 236

I

IBS *see* irritable bowel syndrome
ibuprofen
    premenstrual dysphoric disorder
        (PMDD) 83
    premenstrual syndrome (PMS) 79

Index

IDEA *see* Individuals with Disabilities Education Act
illness-related anxiety, chronic illness 236
impulse control disorder, mental illness stigma 419
indinavir, St. John's wort (*Hypericum perforatum*) 398
individual resilience, overview 435–440
Individuals with Disabilities Education Act (IDEA), depression in children and adolescents 407
infertility
    depression in women 71
    depression triggers 227
inner pharmacy, placebo effect 367
insomnia
    antidepressants 341
    anxiety disorders 197
    atypical depression 31
    bipolar disorder 39
    complementary health approaches 386
    depression 13
    depression screening 323
    disaster responders 468
    major depression 26
    meditation and mindfulness 393
    multiple sclerosis (MS) 288
    pharmacogenomic testing 371
    seasonal affective disorder (SAD) 58
    suicide risk screening 528
insurance
    caregiver stress 176
    depression in men 116
    depression in older adults 121
    finding a therapist 320
    paying for mental health services 413
    psychotherapy 331
    workplace stress 146

International Foundation for Research and Education on Depression (iFred), contact information 567
International OCD Foundation (IOCDF), contact information 567
interpersonal and social rhythm therapy (IPSRT), bipolar disorder 39
interpersonal psychotherapy for depressed adolescents (IPT-A), described 336
interpersonal therapy (IPT), overview 335–336
IPSRT *see* interpersonal and social rhythm therapy
IPT *see* interpersonal therapy
IPT-A *see* interpersonal psychotherapy for depressed adolescents
irinotecan, St. John's wort (*Hypericum perforatum*) 398
irritable bowel syndrome (IBS)
    alcohol use disorder (AUD) 217
    atypical depression 31
    climate change 222
    depression in older adults 118
    depression risk factors 158
    disaster responders 468
    epilepsy 302
    fibromyalgia 243
    human immunodeficiency virus (HIV) 284
    mental illness 4
    premenstrual syndrome (PMS) 78
    suicide risk 508
    workplace stress 143
    youth suicide 517

J

job loss, atypical depression 31
job stress
    first responders 461
    workplace stress 147

joint pain, premenstrual dysphoric disorder (PMDD) 83
juvenile justice system, suicide among young adults 516

K
ketamine, relapsed depression 409
Kristin Brooks Hope Center (KBHC), contact information 567

L
LCSW *see* licensed clinical social worker
leaden paralysis, atypical depression 32
lesbian, gay, bisexual, and transgender (LGBT)
   arthritis 247
   depression prevalence 133
   mental health management 139
   suicide 516
LGBT *see* lesbian, gay, bisexual, and transgender
libido
   disaster responders 469
   hormone imbalance 228
licensed clinical social worker (LCSW)
   diagnosing depression 326
   older adults 120
licensed marriage and family therapist (LMFT), diagnosing depression 326
licensed professional counselors (LPCs), diagnosing depression 326
light therapy
   bipolar symptoms 40
   overview 365–366
liver disease, S-adenosyl-L-methionine (SAMe) 399
LMFT *see* licensed marriage and family therapist
loss of interest
   chronic illness 235
   depression symptoms 25, 110
   diabetes 273
   multiple sclerosis (MS) 287
   older adults 118
   stroke 309
LPCs *see* licensed professional counselors
L-tryptophan, S-adenosyl-L-methionine (SAMe) 399
lupus
   chronic illness 236
   fibromyalgia 244

M
magnetic resonance imaging (MRI)
   magnetic seizure therapy (MST) 363
   multiple sclerosis (MS) 289
magnetic seizure therapy (MST), brain stimulation therapies 355
major depression
   cancer 261
   correctional facilities 149
   fibromyalgia 244
   heart disease 277
   interpersonal therapy (IPT) 335
   lesbian, gay, and bisexual (LBG) youth 134
   magnetic seizure therapy (MST) 362
   men and depression 110
   mental illnesses 4
   multiple sclerosis (MS) 287
   overview 23–30
   rumination cycle 161
   seasonal affective disorder (SAD) 57

Index

major depressive disorder (MDD)
  atypical depression 31
  combination treatment 353
  depression and older adults 119
  men and depression 109
  omega-3 fatty acids 395
  persistent depressive disorder (PDD) 47
  seasonal affective disorder (SAD) 59
  traumatic brain injury (TBI) 258
major depressive episode
  mental and behavioral health 125
  substance use disorder (SUD) 206
mania
  bipolar disorder 39
  men and depression 111
  mood stabilizers 346
  psychiatric disorders 29
manic depression *see* bipolar disorder
manic episodes
  bipolar disorder 35
  seasonal affective disorder (SAD) 59
MAOIs *see* monoamine oxidase inhibitors
marijuana
  major depressive episode 207
  psychotic depression 54
MBRP *see* mindfulness-based relapse prevention
MBSR *see* mindfulness-based stress reduction
MDD *see* major depressive disorder
MDFT *see* multidimensional family therapy
medications
  alcohol use disorder (AUD) 213
  bipolar disorder 39
  chronic illness 236
  depression and older adults 121
  electroconvulsive therapy (ECT) 359
  finding therapist 320
  genetic and environmental factors 158
  heart disease 278
  kava 387t
  major depressive disorder (MDD) 25
  men and depression 110
  mental health 341
  Parkinson disease (PD) 300
  persistent depressive disorder (PDD) 49
  placebo effect 370
  psychotherapy 332
  seasonal affective disorder (SAD) 60
  substance use disorder (SUD) 203, 381
  suicide 515
  trauma 456
  treatment-resistant depression (TRD) 409
  workplace stress 146
MedlinePlus
  publications
    depression 158n
    depression screening 326n
    suicide risk screening 531n
    teen depression 107n
melancholic depression, major depressive disorder (MDD) 31
melatonin, seasonal affective disorder (SAD) 59
memory loss
  depression and older adults 121
  electroconvulsive therapy (ECT) 357
menopause
  overview 96–97
  premenstrual syndrome (PMS) 78

menopause, *continued*
  serotonin norepinephrine reuptake inhibitors (SNRIs) 267
  women and depression 65
mental disorders
  acupuncture 385
  anxiety 193
  brain stimulation therapies 355
  correctional facilities 149
  depression treatment 403
  human immunodeficiency virus (HIV) 284
  magnetic seizure therapy (MST) 362
  men and depression 109
  mental illness 421
  persistent depressive disorder (PDD) 48
  psychotherapy 333
  seasonal affective disorder (SAD) 59
  smoking 208
  suicide 496, 522
mental health
  acceptance and commitment therapy (ACT) 338
  adverse childhood experiences (ACEs) 185
  atypical depression 33
  chronic pain 239
  depression 404
  diabetes 273
  epilepsy 302
  finding therapist 320
  human immunodeficiency virus (HIV) 283
  individual resilience 438
  LGBT youth 134
  men and depression 112
  menopause 97
  mental illness 421
  overview 3–5
  persistent depressive disorder (PDD) 48
  posttraumatic stress disorder (PTSD) 220
  pregnancy and depression 84
  rumination cycle 164
  seasonal affective disorder (SAD) 60, 365
  stress 468
  substance use disorder (SUD) 205, 382
  suicide 498
  trauma 455
  workplace stress 146
Mental Health America (MHA), contact information 567
mental health disorders
  heart disease 277
  omega-3 fatty acid 398
  overview 7–10
  persistent depressive disorder (PDD) 48
  smoking 209
  suicide 516
  traumatic brain injury (TBI) 258
mental illness
  adverse childhood experiences (ACEs) 186
  Alzheimer disease (AD) 297
  antipsychotics 346
  bipolar disorder 35
  cognitive-behavioral therapy (CBT) 28
  finding a therapist 320
  mindfulness meditation 386
  postpartum depression 87
  posttraumatic stress disorder (PTSD) 220
  psychotic depression 54
  smoking 208
  stigma 420
  suicide 507, 532

Index

mental illness, *continued*
  teen and depression 104
  traumatic brain injury (TBI) 258
  treatment-resistant depression
    (TRD) 409
  workplace stress 145
  see also mental health
Mental Illness Research, Education
  and Clinical Centers (MIRECC)
  publication
    acceptance and commitment
      therapy (ACT) 337n
    major depression 30n
MentalHealth.gov
  publications
    mental health 5n
    myths and facts 10n
    suicidal behavior 507n
messenger RNA (mRNA), Alzheimer
  disease (AD) 296
methylphenidate, disruptive mood
  dysregulation disorder (DMDD) 45
migraine
  antidepressants 342
  bladder pain syndrome (BPS) 78
  brain biofeedback 377
  fibromyalgia 243
mild traumatic brain injury (mTBI),
  mental health disorders 258
mindfulness
  children and depression 102
  multiple sclerosis (MS) 290
  overview 389–395
  persistent depressive disorder
    (PDD) 50
  psychotherapy 332
  rumination cycle 163
  substance use disorder (SUD) 204
  workplace stress 147
mindfulness-based relapse prevention
  (MBRP), substance use disorder
  (SUD) 394

mindfulness-based stress reduction
  (MBSR) *see* mindfulness
minor depression, men 111
mobility
  anxiety 248
  suicide 519
monoamine oxidase inhibitors
  (MAOIs)
  anxiety disorders 197
  atypical depression 33
  cancer 267
  kava 387t
  mental health 341
monoamines, treatment-resistant
  depression (TRD) 410
mood disorders
  chronic pain 239
  heart disease 277
  traumatic brain injury (TBI) 257
  treatment-resistant depression
    (TRD) 410
mood swing
  bipolar disorder 41
  hormone imbalance 229
  postpartum psychosis 92
  premenstrual dysphoric disorder
    (PMDD) 82
  premenstrual syndrome
    (PMS) 67
  suicide 496, 517, 530
movement disorder
  magnetic seizure therapy
    (MST) 363
  Parkinson disease (PD) 298
movement therapy, acupuncture 385
MRI *see* magnetic resonance
  imaging
mRNA *see* messenger RNA
MS *see* multiple sclerosis
MST *see* magnetic seizure therapy
MST *see* multisystemic therapy
mTBI *see* mild traumatic brain injury

multidimensional family therapy (MDFT), substance use disorder (SUD) 205
multiple sclerosis (MS)
　chronic illness 236
　depression and older adults 119
　overview 287–291
Multiple Sclerosis Association of America (MSAA), contact information 568
multisystemic therapy (MST), substance use disorder (SUD) 205
μ-opioid receptor, placebo effect 369
muscle pain
　premenstrual dysphoric disorder (PMDD) 82
　premenstrual syndrome (PMS) 67
muscle relaxant, electroconvulsive therapy (ECT) 356
muscle tension
　anxiety disorders 195
　arthritis 247
　brain biofeedback 377
　stress 170
muscle twitches, antidepressants 342
music therapy, described 400

N

naproxen
　premenstrual dysphoric disorder (PMDD) 83
　premenstrual syndrome (PMS) 79
National Alliance on Mental Illness (NAMI), contact information 568
National Association of Anorexia Nervosa and Associated Disorders (ANAD), contact information 568
National Association of School Psychologists (NASP), contact information 568
National Cancer Institute (NCI)
　contact information 562
　publication
　　depression 272n
National Center for Complementary and Integrative Health (NCCIH)
　contact information 562
　publications
　　complementary health approaches 401n
　　meditation and mindfulness 395n
National Center for Health Statistics (NCHS), contact information 562
National Center for Posttraumatic Stress Disorder (NCPTSD)
　contact information 562
　publications
　　depression, trauma, and PTSD 185n
　　family support 491n
National Eating Disorders Association (NEDA), contact information 568
National Federation of Families for Children's Mental Health (NFFCMH), contact information 568
National Human Genome Research Institute (NHGRI)
　publication
　　attention deficit hyperactivity disorder (ADHD) 252n
National Institute of Mental Health (NIMH)
　contact information 562
　publications
　　bipolar disorder 41n
　　brain stimulation therapies 364n
　　child and adolescent mental health 405n, 407n
　　depression 15n

Index

National Institute of Mental Health
(NIMH)
publications, *continued*
disruptive mood dysregulation
disorder (DMDD) 45n
ketamine 412n
major depression 20n
medications 349n
men and depression 116n
mental illnesses 322n
psychosis 56n
psychotherapies 320n, 333n
seasonal affective disorder
(SAD) 61n
substance use 205n
suicide 498n, 505n
suicide prevention 534n
National Institute on Aging (NIA)
contact information 563
publications
genetic risk factors 296n
older adults 122n
National Institute on Alcohol Abuse
and Alcoholism (NIAAA)
publication
alcohol use disorder
(AUD) 214n
National Institutes of Health (NIH)
contact information 563
publications
chronic pain 242n
depression risk factors 160n
self-esteem 453n
teen suicide 516n
National Suicide Prevention
Lifeline
dealing with trauma 457
suicide risk screening 529
teen suicide 515
National Survey of Drug Use and
Health (NSDUH), depression
prevalence 17

naturopathy, complementary health
approaches 382
nausea
alcohol use disorder (AUD) 213
anxiety disorders 194
depression in men 113
depression in older adults 121
ectopic pregnancy 86
placebo effect 367
S-adenosyl-L-methionine
(SAMe) 399
NDRIs *see* norepinephrine-dopamine
reuptake inhibitors
The Nemours Foundation, contact
information 568
nerve blocks, pain 239
nervous system
acupuncture 400
human immunodeficiency virus
(HIV) 283
Parkinson disease (PD) 298
neurodegenerative disorders,
Alzheimer disease (AD) 296
neurofeedback, brain
biofeedback 377
neuropathy, cancer 267
neuroreceptor, atypical depression 32
neurotransmitters
atypical depression 31
brain stimulation therapies 358
cancer 267
depression genetic causes 158
depression triggers 225
major depression 29
treatment-resistant depression
(TRD) 410
News and Events
publications
African Americans and
Latinos 132n
mild head injury 260n
placebo effect 370n

593

nicotine
    acupuncture 385
    meditation and mindfulness 391
    smoking 209
    substance use disorder (SUD) 205
nicotine relapse prevention,
    acupuncture 385
nicotine withdrawal, mood
    changes 209
NIH News in Health
    publications
        coping with grief 478n
        dealing with trauma 457n
        nurturing resilience 437n
        postpartum depression 94n
        powerful placebo 368n
988 Suicide and Crisis Lifeline, contact
    information 568
nonpharmacological therapies,
    combination treatment 352
norepinephrine
    cancer 267
    major depression 24
    medications 341
    treatment-resistant depression
        (TRD) 410
    vagus nerve stimulation (VNS) 358
norepinephrine-dopamine reuptake
    inhibitors (NDRIs)
    antidepressants 341
    cancer 267
NSDUH *see* National Survey of Drug
    Use and Health

O

obesity
    body image 447
    caregiver stress 174
    depression 69
    depression triggers 229
    fibromyalgia 244
    mental health disorders 278

obsessive-compulsive disorder (OCD)
    acceptance and commitment
        therapy (ACT) 338
    anxiety disorders 199
occupational therapy, biofeedback 378
OCD *see* obsessive-compulsive
    disorder
ODD *see* oppositional defiant
    disorder
Office of Disability Employment Policy
    (ODEP), contact information 563
Office of Minority Health (OMH)
    contact information 563
    publications
        mental and behavioral health–
            African Americans 125n
        mental and behavioral health–
            American Indians/Alaska
            natives 127n
        mental and behavioral health–
            Asian Americans 128n
        mental and behavioral health–
            Hispanics 130n
Office of the Assistant Secretary
    for Preparedness and Response
    (ASPR)
    publication
        individual resilience 440n
Office on Women's Health (OWH)
    publications
        anxiety disorders 197n
        body image 450n
        caregiver stress 176n
        depression 67n, 68n
        holiday blues 481n
        menopause symptoms and
            relief 96n
        postpartum depression 92n
        premenstrual dysphoric
            disorder (PMDD) 83n
        premenstrual syndrome
            (PMS) 81n

Index

older adults
    alcohol use disorder (AUD) 214
    antipsychotic medications 345
    depression 13
    music therapy 401
    overview 117–122
    suicide 518
    traumatic brain injury (TBI) 255
omega-3 fatty acids
    alternative and complementary therapies 397
    complementary health approaches 386
opioids
    acupuncture 384
    chronic pain 239
    placebo effect 368
    traumatic brain injury (TBI) 258
oppositional defiant disorder (ODD), disruptive mood dysregulation disorder (DMDD) 44
orthopedic trauma *see* traumatic brain injury (TBI)
orthostatic hypotension, Parkinson disease (PD) 300
osteoarthritis
    biofeedback 377
    fibromyalgia 244
osteoporosis
    biofeedback 377
    fibromyalgia 244
OTC *see* over-the-counter
overeating
    diabetes 274
    men and depression 110
    seasonal affective disorder (SAD) 58
oversleeping
    atypical depression 31
    chronic illnesses 235
    depression 12
    older adults 118
    seasonal affective disorder (SAD) 58
over-the-counter (OTC)
    alcohol use disorder (AUD) 215
    bipolar disorder 39
    premenstrual syndrome (PMS) 79

P

Pacific Islanders, racial and ethnic minorities 127
pain *see* chronic pain; joint pain; muscle pain; pain relievers
pain relievers
    anxiety disorders 197
    fibromyalgia 245
    major depression 29
    premenstrual syndrome (PMS) 79
    suicide risk 541
pancreatic cancer, depression 262
panic attack
    antianxiety medications 343
    anxiety disorders 195
    premenstrual dysphoric disorder (PMDD) 82
panic disorder
    anxiety disorders 193
    heart disease 277
    seasonal affective disorder (SAD) 59
    see also panic attack
paranoia, postpartum psychosis 92
paranoid delusions, major depression 27
parental burnout, overview 177–179
Parkinson disease (PD)
    brain stimulation therapy 362
    chronic illness 236
    men and depression 109
    overview 298–302
    women and depression 66

parkinsonian gait *see* Parkinson disease (PD)
Parkinson's Foundation, contact information 568
paroxetine, premenstrual dysphoric disorder (PMDD) 83
PD *see* Parkinson disease
PDD *see* persistent depressive disorder
peer support
    alcohol use disorder (AUD) 213
    depression and first responders 463
    major depression 29
    mental illness 421
    overview 483–485
    workplace stress 147
pelvic floor muscle training (PFMT), biofeedback 378
perimenopause
    women and depression 65
    see also menopause
perinatal depression
    described 67
    herbs and supplements 397
    see also postpartum depression
persistent depressive disorder (PDD)
    overview 47–51
    see also dysthymia
PET *see* positron emission tomography
PFMT *see* pelvic floor muscle training
pharmacogenomic testing, genes 371
pharmacotherapy, psychotic depression 55
phobia
    antianxiety medications 343
    anxiety disorders 195, 277
    see also social phobia
phototherapy *see* light therapy
physical abuse *see* sexual abuse
Pilates, movement therapy 386
placebo effect, overview 367–370
PMDD *see* premenstrual dysphoric disorder

PMS *see* premenstrual syndrome
pneumonia, family support 489
positive emotions, well-being concepts 425
positive parenting, lesbian, gay, bisexual, and transgender (LGBT) 140
positron emission tomography (PET), placebo effect 369
postpartum depression (PPD)
    mood stabilizers 348
    omega-3 fatty acid 397
    overview 86–95
    premenstrual syndrome (PMS) 68
postpartum period, women and depression 65
postpartum psychosis, described 92
Postpartum Support International (PSI), contact information 569
posttraumatic amnesia, mild traumatic brain injury (mTBI) 259
posttraumatic stress disorder (PTSD)
    anxiety disorders 194
    fibromyalgia 243
    mental and behavioral health 127
    multiple sclerosis (MS) 289
    rumination cycle 161
    trauma 455
poverty
    adverse childhood experiences (ACEs) 187
    epilepsy 302
    mental illness 420
    women and depression 65
prefrontal cortex
    cognitive development 442
    traumatic brain injury (TBI) 256
pregnancy
    adverse childhood experiences (ACEs) 186
    depression 12, 65
    human immunodeficiency virus (HIV) 283

Index

pregnancy, *continued*
   mood stabilizers 347
   omega-3 fatty acid 397
   persistent depressive disorder (PDD) 47
premenstrual dysphoric disorder (PMDD), overview 81–83
premenstrual syndrome (PMS), overview 75–81
prescription medications *see* medications
procarbazine, cancer 262
progesterone
   postpartum depression 87
   women and depression 65
prostatectomy, biofeedback 377
pseudodementia, depression 13
psychoeducation
   interpersonal therapy (IPT) 336
   mindfulness meditation 391
psychomotor agitation, major depression 26
psychomotor retardation, major depression 26
psychosis
   antipsychotics 344
   climate change 221
   major depressive disorder (MDD) 12
   overview 53–56
   repetitive transcranial magnetic stimulation (rTMS) 360
   treatment-resistant depression (TRD) 410
psychotherapy
   anxiety disorder 196
   chronic illness 238
   depression 14, 112
   disruptive mood dysregulation disorder (DMDD) 44
psychotic depression *see* psychosis
PTSD *see* posttraumatic stress disorder
pulse generator, vagus nerve stimulation (VNS) 358

Q

QOL *see* quality of life
quality of life (QOL)
   arthritis–mental health connection 247
   combination treatment 351
   complementary and alternative therapies 386
   diabetes 274
   epilepsy 303
   mental health disorders 10
   mental illness 419
   peer support and social inclusion 484
   smoking 209

R

RA *see* rheumatoid arthritis
RAISE *see* Recovery After an Initial Schizophrenia Episode
randomized controlled trial (RCT), complementary health approaches 383
rasa shastra, complementary health approaches 388
RCT *see* randomized controlled trial
Recovery After an Initial Schizophrenia Episode (RAISE), psychosis 55
recreational drugs
   assertive community treatment (ACT) 29
   chronic pain 241
   multiple sclerosis (MS) 288
   stroke 310
relapse
   acupuncture 385

relapse, *continued*
    alcohol counseling 213
    alcohol use disorder (AUD) 211, 214
    antidepressants 114
    correctional facilities 149
    electroconvulsive therapy (ECT) 29, 356
    mutual-support groups 214
relaxation
    cancer 266
    cognitive-behavioral therapy (CBT) 196
    compassion fatigue (CF) 466
    complementary treatments 70, 384
    depression 291
    depression in children 102
    meditation and mindfulness 391
    menopause 97
    music therapy 400
    premenstrual dysphoric disorder (PMDD) 83
    psychotherapy 332
    self-management interventions 430
    workplace stress 147
repetitive transcranial magnetic stimulation (rTMS)
    bipolar disorder 40
    brain stimulation therapies 355
    older adults 121
resilience
    meditation and mindfulness 390
    overview 435–444
    psychotic depression 55
    well-being 425
    workplace stress 145
rheumatoid arthritis (RA)
    chronic illness 236
    fibromyalgia 243, 244
rTMS *see* repetitive transcranial magnetic stimulation
rumination-depression cycle, overview 161–165

S

SAD *see* seasonal affective disorder
safety plan
    psychotherapy 332
    suicidal thoughts 533
    teens safe 515
schizoaffective disorder
    depression symptoms 25
    mood stabilizers 346
    postpartum psychosis 92
    suicidal thoughts 534
schizophrenia
    antipsychotics 344
    correctional facilities 149
    epilepsy 302
    mental illnesses 4
    psychotic depression 54
    substance use 203
    suicidal thoughts 534
    traumatic brain injury (TBI) 257
    treatment-resistant depression (TRD) 410
Schizophrenia & Psychosis Action Alliance (S&PAA), contact information 569
seasonal affective disorder (SAD)
    holiday blues 480
    light therapy 365
    men and depression 111
    overview 57–61
    psychotherapy 40
seizures
    epilepsy 303
    repetitive transcranial magnetic stimulation (rTMS) 361
selective serotonin reuptake inhibitors (SSRIs)
    antidepressant 341
    cancer 267
    depression treatments 27
    older adults 121
    persistent depressive disorder (PDD) 49

Index

selective serotonin reuptake inhibitors (SSRIs), *continued*
   premenstrual dysphoric disorder (PMDD) 83
   premenstrual syndrome (PMS) 79
self-esteem
   cancer 261
   depression triggers 226
   major depression 25
   mental illness stigma 420
   overview 450–453
   rumination cycle 165
   suicide risk 527
   teen depression 104
serious mental illness
   correctional facilities 149
   epilepsy 304
   mental health disorders 7
   postpartum depression 87
   smoking 208
serious psychological distress, racial and ethnic minorities 123
serotonin and norepinephrine reuptake inhibitors (SNRIs)
   antidepressant 341
   cancer 267
   depression treatments 27
   persistent depressive disorder (PDD) 49
serotonin syndrome
   herbs and supplements 398
   medications 342
sertraline, premenstrual dysphoric disorder (PMDD) 83
sexual abuse
   environmental risk factors 157
   suicide 496
sexual assault
   anxiety disorders 194
   mental illness 4
   multiple sclerosis (MS) 289
   women and depression 66

sexual dysfunction
   medications 342
   Parkinson disease (PD) 301
sexual orientation, gender-diverse populations 134
sexually transmitted infections (STIs), adverse childhood experience (ACE) 186
shaken baby syndrome, traumatic brain injury (TBI) 255
shamanism, complementary health approaches 382
side effects
   anxiety disorder 197
   attention deficit hyperactivity disorder (ADHD) 253
   bipolar disorder 39
   complementary and alternative therapies 381
   depression 11
   epilepsy 303
   medications 341
   men and depression 110
   postpartum depression 91
   psychotic depression 56
   repetitive transcranial magnetic stimulation (rTMS) 361
   suicidal thoughts 534
   treatment-resistant depression (TRD) 409
SLE *see* systemic lupus erythematosus
sleep deprivation, psychotic depression 54
sleep problems
   attention deficit hyperactivity disorder (ADHD) 252
   disaster responders 468
   fibromyalgia 242
   older adults 118
   Parkinson disease (PD) 300
   premenstrual syndrome (PMS) 76
   self-management intervention 431

Smokefree.gov
   publication
      smoking and depression 210n
smoking
   caregiver stress 173
   heart disease 278
   individual resilience 439
   mental illness stigma 420
   overview 208–210
   racial and ethnic minorities 313
   suicide risk screening 527
   workplace stress 145
SNRIs *see* serotonin and
   norepinephrine reuptake inhibitors
social exclusion, mental illness
   stigma 420
social inclusion, described 485
social isolation
   atypical depression 31
   epilepsy 302
   nongenetic factors 158
   older adults 118, 518
   relationship risk factors 508
social media
   body image 447
   depression triggers 229
   holiday blues 480
   suicide 498
social phobia
   anxiety disorders 193
   depression 13
SPD *see* serious psychological distress
SSRIs *see* selective serotonin reuptake
   inhibitors
St. John's wort
   complementary and alternative
      therapies 386
   herbs and supplements 399
   medications 342
stigma
   adverse childhood experiences
      (ACEs) 189

   climate change 222
   epilepsy 302
   firefighters 461
   gender-diverse populations 134
   human immunodeficiency virus
      (HIV) 284
   overview 419–422
   peer support 485
   suicide risk 508
   workplace stress 147
stimulants
   depression in adolescents 405
   described 344
   disruptive mood dysregulation
      disorder (DMDD) 45
STIs *see* sexually transmitted infections
stress
   adverse childhood experiences
      (ACEs) 187
   atypical depression 31
   cancer 266
   climate change 219
   correctional facilities 149
   depression in children 102, 405
   depression triggers 225
   fibromyalgia 245
   health basics 3
   holiday blues 480
   individual resilience 435
   light therapy 366
   major depressive disorder
      (MDD) 316
   meditation and mindfulness 390
   multiple sclerosis (MS) 289
   older adults 121
   overview 167–179
   premenstrual dysphoric disorder
      (PMDD) 83
   psychotherapy 332
   seasonal affective disorder
      (SAD) 59
   smoking 209

Index

stress, *continued*
    suicidal behavior 508
    suicide attempt 542
    see also caregiver stress; disaster responders; workplace stress
stroke
    brain biofeedback 377
    cancer 262
    caregiver stress 174
    chronic illnesses 236
    deep brain stimulation (DBS) 363
    depression in women 66
    epilepsy 303
    genetic risk factors 157
    medications 345
    mental health basics 3
    older adults 117
    overview 307–311
substance abuse
    acupuncture 384
    anxiety 199
    major depression 24
    rumination cycle 161
    teen suicide 513
    workplace stress 146
Substance Abuse and Mental Health Services Administration (SAMHSA)
    contact information 563
    publications
        alcohol use disorder (AUD) 217n
        childhood resilience 444n
        compassion fatigue (CF) 467n, 471n
        complementary health approaches 388n
        family support 489n
        first responders 463n
        major depressive disorder (MDD) 53n, 317n
        social inclusion 485n

        substance use and mental health indicators 207n
        suicide 523n, 543n, 552n
        trauma triggers 479n
        traumatic brain injury (TBI) 256n
substance use disorder (SUD)
    complementary and alternative therapies 381
    depression 13
    overview 203–208
    suicide 496
SUD *see* substance use disorder
suicide
    adverse childhood experiences (ACEs) 185
    cancer 270
    epilepsy 303
    gay and bisexual men 134
    individual resilience 437
    mental health disorders 7
    older adults 118
    overview 495–498
    protective factors 509
    recovery 545
    statistics 499
    substance use disorder (SUD) 204
    teens 513
    warning signs 525
Suicide Awareness Voices of Education (SAVE), contact information 569
Suicide Prevention Resource Center (SPRC), contact information 569
suicide risk
    bipolar disorder 40
    cancer 270
    electroconvulsive therapy (ECT) 356
    individual resilience 437
    older adults 519
    overview 507–510
    warning signs 530

support groups
    depression triggers 227
    family support 491
    finding help 15
    gender-diverse populations 139
    psychotherapy 331
    stroke 310
supported employment and education, psychotic depression 56
synapse, genetic factors 158
synaptic plasticity, genetic factors 158
systemic lupus erythematosus (SLE)
    chronic illnesses 236
    fibromyalgia 244

T

tai chi
    complementary health approaches 386
    major depressive disorder (MDD) 316
    multiple sclerosis (MS) 291
    workplace stress 148
talk therapy *see* psychotherapy
tardive dyskinesia (TD), mental health medications 345
Targeted Self-Management for Epilepsy and Mental Illness (TIME), epilepsy 304
TBI *see* traumatic brain injury
TCs *see* therapeutic communities
TD *see* tardive dyskinesia
telemental health, finding therapist 320
temporal lobes, traumatic brain injury (TBI) 256
temporomandibular joint syndrome (TMJ), fibromyalgia 243
tetracyclics, major depression 28
TF *see* treatment failure
therapeutic communities (TCs), substance use disorder (SUD) 205

therapist
    depression in children 406
    depression in teens 105
    depression in women 70
    depression signs 316
    holiday season 481
    interpersonal therapy (IPT) 336
    major depression 28
    overview 319–322
    persistent depressive disorder (PDD) 49
    postpartum depression 90
    suicidal ideation 533
therapy
    attention deficit hyperactivity disorder (ADHD) 253
    bipolar disorder 39
    cancer 266
    depression 185, 489
    depression during pregnancy 84
    depression in children 102
    depression in older adults 121
    depression in women 69
    depression signs 316
    diabetes 273
    divorce 227
    eating disorders 200
    mental health disorders 9
    multiple sclerosis (MS) 290
    psychotherapy 330, 533
    rumination cycle 164
    selective serotonin reuptake inhibitors (SSRIs) 351
    trauma effects 456
    see also cognitive-behavioral therapy (CBT); light therapy; music therapy
thyroid
    cancer 263
    depression 14, 229, 325
    depression in women 69

Index

thyroid, *continued*
   genetic and environmental risk factors 158
   major depression 27
   mental health medications 346
   postpartum depression 87
   seasonal affective disorder (SAD) 365
TIA *see* transient ischemic attack
TIME *see* Targeted Self-Management for Epilepsy and Mental Illness
TMJ *see* temporomandibular joint syndrome
tolerance
   childhood resilience 442
   meditation and mindfulness 393
   mental health medications 343
   premenstrual syndrome (PMS) 76
transient ischemic attack (TIA), defined 308
transition
   depression in women 68
   menopause and depression 96
   premenstrual syndrome (PMS) 75
   suicide 516, 547
trauma
   alcohol use disorder (AUD) 211
   bereavement 477
   brain injury 255
   childhood resilience 444
   depression 183
   depression in children 102
   depression in women 66
   environmental risk factors 159
   major depression 24
   mental illness 4
   multiple sclerosis (MS) 289
   overview 455–457
   racial and ethnic minorities 127
   suicidal behavior 508, 523
traumatic brain injury (TBI)
   epilepsy 303
   overview 255–260

TRD *see* treatment-resistant depression
treatment failure (TF), selective serotonin reuptake inhibitors (SSRIs) 352
treatment-resistant depression (TRD)
   overview 409–412
   selective serotonin reuptake inhibitors (SSRIs) 352
tricyclics
   anxiety disorders 197
   depression 28
   mental health medications 341
triggers
   alcohol use disorder (AUD) 214
   complementary health approaches 385
   eating habits 229
   holiday season 479
   major depression 24
   major depressive disorder (MDD) 316
   rumination cycle 162
   seasonal affective disorder (SAD) 365

U

U.S. Department of Education (ED), contact information 563
U.S. Department of Health and Human Services (HHS)
   contact information 563
   publication
      self-management support 430n
U.S. Department of Veterans Affairs (VA)
   publications
      acceptance and commitment therapy (ACT) 338n, 339n
      biofeedback 378n

U.S. Department of Veterans
    Affairs (VA)
    publications, *continued*
        cognitive-behavioral therapy
            (CBT) 334n
        complementary health
            approaches 389n
        depression 289n, 432n
        ectopic pregnancy 86n
        genetic testing 375n
        menopause 96n
        miscarriage 85n
        multiple sclerosis (MS) 291n
        pregnancy 85n
        seasonal affective disorder
            (SAD) 366n
        stroke 311n
        suicide risk assessment 528n
U.S. Equal Employment Opportunity
    Commission (EEOC), contact
    information 563
U.S. Food and Drug Administration
    (FDA), contact information 564
U.S. National Library of Medicine
    (NLM), contact information 564
unemployment
    epilepsy 302
    grief 473
    mental illness 421
    workplace stress 145
United States Census Bureau
    publication
        mental health struggles 138n
urinary incontinence,
    biofeedback 377

V

vagus nerve stimulation (VNS),
    described 357
vicarious trauma, compassion fatigue
    (CF) 464

violence
    anxiety disorders 196
    climate change 222
    depression and trauma 183
    lesbian, gay, bisexual, and
        transgender (LGBT) 139
    mental illness stigma 4, 422
    peer support workers 484
    suicidal behavior 508
vitamin B_{12}, cancer 263
vitamin D, seasonal affective disorder
    (SAD) 59, 365
VNS *see* vagus nerve stimulation

W

warning signs
    children and adolescents 403
    major depressive disorder
        (MDD) 316
    mental health disorders 7
    older adults 119
    psychosis 54
    psychotherapy 332
    suicide 495, 514
weight gain
    anxiety disorders 197
    complementary health
        approaches 386
    depression 13
    hormonal imbalance 228
    older adults 118
    seasonal affective disorder
        (SAD) 58
    stress 169
weight loss
    body image 449
    complementary and alternative
        therapies 381
    depression 25
    seasonal affective disorder
        (SAD) 58

Index

well-being concepts,
    overview 425–432
winter blues *see* seasonal affective
    disorder (SAD)
winter depression, seasonal affective
    disorder (SAD) 57, 365
withdrawal symptoms
    acupuncture 384
    alcohol use disorder
        (AUD) 213
    antianxiety medications 343
    anxiety disorders 197
    depression in men 114
    major depressive disorder
        (MDD) 317
workplace stress, overview 143–148

Y

yoga
    compassion fatigue (CF) 466
    complementary health
        approaches 383
    hormonal imbalance 229
    mental health and stress 148
    multiple sclerosis (MS) 290
    music therapy 401
    older adults 121
    parenting stress 178
    premenstrual syndrome (PMS) 78
Youth.gov
    publications
        suicide prevention 517n
        youth suicide 517n